P9-CBR-147

STOPPING
KIDNEY DISEASE

LEE HULL

Stopping Kidney Disease

Copyright © 2017, 2018 by Lee Hull and Kidneyhood.org

Limit of Liability/Disclaimer of Medical Advice

While the publisher and author have used their best efforts in writing and preparing this book, no representation or warranties exist with the respect to the accuracy and completeness of this book, or that the contents apply to your current health or form of disease. The advice, research, diet and plan may not be appropriate for all patients. A medical doctor should always assist you in making any treatment decisions and patients should always be under the care and supervision of a physician. You should never make treatment decisions on your own without consulting a physician. Neither the author nor the publisher are liable for any medical decisions made based on the contents of this book. This includes special, incidental, consequential, or any other kinds of damages or liability.

Patients should always be under the care of a physician and defer to their physician for any and all treatment decisions. This book is not meant to replace a physician's advice, supervision, and counsel. No information in this book should be construed as medical advice. All medical decisions should be made by the patient and a qualified physician. This book is for educational purposes only.

Published by Kidneyhood.org

No part of this publication may be reproduced, stored in retrieval systems, or transmitted in any form or by any means, electronic, mechanical, photocopying, recording or otherwise without written permission of the publisher.

First edition, January 2019

All rights reserved.

ISBN: 978-0-692-90115-1

Table of Contents

About the Author

Lee Hull has been a kidney patient for the past twenty-two years, the first twelve of which he spent trying to cure an incurable kidney disease. Lee went into remission ten years ago and has stayed in remission using the treatment and diet plan in this book.

INTRODUCTION

I was lying on my side, waiting for the doctor to use a spring-loaded biopsy gun to take a sample from my right kidney. He could see I was worried after they asked me not to move when the biopsy gun made a loud noise.

Right.

It was just a gun thrusting a large needle deep into my kidney. No need to be alarmed.

The doctor reassured me that I shouldn't worry. After the biopsy, they would know what kind of kidney disease I had and would be able to treat it. With just one exception—something called FSGS would be very bad. But don't worry, he went on, we rarely see that one.

Jinx.

I was diagnosed with Focal Segmental Glomerulosclerosis—or FSGS—in 1998. Even worse, I was one of the unlucky ones who did not respond to traditional treatments like Cyclosporine or Prednisone. To date, I have been living with treatment-resistant FSGS for more than twenty years. I had symptoms for years before diagnosis. Our best guess is 2019 marks my 25th year with kidney disease.

After traditional treatments failed, my doctor's only response was "Now go live your life like a normal person. I can't do anything more for you until dialysis or transplant; then we can help you again." Shocked at the lack of other options, I asked "What happens to people like me? The ones who don't respond to treatment?"

He calmly explained that I would continue to decline until dialysis and that hopefully a good transplant kidney could be found. However, there was a good chance that my transplanted kidney would also contract FSGS and would, therefore, have a relatively short life as well. He added, help-fully, that the life expectancy for FSGS patients is typically reduced by twenty to forty years.

The ten-year survival rate for FSGS patients who don't go into remission using drugs is around 30%, and the twenty-year survival rate is around 9%.[1]

I had a 9% chance of making it to fifty-three years old.

Coincidentally, I am writing this at fifty-three years old.

As if my expected survival rate wasn't depressing enough, the thought of spiraling downward in my reduced lifespan was even worse. Each year would be worse than the last as my kidney function declined. I would feel worse, have more symptoms like edema, nausea, and muscle cramps, and I would feel tired all time. I would likely get other ailments such as heart disease, which is what kills most people with kidney disease.

People with kidney disease results have the highest rates of heart disease of any group of people. So, while the official cause of death might be heart disease, it's the kidney disease that leads to the disease–and death.[2]

Adding more misery to the situation for FSGS patients is the fact that medical science doesn't really understand what causes some kidney diseases or why some treatments work while others don't. No one knows why some patients go into remission with steroids or immune-suppressing drugs and others don't. We don't know why some respond to a strict diet and supplements and others don't.

As a father and someone who didn't want to die young, I was angry, frustrated, and somewhat in disbelief at what happens to people with kidney disease who are not cured initially by a pill. We should be outraged at the lack of support and treatment options for people with kidney disease who are not on dialysis.

We are a third world country when it comes to kidney disease care. The World Health Organization ranks countries by outcomes of kidney disease patients. The United States is ranked 66th out of 172 countries–it sits right between Venezuela and Uruguay![3]

In other words, you might be better off living in countries like Venezuela, Qatar, Albania, Cambodia, the Central African Republic, or Tajikistan if you have kidney disease and are waiting on the medical practices in your country to save you.

If you don't believe me, check out the titles of some studies on the same issue:

Pre-end-stage renal disease care in the United States: a state of disrepair.[4]

Prevalence of and factors associated with suboptimal care before initiation of dialysis in the United States.[5]

Patterns of care for patients with chronic kidney disease in the United States: dying for improvement.[6]

Chronic kidney disease: why is current management uncoordinated and suboptimal?[7]

While kidney disease is an epidemic worldwide, survival rates in the U.S. are worse than those in similarly economically developed nations. A 2007 report shows that mortality risk in the U.S. was 15% higher than in Europe and 33% higher than in Japan on comparable treatment modalities.[8] Again, we should be concerned, maybe even outraged, that, as people with kidney disease, our odds are not as good as they are in other economically developed countries.

Twentysix million Americans have kidney disease, and 600,000+ are on dialysis.[9] That leaves 25.4 million of us with no real plan to slow or stop the progression of our disease. Let's further assume that 60% of people with kidney disease will go into remission using some form of drug therapy.[10] That leaves 10 million people just like me who have nowhere to go but down if we rely on traditional advice. I don't know the real number, but you get the idea. There are millions of us who have almost no alternatives after initial treatments fail.

Tremendous resources exist at either end of the kidney disease spectrum. For people at one end, a biopsy can lead to initial diagnosis, and medication can potentially cure them. At the other end of the spectrum, for people whose kidneys are at end-stage renal disease, there is dialysis and transplant, for which tremendous resources exist. So, if you are not cured quickly by drugs, you begin the long decline into kidney failure, dialysis, and transplant. Your kidney function may decline slowly over five to twenty years, yet almost no resources exist for you during this declining period. You are just expected to live with the decline and accept the fact that someday you will be on dialysis and die younger than your peers, probably from heart disease.

If this sounds overly dramatic to you, remember that thirteen people in this country die every day waiting for a kidney transplant.[11]

Why This Gap Exists

Medical and pharmaceutical companies can make a lot of money during the initial diagnosis on biopsies and drug treatments. A lot of money can be made with dialysis and transplants. Not much money can be made by educating patients on how to eat right and adjust their diets based on their blood and urine tests.

Another part of this mess is the slow pace of change and information for us as people with kidney disease. Some well-proven treatments are available in over fifty countries, but not in the U.S. Some treatments that are considered the standard of care in other countries are unheard of in the U.S. This further adds to the chaos.

If we, as patients, are waiting for answers to come from the medical community, we may die waiting for new information that is already at our fingertips.

Cigarettes are a good example. Over 7,000 studies proved cigarettes are bad for you before the Surgeon General took a stand against smoking.[12] Hundreds of studies show certain foods are bad for people with kidney disease, but these foods are included in almost every renal or kidney diet plan. We won't hear about this from our doctor, but the information is widely accepted as medical fact. Will it take 7,000 studies and forty years for us to get a diet and treatment plan that could protect our kidneys?

If you were not cured by a pill and still have kidney disease, this book is for you. I say screw the downward spiral and to hell with each year being worse than the last. I have been fighting and plan to continue fighting my disease all the way. What can be done during this period between diagnosis and dialysis?

Not one thing in this book is a cure by itself, but put all the pieces together and you have a way to control the workload on your kidneys and the factors that leading to kidney disease progression.

Delaying any decline in kidney function is a smart move. Ten or fifteen years from now, we will have better treatments and maybe some cures. If you can make your kidneys last fifteen years instead of seven, your odds of a normal lifespan will go up dramatically.

Not to mention, your quality of life will be much better for those 5,476 days that make up the next fifteen years.

Over the next decade, new treatments will be found, and overall medical care will get better for people with kidney disease. For example, the mortality rate for first-year dialysis patients dropped from 35% to 25% over the past twenty years.[13]

Advancements that will appear in the future include new drugs, 3D-printed kidneys, stem cells to grow a new kidney for you, better methods of transplants, better diets, and the list goes on and on. Slowing the progression of kidney disease may have tremendous benefits down the road.

Your quality of life will be dramatically better, and you will be able to do most, if not all, of the fun activities by avoiding the downward spiral. I go to the gym most days and snowboard with my kids in the winter. We stay out all day and try to ride the last lift. You can have strength, stamina, and the same health as your peers if you know what to do.

I haven't had cramps, nausea, or edema (swelling) in almost a decade. You will not only will feel better but look better, too. I remember how I looked with a round face from steroid use. My face was additionally swollen due to edema, as were my feet, ankles, and hands.

Kidney disease causes specific kinds of nutritional problems for us. Many foods accelerate the speed of kidney decline, and other foods may actually help protect your kidneys. Our kidneys no longer process certain foods correctly, or those foods cause such a high workload on our kidneys that they can't keep up. When this happens, our kidney disease is accelerated, and our chance of heart disease rises exponentially. The last thing we want to do is to speed up a decline in kidney function.

When you manage your kidney disease in more effective ways, not only will you have the chance of living longer and living better, but our government (which pays for dialysis through Medicare and Medicaid) and insurance companies will also save billions of dollars in kidney disease related costs. Costs for dialysis, heart disease, transplants, other related conditions and more frequent medical care could be delayed by many years or even eliminated in some cases.

The savings for the U.S. would be hundreds of millions of dollars. If 10% of people with kidney disease scheduled or expected to be on dialysis were delayed by twelve months, the government would save over $5 billion in one year!

When people with kidney disease are healthier, they have fewer comorbid conditions. Their risk of future ailments or disease drops. They can live healthier, more active lifestyles and eat a kidney- and heart-healthy diet, further reducing the risk of other diseases.

This is one of the few cases where everybody wins. Patients live longer and feel better; doctors can offer more help managing the disease over the long-term; and governments and insurance companies save billions each year.

In the U.S., the average spending on a dialysis patient is $83,356.[14] The cost of the treatment plan and diet in this book are estimated to be less than $5,000 a year. The $5,000 includes doctor visits, blood and urine tests, drugs, and nutritional supplements. Most of the cost and changes are patient-driven and don't require inpatient treatment or hospital stays.

An insurance company in a large state like California, Texas, Florida, or New York could save many tens of millions of dollars per year advocating for, and helping patients with, the diet and treatment plan in this book. Education is sorely lacking for kidney disease patients.

The human costs are staggering as well. Again, thirteen people die every day in the U.S. waiting for a kidney transplant due to the acute shortage of donors. 600,000+ people with kidney disease spend an average of 18 hours a week hooked to a dialysis machine.[15] Kidney disease is the ninth leading killer in the United States,[16] but this may be low. Most people with kidney disease die from heart disease accelerated by kidney disease. While heart disease may be the legal cause of death, kidney disease greatly contributed to heart disease.[2]

Between 1980 and 2009, the increase in end-stage renal disease (ESRD) increased nearly 600%, from 290 to 1,738 cases per million.[17]

FSGS, the disease I have, may have increased as much as 1,000% over the past twenty years.[18] 1,000% is not a typo. How is this possible if the disease cannot be transmitted from one person to another? Clearly, something is going on we don't yet understand.

How did I develop this treatment plan and diet? I became a human guinea pig for kidney disease treatment and management. I researched and tried all manner of treatments. I read every clinical trial and research paper I could find from all over the globe.

I tried everything, no matter how questionable the science, to cure my disease. From traditional medications like immune-suppressing drugs and steroids to special supplements, to ordering illegal medicines from overseas, to all manner of diets—paleo, vegetarian, vegan, raw food, fasting, cleanses—to trying new doctors for second and third opinions. I even flew back and forth from Dallas to be part of a dietary study at Johns Hopkins in Baltimore.

Successful, long-term management of kidney disease is possible and, as people with kidney disease, we need to be experts on this subject. I hope this book will be a bible for those of us with kidney disease.

Hindsight is 20/20; looking back, the problem is clear. The information about the best way to manage kidney disease long-term is a complete chaos. No clear method or process of long-term management of kidney disease has existed until now.

I started a step-by-step analysis of my disease, the factors that would contribute to my kidneys' decline, and predictive mortality rates, and I read all the research I could find. What I ended up with was a plan to cure my disease and, to my surprise, it worked after ten years of failed treatments.

What I can promise you is this treatment plan and diet are based on science that worked for me and I believe they should be the starting place for everyone diagnosed with kidney disease. Knowing all of your options is always a smart strategy for dealing with any disease. Steroids and autoimmune treatment can be lifesaving for some patients and should be used when appropriate, but other options exist that don't have the same side effects.

Matt Damon's character in *The Martian* says "I'm going to have to science the shit out of this" to survive on Mars after being left behind.

My goal is to show you how to science the shit out of your kidney disease and reduce the impact of other diseases that can accompany long-term kidney disease. After twenty plus years with kidney disease, I have a good idea of what works and doesn't work.

I do have one favor to ask. Please let me know how you are doing with the diet and treatment plan. The only way to improve the program and diet is with input from other people with kidney disease. If you have success or failure, please reach out to me. I will try to help any way I can.

You can email me at: **l.hull@kidneyhood.org**

If you have a friend or other family member with kidney disease, please email or share **www.stoppingkidneydisease.com** with them. It might be life-changing–and even lifesaving.

I wish you the best of luck!

Lee

References

1. Korbet SM. Treatment of primary FSGS in adults. *Journal of the American Society of Nephrology.* 2012;23(11):1769-1776.

2. Ahmed A, Campbell RC. Epidemiology of chronic kidney disease in heart failure. *Heart Failure Clinics.* 2008;4(4):387-399.

3. WHO. World Health Rankings: Kidney Disease. 2014; http://www. worldlifeexpectancy. com/cause-of-death/kidney- disease/bycountry/. Accessed 30th June, 2017.

4. Obrador GT, Arora P, Kausz AT, Pereira B. Pre-end-stage renal disease care in the United States: a state of disrepair. *Journal of the American Society of Nephrology: JASN.* 1998;9(12 Suppl):S44-54.

5. Obrador GT, Ruthazer R, Arora P, Kausz AT, Pereira BJ. Prevalence of and factors associated with suboptimal care before initiation of dialysis in the United States. *Journal of the American Society of Nephrology.* 1999;10(8):1793-1800.

6. Owen WF. Patterns of care for patients with chronic kidney disease in the United States: dying for improvement. *Journal of the American Society of Nephrology.* 2003;14(suppl 2):S76-S80.

7. Valderrábano F, Golper T, Muirhead N, Ritz E, Levin A. Chronic kidney disease: why is current management uncoordinated and suboptimal? *Nephrology Dialysis Transplantation.* 2001;16(suppl_7):61-64.

8. Lameire N, Van Biesen W, Vanholder R. Did 20 years of technological innovations in hemodialysis contribute to better patient outcomes? *Clinical Journal of the American Society of Nephrology.* 2009;4(Supplement 1):S30-S40.

9. Manchin III J, Walker MY, Thoenen E. *The Impact of Chronic Kidney Disease in West Virginia.* West Virginia: Department of Health and Human Resources 2006.

10. Appel GB, Crew RJ. Focal Segmental Glomerulosclerosis. In: Greenberg A, ed. *Primer on Kidney Diseases.* Philadelphia, Pennsylvania: Elsevier Saunders; 2005:178-182.

11. NKF. Organ Donation and Transplantation Statistics. 2016; https://www.kidney.org/news/newsroom/factsheets/Organ-

12. Donation-and-Transplantation-Stats. Accessed 25th June, 2017. 12. General US. The reports of the Surgeon General: the 1964 report on smoking and health; 1964. Bethesda, Maryland: *National Institutes of Health.* 1964.

13. USRDS. *USRDS Annual Data Report, Chapter 6: Mortality.* Ann Arbor, Michigan: USRDS Coordinating Center;2016.

14. UCSF. The Kidney Project > Statistics > Cost. 2013; https:// pharm.ucsf.edu/kidney/need/ statistics. Accessed 24th June, 2017.

15. Eichenwald K. Death and Deficiency in Kidney Treatment. 1995; http://www.nytimes.com/1995/12/04/us/death-and-deficiencyin- kidney-treatment.html?pagewanted=all. Accessed 25th May, 2017.

16. Albright A, Burrows NR, Jordan R, Williams DE. The kidney disease initiative and the division of diabetes translation at the centers for disease control and prevention. *American Journal of Kidney Diseases*. 2009;53(3):S121-S125.

17. Capron AM. Six decades of organ donation and the challenges that shifting the United States to a market system would create around the world. *Law and Contemporary Problems*. 2014;77:25-69.

18. Kiffel J, Rahimzada Y, Trachtman H. Focal segmental glomerulosclerosis and chronic kidney disease in pediatric patients. *Advances in chronic kidney disease*. 2011;18(5):332-338.

CHAPTER 1

Why You Should Aggressively Manage Kidney Disease

I assume you or someone you care about has been diagnosed with kidney disease. Perhaps you have already tried steroids and immune-suppressing drugs. You may be reading this book because other treatments have failed. If so, you are in the right place. My goal is to help you or your loved one slow or stop any further decline in kidney function by sharing what I have learned over the past twenty years as a fellow kidney patient.

Being diagnosed with a potentially deadly disease is bad enough, but it is only part of our story, as you will see. When kidney function is lost, it is lost forever. Kidneys don't regrow like other organs. This is important to remember when managing a progressive disease that advances slowly and often painlessly each day. You don't feel it or see it happening, so it's easy to dismiss or forget about for a while. Panic sets in after years of invisible decline when symptoms suddenly appear and become hard to control. You can't get back the kidney function that has been slipping away over the prior years.

So, I will begin with the reasons why you should manage your kidney disease very aggressively over the long term. By aggressive management, I mean doing everything possible to extend the life of your kidneys–going overboard, the full-court press, hardcore and so on. I am living proof that going hard is the right approach.

First, let's agree on some terminology. The chart below shows the generally accepted stages of kidney function and disease. Note that GFR, or "glomerular filtration rate," is how your doctor will measure your renal (kidney) function.

TABLE 1.1: **Stages of Chronic Kidney Disease (CKD) of All Types**[1]

Stage	Qualitative Description	Renal Function (mL/min/1.73 m2)
1	Kidney damage – normal GFR	≥90
2	Kidney damage – mild ↓ GFR	60-89
3	Moderate ↓ GFR	30-59
4	Severe ↓ GFR	15-29
5	End-stage renal disease	<15 (or dialysis)

The most common test for GFR is called "estimated GFR," or eGFR, which measures the amount of creatinine in your blood. Creatinine is a waste by-product of muscle breakdown and it is created at a fairly constant rate. Your kidneys filter creatinine out of your bloodstream and excrete it in your urine; the higher the amount of creatinine in your blood, the less effectively your kidneys are working, and the lower your eGFR.[2]

Alternatively, GFR can be calculated using a 24-hour urine collection. That's right every time you have to urinate over the course of twenty-four hours, you must do so into a container, and then drop it off at the doctor's office. The eGFR, on the other hand, is a simple blood test. You can see why eGFR is so widely used today.[3]

A low GFR or falling GFR does not necessarily mean you have kidney disease. As we age, our kidney function declines. My eighty-three-year-old father, for example, technically has kidney disease because his GFR is in the low 70s. In fact, though, his count is within the normal range for someone his age, as shown in the chart below.

TABLE 1.2: **Average Measured GFR By Age in People Without Chronic Kidney Disease (CKD)[4]**

Age (Years)	Average Measured GFR (mL/min/1.73 m2)
20-29	116
30-39	107
40-49	99
50-59	93
60-69	85
70+	75

> Almost all kidney disease patients in medical trials are at stage 5; a few are at stage 4 of the disease. Most of the kidney function is lost at this point.[5] So why don't we treat kidney disease earlier? The answer is simply: it's because we don't know what to do and patients are not motivated when symptoms are mild. Once initial drug treatments fail, there is not much they can do for us. The standard advice is to wait until our kidneys get worse, start dialysis, and get on the transplant list.Why do we give up at such an early stage? Here are some reasons your doctor or dietician might not recommend aggressive management of your disease after drugs have failed:

- Your kidney function is still not that bad. Your doctor may take a "wait and see" attitude. It's hard to justify aggressive treatment for stage 2 or stage 3 kidney disease, but this is an incredibly bad decision. You are waiting until you lose much of your kidney function before taking other steps to *preserve* your kidney function. This is the road to hell in my eyes. Kidney disease is called the "silent killer" for a reason.

- Diets are not completely proven to cure or slow kidney disease. Too many variations exist, and the studies on them are largely flawed, so it's easy to argue both sides of any diet's perceived benefits. From a medical point of view, who wants to recommend a treatment plan, or diet, that's not proven?

— Dietary compliance is very low. How many times have you or someone you know gone on a diet and stayed with it for a short time before quitting? 99% of us fall into this category. Strict diets are hard for patients to stay with long term. If it can cure you, but you can't stick with it, then it's not a cure at all.

— Dietary plans can be complicated, and it takes a lot of time and resources to educate patients and help keep them on the right track. Patients initially need a lot of support. Our system of medical care is not designed for intensive patient support.

— Doctors are not trained to treat disease with nutrition. They are trained to use drugs or surgery in most cases. Today, a new category of doctors is focusing on diet and lifestyle as preventive medicine or even cures. However, these doctors are still very rare.

— Your doctor personally believes nothing can be done based on his or her training X years ago. This has happened to me more than once.

And lastly, and probably most important of all, patients don't ask for help. We accept the verdict and go about our lives. We don't know to ask for help with long-term management of disease. We don't know what do after drugs fail. We don't know that we can slow or maybe even stop the disease, so we don't even try.

All my doctors, dieticians, and nutritionists have been pretty fantastic, but they work in a system that is broken. In today's liability-prone environment, it's risky to recommend something unproven or out of the ordinary, so they focus primarily on treating symptoms until their patients are close to full-scale kidney failure. It's not their fault; they are good people trying to do a good job. But this means that you are in charge of your treatment options. Treating only the symptoms of kidney disease does very little to keep you living longer.

We know so many things today that we didn't know in 1998, when I was diagnosed. Back then, the advice given to me was based on information primarily from the 1970s and 80s, with only a small amount from the 1990s. One thing I didn't comprehend is what happens in your body as kidney disease progresses. I didn't understand all the things that were going to happen to me over the next ten years if I didn't get my disease under control. Today, we know that the side effects and nutrition problems of kidney disease start very early–even when things look pretty good on the outside. Changes start happening in Stages 2 and 3, and the effects of these small changes accumulate over time.

We now know that heart disease starts early–very early–in people with kidney disease.[6] We also know that up to 48% of patients who have stage 2, 3, and 4 kidney disease don't get enough protein, despite consuming normal amounts of protein.[7] (It's not the kind of protein malnutrition you might be thinking of; we will cover this in detail later.)

When to Start Aggressively Treating Your Kidney Disease

Most aggressive management does not start until late–stage 4 or stage 5–but waiting until things go from bad to worse is mistake number one. A survey of Italian nephrologists[8] suggests that starting treatment in stage 3 is the best time to begin. Basically, earlier is always better, because early in your disease is when you still have good kidney function, with GFRs in the 40 to 70 range. Your best chance of slowing or stopping the progression of your disease is when you still have adequate kidney function.

In the early stages, all the advice you will hear is to limit a few things, like phosphorus and sodium, and to take blood pressure and cholesterol medication. That's about the extent of treatment after drugs fail. But kidney disease is a downward spiral–there is no other way to describe it. However, this downward spiral can be slowed or even stopped if you are willing to do the work and follow a plan.

As people with kidney disease, we are at risk for a large number of other diseases and conditions. When our kidneys stop working correctly, every part of our bodies is affected. "Crosstalk" is a term used to describe the interaction between body parts and organs. This crosstalk has the power to accelerate a decline in kidney function and can lead to other ailments and diseases. You will hear a lot about crosstalk in this book.

> I have put together a partial, but very sobering list of the risks early-stage kidney disease patients face. After reading this section, I hope you will be motivated to manage your disease aggressively over the long term.

> Risk of cardiovascular diseases, or CVD, is the highest of any group ever studied. You read that right. Of any group or population ever studied in the world, people with kidney disease have the highest rates of cardiovascular disease.[9]

> Risk of developing cancer rises from 10% to 80%, depending on the study. If you do get a kidney transplant, your risk of cancer jumps to 300% to 400% higher than the average person.[10]

> Risk of Parkinson's disease increases by over 150%.[11]

> Risk of cognitive decline and dementia increases by over 50%.[12]

> You will age much faster than the average person. Kidney disease in effect accelerates aging. This phenomenon is so prevalent that scientists use kidney disease patients to study aging.[13]

> Your life expectancy will be 20 to 40 years shorter than the average person.[14]

> There is a higher risk of sexual dysfunction, erectile dysfunction, lower libido, and menstrual abnormalities. Erectile dysfunction affects 70% of male patients in end-stage renal diseases.[15]

> For those who go on dialysis, the one-year mortality rate is around 25%.[16]

> Life expectancy after going on dialysis is 4.5 years if you are over 60, and 8 years if you are around 40 years old.[17]

> People with kidney disease have a higher risk of stroke.[18]

> Women with kidney disease are at greater risk for osteoporosis and bone disease.[19]

> You are at greater risk of depression than the average population.[20]

> The crosstalk effect: 96% of people with kidney disease with stage 3 kidney disease (GFR in the 50s) also suffer from other diseases or health conditions.

> You have an 84% higher risk of suicide if you are a kidney patient or have chronic kidney disease (CKD).[21]

> Quality of life and physical abilities decrease with each stage of kidney disease. This is the slow decline or, as I call it, the road to hell.

As a fellow kidney patient, I found it hard to write this list. I wish my doctors had explained some of these facts to me early in my treatment and diagnosis. I might have made different decisions, or at least been more aggressive in my treatment options early on. As depressing as these facts can be, hiding from reality won't help us conquer or slow our disease.

Mild kidney disease is easy to ignore. It's painless, and symptoms are not severe. Most patients won't be spurred to action until their kidney disease has progressed significantly. But I urge you to act now before too much kidney function is lost. The list above is only a partial list of risks you face and it's why I implore you to take your disease and treatment very seriously. The fact is that you are not fighting one disease; you are fighting the possibility of many diseases all at once. This is easier to see visually in the chart below.

FIGURE 1.1: **Survival Rates of End-Stage Kidney Disease Patients With Complications**[22]

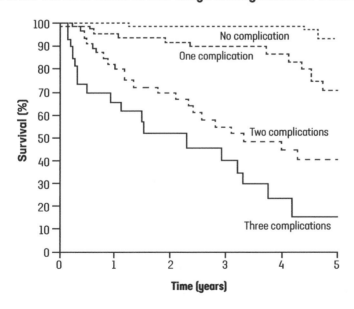

Survival, represented by Kaplan-Meier survival curves (Log Rank 84.2; *P*<0.00001), in 204 end-stage renal disease (ESRD) patients with none, one, two, or all three of the complications malnutrition, inflammation, and atherosclerosis.

As the chart shows, when the number of complications, illnesses, or ailments increases, so does your chance of dying. Your odds of survival drop dramatically over five years as the complications mount. A survival rate of more than 90% versus a 15% survival rate is astounding when you think about it. In the past, doctors have told me "Don't worry about a little high cholesterol or low albumin levels; it's expected with kidney disease, it's okay." This is 100% wrong in every way. We do have to worry about these things. I am a patient who doesn't want to die young and leave his wife and three kids or watch my parents bury another child. We have to worry about other conditions no matter how mild they seem today. These mild issues snowball into multiple issues over years if we are not careful. This causes our mortality rates to skyrocket when compared to rates for someone who keeps even the smallest issue in check. The goal is to stay on top of your health so you can stay in the no-complication or, at worst, one-complication range. You want to treat them before the complications become an unmanageable problem. You should start treating or managing your disease early to avoid related illnesses or complications.

Many people wonder about our odds of survival if we go into total or partial remission. The truth is that total remission is probably not possible for most of us, but partial remission is. The chart below shows how levels of remission can affect survival rates.

FIGURE 1.2: **Survival Rates of Chronic Kidney Disease Patients with Complete, Partial, and No Remission**[23]

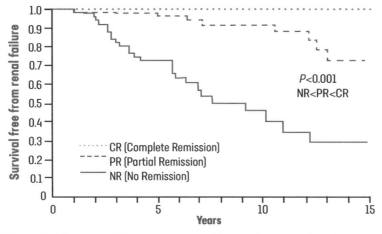

Figure 1.2: Survival from renal failure in patients with complete, partial, and no remission.

As you can see, even partial remission improves your survival rates dramatically. Partial remission usually means a reduction of 50% of the amount of protein in your urine. Other symptoms improve as well. You will still have protein leakage, but it will be much less than before. We could also define remission as the time when your kidney disease stops progressing, but you still have symptoms. I am in the former category. My kidneys are still damaged, but my kidney disease has not progressed in many years.

If we combine the data about complications and remission in a single chart, we get a more realistic picture of what happens to us over time.

FIGURE 1.3: **Survival Rates of Chronic Kidney Disease Patients With Complications in Various States of Remission***

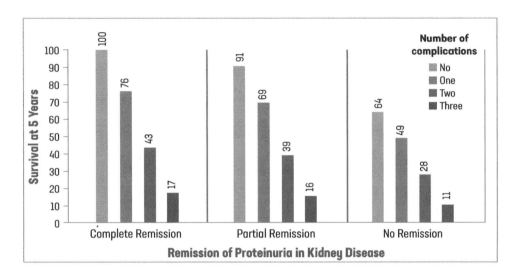

As you can see, 91% of patients are still alive five years after partial remission if they have no other conditions, but only 39% survive if they have two conditions. A little edema (swelling), a little high cholesterol, a little high blood pressure, a little low blood albumin, or a little protein in your urine may seem relatively harmless, and you will be told these are harmless. However, the more of these factors you have today, the worse your outcome over the upcoming years. It is so easy to let these things slide as they don't hurt and most doctors will say not to worry unless your numbers are extreme. But here is a partial list of indicators that are measured as reliable predictors of mortality for kidney disease patients:

> GFR

> Cholesterol

> Statins (cholesterol-lowering medications)

> Smoking

> Body weight index (BMI)

> Magnesium

> Phosphorous

> Protein in urine (*proteinuria*)

> Blood protein or albumin levels

- White blood cell count
- Blood pressure
- Exercise
- Depression
- Body pH (metabolic acidosis)
- Sodium
- Cardiovascular disease
- Inflammation
- Malnutrition

While no studies have examined all of these factors at once, separate studies show each one of these, when unmanaged, is a predictor of mortality in people with kidney disease. Research strongly suggests that, as you add unmanaged conditions, your survival rates start to drop dramatically.[24,25] The "crosstalk" between your kidneys and the rest of your body has profound effects on your health and chance of survival. The source of all of these conditions or abnormal levels is damaged kidneys. I had no idea how many things go wrong when our kidneys are damaged. For me, this "crosstalk" effect was far greater than I ever imagined. It was overwhelming, almost debilitating for me to discover the sheer number of variables to manage. For your part, it may seem impossible right now to manage all of these factors, but as you will see our approach makes it much easier.

In the chart above, you can also see that the number of complications is not as important as getting into some form of remission. Going into remission or partial remission is truly your silver bullet.

Remission rates in kidney disease vary widely depending on not only the form of kidney disease, but also other factors, such as genetics. The best scenario is that you and your doctors catch the disease early and use steroids or autoimmune drugs to put you into remission within a few months. It's hard to know how often this happens and if complete remission is achieved.

Partial remission is also hard to nail down because few studies look at partial remission rates alone.[26] We really don't know how many patients achieve partial remission. In addition, remission might occur for no known reason or cause. Spontaneous remission also happens in some cases. In these cases, no one can explain why a patient goes into remission.

One thing we know for sure is that the more illnesses or complications you have–no matter how minor–the higher your odds of mortality. We also know that getting into any kind of remission matters. Therefore, we must address every issue or complication and work towards remission. This can be done with our treatment plan and diet.

Our treatment plan needs to focus on remission and reducing the number of conditions along the way. This combination gives us the best odds of success.

You Have Control

Now that the bad news is out of the way, let's get to some good news. You have far more control than you ever imagined over your kidney disease and kidney function.

You can control the level of protein, or albumin, in your blood with great accuracy despite the fact you are probably "leaking" a large amount of protein in your urine. Albumin levels are a strong predictor of mortality.[27] In fact, low albumin levels increase your odds of dying by over 400%, but again, this is under your control. (Something I was never told by a doctor or nutritionist.)

You can control–to a large degree–the amount of acid your kidneys process. Metabolic acidosis is common among people with kidney disease.[28] Acidosis is a term used to describe your body's inability to keep your pH in the right range. Even low-grade acidosis accelerates the decline in kidney function. You are twice as likely to die if you have acidosis. (Again, something I was never told.)

You can control your diet. Some proteins are very bad for your kidneys while other proteins may actually be renal-protective. Lowering the amount of the damaging protein in your diet can reduce renal death by as much as 32% compared to a high-protein or unrestricted protein diet. Again, this is in your control.[29]

You can dramatically reduce oxidative stress on your body and kidneys. Oxidative stress and damage is increased in patients with kidney disease, and it accelerates the decline of your kidneys and heart disease.[30] (Yet again, something I was never told!)

You can consider taking certain supplements. It's important to note that most supplements don't have an impact on your kidney disease, but a few might. You need to know which ones may help with the disease, and which ones could make it worse.[31]

In short, you can regulate the amount of work your kidneys have to do on a daily basis. It's completely in your control. All manner of variations exists to control your kidneys' workload. Reducing the workload on your kidneys can slow or even stop the progression of kidney disease. If we keep taxing our kidneys, we accelerate our disease. Most of us are driving 100 mph towards dialysis and don't even know it.

The weight of scientific evidence has identified the best foods to eat (and which to avoid) for people with kidney disease to slow or stop their decline in kidney function. But not one kidney diet or recipe book follows the latest research, which is very frustrating from the patient's point of view. The right diet–the one I will outline in this book–will improve edema, muscle cramps, and oxidative stress; improve your kidney function; and may slow or stop your decline in kidney function.

So, you have far more control of your kidney disease progression, symptoms, and outcome than anyone has ever told you. This translates to a longer lifespan, fewer health conditions, and a higher quality of life.

I know many of you have given up–I did, too, for a while. But I am here to tell you that it is not hopeless. Remember, I went into remission after ten years of slow decline. It is never too late to try to slow or stop your kidney disease.

I hope that you will fight the good fight along with me and not go quietly into the downward spiral. I refused to give up and was eventually able to put my kidney disease into remission. It won't always be easy, and you will have to be on top of things, but it is possible to greatly extend the useful life of your kidneys.

References

1. Levey AS, Eckardt K-U, Tsukamoto Y, et al. Definition and classification of chronic kidney disease: a position statement from Kidney Disease: Improving Global Outcomes (KDIGO). *Kidney international.* 2005;67(6):2089-2100.

2. Rule AD, Larson TS, Bergstralh EJ, Slezak JM, Jacobsen SJ, Cosio FG. Using serum creatinine to estimate glomerular filtration rate: accuracy in good health and in chronic kidney disease. *Annals of internal medicine.* 2004;141(12):929-937.

3. Waller D, Fleming J, Ramsey B, Gray J. The accuracy of creatinine clearance with and without urine collection as a measure of glomerular filtration rate. *Postgraduate medical journal.* 1991;67(783):42-46.

4. NKF. Glomerular Filtration Rate (GFR) > What are the Stages of Chronic Kidney Disease (CKD)? > What is a normal GFR number? 2015; https://www.kidney.org/atoz/content/gfr. Accessed 20th May, 2017.

5. Abbasi MA, Chertow GM, Hall YN. End-stage renal disease. *BMJ Clinical Evidence.* 2010;2010(07:2002):1-16.

6. Silverberg D, Wexler D, Blum M, Schwartz D, Iaina A. The association between congestive heart failure and chronic renal disease. *Current opinion in nephrology and hypertension.* 2004;13(2):163-170.

7. Kuhlmann MK, Kribben A, Wittwer M, Hörl WH. OPTA— malnutrition in chronic renal failure. *Nephrology Dialysis Transplantation.* 2007;22(suppl_3):iii13-iii19.

8. Trifirò G, Fatuzzo PM, Ientile V, et al. Expert opinion of nephrologists about the effectiveness of low-protein diet in different stages of chronic kidney disease (CKD). *International journal of food sciences and nutrition.* 2014;65(8):1027-1032.

9. Shiba N, Shimokawa H. Chronic kidney disease and heart failure—Bidirectional close link and common therapeutic goal. *Journal of cardiology.* 2011;57(1):8-17.

10. Bordea C, Wojnarowska F, Millard P, Doll H, Welsh K, Morris P. Skin cancers in renal-transplant recipients occur more frequently than previously recognized in a temperate climate. *Transplantation.* 2004;77(4):574-579.

11. Wang I-K, Lin C-L, Wu Y-Y, et al. Increased risk of Parkinson's disease in patients with end-stage renal disease: a retrospective cohort study. *Neuroepidemiology.* 2014;42(4):204-210.

12. Bugnicourt J-M, Godefroy O, Chillon J-M, Choukroun G, Massy ZA. Cognitive disorders and dementia in CKD: the neglected kidney-brain axis. *Journal of the American Society of Nephrology.* 2013;24(3):353-363.

13. Anand S, Johansen KL, Kurella Tamura M. Aging and chronic kidney disease: the impact on physical function and cognition. *Journals of Gerontology Series A: Biomedical Sciences and Medical Sciences.* 2013;69(3):315-322.

14. Neild GH. Life expectancy with chronic kidney disease: an educational review. *Pediatric Nephrology.* 2017;32(2):243–248.

15. Ayub W, Fletcher S. End-stage renal disease and erectile dysfunction. Is there any hope? *Nephrology Dialysis Transplantation.* 2000;15(10):1525-1528.

16. Wingard RL, Chan KE, Lazarus JM, Hakim RM. The "right" of passage: surviving the first year of dialysis. *Clinical Journal of the American Society of Nephrology.* 2009;4(Supplement 1):S114-S120.

17. Stokes JB. Consequences of frequent hemodialysis: comparison to conventional hemodialysis and transplantation. *Transactions of the American Clinical and Climatological Association.* 2011;122:124.

18. Olesen JB, Lip GY, Kamper A-L, et al. Stroke and bleeding in atrial fibrillation with chronic kidney disease. *New England Journal of Medicine.* 2012;367(7):625-635.

19. Miller PD. Chronic kidney disease and osteoporosis: evaluation and management. *Bone Key Reports.* 2014;3(542):1-7.

20. Bautovich A, Katz I, Smith M, Loo CK, Harvey SB. Depression and chronic kidney disease: A review for clinicians. *Australian & New Zealand Journal of Psychiatry.* 2014;48(6):530-541.

21. Chen C-K, Tsai Y-C, Hsu H-J, et al. Depression and suicide risk in hemodialysis patients with chronic renal failure. *Psychosomatics.* 2010;51(6):528-528. e526.

22. Rao P, Reddy G, Kanagasabapathy A. Malnutrition-inflammation- atherosclerosis syndrome in Chronic Kidney disease. *Indian Journal of Clinical Biochemistry.* 2008;23(3):209-217.

23. Troyanov S, Wall CA, Scholey JW, Miller JA, Cattran DC, Group FTTGR. Idiopathic membranous nephropathy: definition and relevance of a partial remission. *Kidney international.* 2004;66(3):1199-1205.

24. CDC. Prevalence of chronic kidney disease and associated risk factors--United States, 1999-2004. *Morbidity and Mortality Weekly Report* (MMWR). 2007;56(8):161.

25. Goldwasser P, Mittman N, Antignani A, et al. Predictors of mortality in hemodialysis patients. *Journal of the American Society of Nephrology.* 1993;3(9):1613-1622.

26. Chen YE, Korbet SM, Katz RS, Schwartz MM, Lewis EJ, Group CS. Value of a complete or partial remission in severe lupus nephritis. *Clinical Journal of the American Society of Nephrology.* 2008;3(1):46-53.

27. Iseki K, Kawazoe N, Fukiyama K. Serum albumin is a strong predictor of death in chronic dialysis patients. *Kidney international.* 1993;44(1):115-119.

28. Kovesdy CP. Metabolic acidosis and kidney disease: does bicarbonate therapy slow the progression of CKD? *Nephrology Dialysis Transplantation.* 2012;27(8):3056-3062.

29. Piccoli GB, Capizzi I, Vigotti FN, et al. Low protein diets in patients with chronic kidney disease: a bridge between mainstream and complementary-alternative medicines? *BMC nephrology.* 2016;17(1):76.

30. Montesa MP, Rico MG, Salguero MS, et al. Study of oxidative stress in advanced kidney disease. *Nefrologia.* 2009;29(5):464-473.

31. Handelman GJ, Levin NW. Guidelines for vitamin supplements in chronic kidney disease patients: what is the evidence? *Journal of Renal Nutrition.* 2011;21(1):117-119.

CHAPTER 2

Why is My Body Trying to Evict My Kidneys?

After thirty-three years of getting along very well with my kidneys, my body began to attack them slowly. At first, the symptoms were minor; a few bubbles in my urine, an almost unnoticeable amount of swelling in my ankles and face in the morning, the occasional nighttime cramp, but everything was so trivial that I barely noticed. I had slight but constant symptoms for three or four years before I was finally diagnosed with kidney disease. My doctors explained to me that my body was attacking my kidneys and that the standard treatment was the same drugs used for organ transplant patients. These drugs suppress the immune system to such an extent that your body will not reject an organ that is not an original part–in other words, a new organ. The significance of this treatment option was lost on me at the time, but it became my inspiration later.

I tried a combined thirteen months of prednisone and cyclosporine to put my disease in remission. No change. My disease progressed unabated during this period. The side effects were, well, not pleasant for my family or me.

My specific diagnosis in 1998 was Focal Segmental Glomerulosclerosis (FSGS), the fastest growing form of kidney disease. FSGS cases have risen by 1,100% from 1980 to 2000. An elevenfold increase in a non-communicable disease.[1] Again, we can't give FSGS to each other, so why the hell is this disease spreading so fast and across all groups?

What could cause kidney disease to grow at more than 1,000% over a twenty-year period?

I set out to try to figure out both why I had been diagnosed with this disease and why there has been such an enormous uptick in diagnoses. At the time of my diagnosis, I was working more than sixty hours a week at a Fortune 500 company in Dallas, and generally not eating or living a healthy lifestyle. I am human, and I eat when stressed. Maybe it was stress and diet? I also wondered if maybe it was genetic. Nope, no family history of kidney disease. Furthermore, I hadn't had any surgeries or other medical events that could have damaged my kidneys. I wasn't diabetic, and I didn't have high blood pressure.

Looking for a Cause

Many years later, I restarted the quest to find a cause and cure. I went back over medications, diets, and anything I could find to give me a direction; I came upon my records from Johns Hopkins. No medications provided any relief or improvement. However, I did have some improvement on a low-protein diet referred to as the "Walser" diet, after the late Dr. Mackenzie Walser, who treated me at Johns Hopkins. I was part of a dietary intervention study Dr. Walser was running. Dr. Walser believed that a very low-protein diet could stop or slow the progression of kidney disease. Dr. Walser had been working in this area for over thirty years. Studies on low-protein diets, as a group, are inconclusive. Some patients respond, and some don't, and no one knows why. The diet didn't put me into remission or slow my disease. However, a few symptoms did get better. My edema, cramps, and nighttime nausea improved. On the other hand, I was still leaking a massive amount of protein in my urine, and my GFR, creatinine, and albumin didn't budge. On a personal basis, I really liked Dr. Walser and felt he was a sincere, honest, and caring guy. I really wanted the diet to work for the both of us.

We were both very frustrated when the diet didn't work for me. I followed the diet plan to the letter and made every appointment, but with very limited success. However, Dr. Walser's comments changed the way I thought about kidney disease.

Dr. Walser felt diet was to blame for the incredible increase in kidney disease cases. Nothing else could explain the increase in kidney disease rates. He felt diet might be the cause **and** cure of some forms of kidney disease.

During my last appointment with Dr. Walser, he encouraged me to keep trying to improve my diet. He also encouraged me to try to get my hands on something called keto acids, even though they were not available in the United States. He wondered if keto acids would have improved my response better than an amino acid supplement. Keto acids slowed kidney disease progression more effectively than amino acids but, again, are not available to U.S. patients. More on keto and amino acids and the new availability of keto acids to U.S. patients later.

I was depressed after trying the Walser diet. I added a special diet to the list of things that failed to cure my disease. I didn't know what to do next, and my nephrologist said waiting until my kidneys got bad enough to go on dialysis was the next step.

I played with diets from 2001-2007 with no real success. I would get motivated and to stay on a new version of a low-protein diet and then fall off the wagon again after getting bad test results. It's was a brutal cycle full of highs and lows.

After playing with low-protein diets for almost ten years, I gave up, but then something happened in my life that caused me to back up and take another shot at trying to stop or slow the progression of my disease. I thought back and realized that the Walser diet led to a small improvement. I began to wonder if Dr. Walser could, in fact, be right about a low-protein diet. But maybe protein was only part of the problem. Maybe my diet hadn't been extreme enough. Maybe I did something wrong. What made me think about this was reading books by Dean Ornish[2] and Caldwell Esselstyn.[3] Dr. Dean Ornish had shown the amount of lifestyle change was correlated with the success of a diet and lifestyle treatment for prostate cancer. The more extreme the change, the better the results.

This chart shows the reduction percentage in cancer cells based on lifestyle change. The bigger the change, the better the results.

FIGURE 2.1: **Mean Relationship ± SEM of Degree of Lifestyle Change and Changes in LNCaP Cell Growth Across 2 Groups by Tertiles**

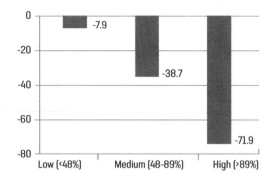

A little bit of change got a little result. It takes a big change to get big results. I began to wonder if the Walser diet was not "extreme" enough or if more lifestyle changes were needed.

Dr. Caldwell Esselstyn wrote that "moderation kills" when it comes to diets for heart disease. His example is that hitting a brick wall at 100 mph kills all the occupants. The same is true for 90 mph, 80 mph, 70 mph and so on. The occupants will only survive unscathed when the speed drops to 10 mph. Moderating the speed from 100 to 70 didn't work. We need to slow down from 100 to 10 to get the desired result.

From *Prevent and Reverse Heart Disease*[3]

"Every mouthful of oils and animal products, including dairy foods, initiates an assault on these membranes and, therefore, on the cells they protect. These foods produce a cascade of free radicals in our bodies—especially harmful chemical substances that induce metabolic injuries from which there is only partial recovery. Year after year, the effects accumulate. And eventually, the cumulative cell injury is great enough to become obvious, to express itself as what physicians define as disease. Plants and grains do not induce the deadly cascade of free radicals. Even better, in fact, they carry an antidote. Unlike oils and animal products, they contain antioxidants, which help to neutralize the free radicals and also, recent research suggests, may provide considerable protection against cancers."

What if Dr. Esselstyn was right? One mouthful of something bad could negate an entire meal of good foods. We could eat right all week long and then negate the effects with one or two bad meals.

Maybe they were right; maybe my diet was not extreme enough. Maybe the approach to the diet was the problem. The Walser diet focused on eating a very low-protein diet but used familiar and "fake" foods to keep cravings at bay or to make the transition easier. Fake foods were designed to taste, look and feel like regular foods, but have very low levels of protein. These include cheese made from oils or spaghetti noodles made from cornstarch. Maybe eating even a little bit of bad food was enough to derail any progress. Maybe the entire concept of fake foods was wrong.

Fake cheese, fake bread, fake spaghetti, and so on were the norm. The hope was that these fake foods would reduce protein intake while ensuring patients would not feel too deprived of their "normal" foods.

Here are a few examples of the recipes and processed foods that patients on low-protein diets in America are encouraged to eat:

Orange Cream Shake

> 1/2 cup liquid nondairy creamer

> 1/2 cup orange sherbet

> 1 tablespoon sugar

> 1 tablespoon vegetable oil

[Nutritional analysis: 461 calories / 1.4 grams of protein]

And here are the ingredient lists from specialized low-protein foods :

Low-Protein Cheese Product

Water, food starch, partially hydrogenated soybean oil, modified food starch, milk protein concentrate, salt, natural flavor, sodium phosphate, stabilizers (xanthan, locust bean, guar gums), sorbic acid (preservative), lactic acid, artificial color. Contains milk and soy.

[Nutritional analysis, per slice: 35 calories / 1.4 grams of protein]

Low-Protein Spaghetti

Cornstarch, pregelatinized potato starch, pregelatinized cornstarch, emulsifier (mono- and diglycerides), stabilizer (methylcellulose), artificial color (beta carotene), antioxidant (L-ascorbic acid).

[Nutritional analysis, per 1 cup 363 calories / 0.5 gram of protein]

These ingredients don't even sound like food. They sound like a science experiment. Could they really be good for me? I doubt it.

A 2004 edition of *Nutritional Management of Renal Disease, 2nd edition* (the book used to train doctors in medical school) recommends the following for lunch:

> 2 slices white bread

> 2 oz. chicken

> 2 tsp mayonnaise

> Lettuce leaf

> 1/2 medium pear

> 1 can regular soda

A white bread chicken sandwich with a Coke. This is what is being taught to doctors, nutritionists, and dieticians today.

The people behind these recipes and products are doing the best they can given the restrictions of the certain diets. A lot of time, ingenuity, and effort goes into making these products and recipes. I mean no disrespect when I question the wisdom of these foods or diets.

However, if I have a deadly disease, should I be eating pasta that is mostly cornstarch with zero nutritional value in the name of protein restriction? Maybe that nondairy creamer has no protein, but being made from corn syrup and cottonseed oil, the creamer created as many problems as it solved for me. Should I be eating pregelatinized potato starch, sugar, and vegetable oil for my calories? What does eating these foods do to the rest of my body and health?

Remember, chronic kidney disease patients are the highest risk group for heart attacks.[4] Sugar, vegetable oil, and processed starches may help with our kidney disease, but they may add to our risk for heart disease and diabetes.

So maybe Dr. Walser was on the right track, and diet was the issue. I just had to figure out the right diet. Maybe protein restriction helps, but its success depends on what we replace the protein with. Perhaps when we replace the protein with unhealthy foods, the diet doesn't work. Could the replacement foods be just as bad for my kidneys? Could eating "bad" calories negate the benefits of a low-protein diet?

A study from Japan[5] and another on red meat convinced me to try a different approach. I found this study after reading Ornish and Esselstyn. Maybe our bodies are attacking our kidneys because our kidneys are not working properly anymore.

Effects of Acute Protein Loads of Different Sources on Renal Function of Patients with Diabetic Nephropathy[5]

The study compared the effect on kidney function when eating tuna versus bean curd (soybean) in four groups: N (normal, no kidney disease), and groups A, B, and C, which each have a form of kidney disease called diabetic neuropathy. Group A is a mild or early form of the disease, group B is more severe, and group C is more severe than group B.

FIGURE 2.2: **Changes in GFR Following Protein Loads**

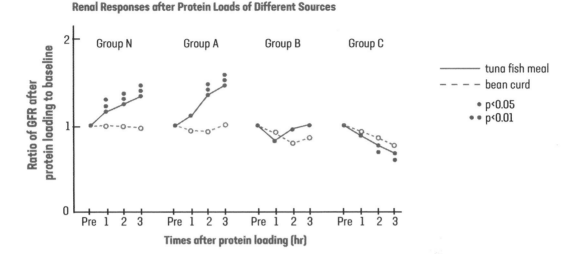

Group N shows a spike in GFR (glomerular filtration rate) following the tuna meal, as does the group with mild kidney disease, group A. However, groups B and C, whose kidney function is much lower, do not have the hyperfiltration effect or spike in GFR after the tuna meal. Hyperfiltration is a body response to eating foods with a high acid load that we need our kidneys to process. Hyperfiltration increases blood pressure in the kidneys to increase the amount of blood our kidneys can filter.

A few pertinent notes about tuna and bean curd: They are matched for amino acid content and protein content. However, potential renal acid load (PRAL) is -3.4 for soybeans and 11 for tuna. Antioxidants are also in soybeans, but not in tuna. (See Chapter 4 for more on potential renal acid load.)

This chart shows that as our disease progresses, our ability to handle the dietary acid load and protein waste products drops. Our kidneys are no longer able to kick into high gear to offset a high workload of acid and protein. This means we can't eat these foods because our bodies cannot respond correctly.

Eating bean curd showed little effects on GFR in all groups. None of the groups needed their kidneys to kick into hyperfiltration mode after a bean curd meal.

Above 60 GFR, kidney function is likely good enough to still process a normal workload. By the way, a GFR of 60 is not a magic number, but a representation of mild kidney disease. Our body's mechanisms for dealing with high protein and/or high acid loads are impaired or reduced in kidney disease. The problem is most, if not all, diets to improve kidney function act as if this impairment does not exist. If we can't process certain foods anymore, then we shouldn't be eating them. This isn't rocket science.

Another study shows that just two servings of red meat a week has an impact on kidney disease.

| Study 2.1 | Associations of diet with albuminuria and kidney function decline[6] |

RESULTS:

Compared with the lowest quartile, the highest quartile of animal fat (odds ratio (OR): 1.72; 95% confidence interval (CI): 1.12 to 2.64) and two or more servings of red meat per week (OR: 1.51; 95% CI: 1.01 to 2.26) were directly associated with microalbuminuria. After adjustment for other nutrients individually associated with eGFR decline > or = 30%, only the highest quartile of sodium intake remained directly associated (OR: 1.52; 95% CI: 1.10 to 2.09), whereas beta-carotene appeared protective (OR: 0.62, 95% CI: 0.43 to 0.89). Results did not vary by diabetes status for microalbuminuria and eGFR outcomes or in those without hypertension at baseline for eGFR decline. No significant associations were seen for other types of protein, fat, vitamins, folate, fructose, or potassium. Just two servings of red meat with the associated animal fat may have an impact on our kidney health and kidney disease progression.

CONCLUSIONS:

Just two servings of red meat with the associated animal fat may have an impact on our kidney health and kidney disease progression.

> Think about the tuna/bean curd study combined with the second study on red meat. The waste products of protein digestion, urea, and ammonia are still hanging around in our bodies for hours or days after a meal if we can't process them in a timely manner anymore.
>
> One, two, or three servings of something bad for us might negate the benefit of eating well for the rest of the week.
>
> My thinking changed to "Don't eat anything my kidneys cannot process easily," and "One or two bad meals a week could stop my progress."
>
> My body may have been trying to evict my kidneys because they had stopped working correctly. I had lost the ability to process or deal with any extra load on my kidneys. Only my body knew that something was very wrong with my kidneys. My kidneys could not handle my current diet, so my body went to war with my kidneys trying to fix the problem. No one really knows why our bodies attack organs in autoimmune diseases. My guess (only a guess) is our bodies are trying some last-ditch effort to solve a life-threatening problem.
>
> Maybe my kidneys were more like a cesspool than a pristine body part—a holding place for toxic wastes that I couldn't get rid of fast enough. Toxic substances just kept piling up. Maybe my body saw my kidneys as a toxic waste dump that could never be cleaned up. Therefore, they had to be evicted.
>
> I no longer had the ability to handle the bad aspects of protein waste products. However, it didn't explain why so many other things went wrong along with protein processing. My view became

that protein restriction solved only one problem and, therefore, it needed to be only one aspect of treatment.

However, when I stopped eating foods that caused those waste products and other factors contributing to my disease, things started getting better for me. My kidneys and I have a long-lasting truce as long as I don't break the treaty and start eating bad foods again. I also live with the knowledge that my disease could come back at any time.

Think about it people with heart disease can digest and process food normally in most cases. People with kidney disease can't. For example, free radicals are much higher in people with kidney disease.[7] We have metabolic disorders, too many waste products in our bloodstreams, low blood protein, and so on. If an extreme diet is important for heart disease, it's got to be doubly important for kidney disease.

Diet was the only legal course of action I had left and necessity is the mother of invention, so I had to invent a diet-based plan to cure myself.

I decided to take another crack at trying to cure my disease through diet and supplements. This time, I would do my own research and design my own diet and treatment plan. I had plenty of experience with diets for kidney disease before; I would go more extreme this time.

The epidemic of kidney disease has to do with multiple factors. Diabetes is the number one cause, followed by high blood pressure. However, the incredible increase in FSGS can't be explained by diabetes or high blood pressure alone.[8]

According to the World Health Organization (WHO), the leading cause of all death is diet-related.[9] Obesity, nutrition, and lack of exercise all contribute to the leading causes of death all over the world. Inadequate diets have given us the first generation in two hundred years that is expected to have a shorter lifespan than their parents. Think about that for a moment. Diet is causing an explosion in kidney disease rates around the world. If diet can cause us problems, perhaps diet may be able to cure us.

My first step was to find out everything I could about what foods, medicines, supplements, and even lifestyles could hurt my kidneys. I thought I would never go into remission, so I took the approach of trying to identify and stop every condition that was contributing to disease progression. I would cure or manage every condition that contributed to my disease and add every factor that might slow my disease.

At the time, I used the following analogy: I was the home team and my disease was the hated rival team from another town. If I had ten blood tests outside the normal range or comorbid conditions and I was doing nothing to slow my disease, the score was 0-10. I was getting killed by the rival team. If this continued my future was not going to look very good.However, if I could change the score to 2-2 by reducing the number of problems to two and adding two things that slowed my disease, the score would be tied. I might have a fighting chance if I could tie the score.My disease progression would definitely slow, I thought. What if I could get the score to 3-1? What would happen to my disease? This process took some time, but ended with my disease going into remission. I went from losing the battle to tying the score, and then to a decisive victory.

Before I go any further, I want to say that I am not a vegan, vegetarian, paleo, Atkins, or other diet advocate. I have no food politics agenda. I grew up in Louisiana and Texas and served in the military. I am about as far away from a pretty girl holding a basket of brightly colored veggies on a book cover as you can get. I say this because I have accumulated dozens of diet guides over the years that are written just to sell, not to use real science and help people with their health. Take a walk over to the diet section of your local bookstore and see what you find. There must be a hundred different kinds of diets, all claiming to be the best or healthiest. This means that either most are lying, or that science knows absolutely nothing about nutrition. You can come to your own conclusion, but I implore you not to get sucked into the diet hell I was in for years, trying everything in the world to help my kidneys, no matter how crazy.

This is painstaking work, which is why you never see it in books designed for everyday readers. However, we have a deadly disease. We are not everyday people anymore. We need to understand the research and our doctors need to understand it as well. My plan is the result of years of experience and research. Note, though, that I am only looking at diet and health from only a kidney and heart point of view. I went where the science and research took me, and I have based my plan on it, not on what we grew up with, or what is the custom in our area. Science has spoken on what is best and worst for our kidneys and heart. No doubt, in the future new facts will be discovered that will change the diet. That's okay. As of 2019, we know what science has said to date.

References

1. Kitiyakara C, Eggers P, Kopp JB. Twenty-one-year trend in ESRD due to focal segmental glomerulosclerosis in the United States. *American Journal of Kidney Diseases.* 2004;44(5):815-825.

2. Dean O. *Dr. Dean Ornish's Program for Reversing Heart Disease- The Only System Scientifically Proven to Reverse Heart Disease.* New York: Ivy Books; 1995:672.

3. Esselstyn CB. *Prevent and Reverse Heart Disease: The Revolutionary, Scientifically Proven, Nutrition-based Cure.* New York: Penguin Books/ Avery; 2008.

4. Ahmed A, Campbell RC. Epidemiology of chronic kidney disease in heart failure. *Heart Failure Clinics.* 2008;4(4):387-399.

5. Nakamura H, Takasawa M, Kasahara S, et al. Effects of acute protein loads of different sources on renal function of patients with diabetic nephropathy. *The Tohoku journal of experimental medicine.* 1989;159(2):153-162.

6. Lin J, Hu FB, Curhan GC. Associations of diet with albuminuria and kidney function decline. *Clinical Journal of the American Society of Nephrology.* 2010;5(5):836-843.

7. Salahudeen AK. Free radicals in kidney disease and transplantation. *Saudi Journal of Kidney Diseases and Transplantation.* 1999;10(2):137.

8. Jones CA, Krolewski AS, Rogus J, Xue JL, Collins A, Warram JH. Epidemic of end-stage renal disease in people with diabetes in the United States population: do we know the cause? *Kidney international.* 2005;67(5):1684-1691.

9. Kaczorowski J, Campbell NR, Duhaney T, Mang E, Gelfer M. Reducing deaths by diet. *Canadian Family Physician.* 2016;62(6):469-470.

CHAPTER 3

The Concept of Kidney Workload and Factors

While working on the different issues that affected my kidneys, one day I had an epiphany one day that changed the way I thought about kidney disease and special diets. As I reviewed kidney diets and the latest research, it hit me that we are always treating the symptoms of kidney disease rather than the real problem or root cause.

For example, potassium was not a problem for me, so I had no dietary potassium restriction at first. Sodium was a problem, so I had a sodium restriction. These kinds of restrictions are all well and good,[1] but we are basically saying, "If you have a symptom let's manage it." Most modern kidney disease diets and treatments should be called "symptom management." In most cases, we have stopped trying to slow or stop the disease in most cases. Maybe I should be thinking about curing the underlying need for a salt restriction. Salt restriction is a cure for a symptom, not for the disease itself.

We have forgotten about stopping or slowing a deadly disease. If we want to live a long time and have a better quality of life, we need to keep trying to treat the disease, not just manage symptoms. Plus, as your kidney function declines, your dietary restrictions will grow because the disease gets harder to manage.[2] New symptoms equal new restrictions, but no attempt is made to slow or stop the disease. I think this approach is one of the reasons why outcomes for people with kidney disease are so poor in the U.S. compared to other countries.

So, I sat back one day and thought about treating the factors driving my disease instead of just managing my symptoms. I asked myself what remission would look like. How could I get there? How could I stop or slow the pace of my disease when drugs and many diets had failed? Remission typically means your kidneys go back to normal. That wasn't realistic for me after more than ten years of disease progression. At this stage, my kidneys would still be damaged even in the best scenario, but partial remission or a dramatic slowdown in the progression of my disease might be possible.

My epiphany was the thought that maybe my body would stop attacking my kidneys if everything looked normal again. I needed to find a way to reduce the total workload on my kidneys so much that I would have excess capacity like the old days, when I was healthy. In addition to reducing protein workload, I had to treat all of the other factors that were causing me to drive 100 mph toward kidney failure.

Low-protein diets did reduce the workload on my kidneys, but the theory behind these diets seemed to be that all our kidneys do is deal with protein wastes.[3] However, when you lose kidney function, you lose it across the board. Your whole body goes haywire. Low-protein diets take part of the workload off our kidneys, but they still have plenty of work to do. I needed to treat all of the functions of my kidneys, not just the protein workload. I also needed to eat foods that helped or protected my kidneys, if possible.

I would eat only foods that required very little work or foods that might even protect my kidneys. Combined with this was the knowledge that I needed to treat every factor of kidney disease I could, not just the protein processing part. This is why I refer to my plan as the "Kidney Factors" diet. I wanted to address all of the factors driving my disease. Low-protein diets should be called "protein workload" diets.

After trying dozens of diets, I can tell you that, to have real success, you have to treat the whole kidney, not just part of kidney function. It makes sense and science backs up this approach. The problem is, no one does it or educates patients on this approach. Look at it this way: Healthy kidneys can handle anything we throw at them, regardless of what we eat. Our kidneys have excess capacity to handle the waste products, keep our pH balances, and so on. Even if you eat the worst foods in the world for your kidneys, they will dutifully do their job and will keep your metabolic numbers in the normal ranges. But as you lose kidney function to disease, your kidneys' capacity for all workloads fall, not just handling protein wastes.[4]

So, we have to reduce the total workload of kidneys to slightly below what they can actually handle. I will use GFR (glomerular filtration rate) as an example. You can roughly define the capacity of the workload of your kidneys by using GFR or eGFR (estimated glomerular filtration rate). Your GFR could be as high as 100 or even 120 when you are healthy. You have 100% of your normal capacity plus 20% of excess capacity at 120 GFR, in this example. In addition, healthy kidneys can kick into high gear (hyperfiltration) when needed to effectively increase GFR temporarily. But when patients go on dialysis, GFRs tend to be around 15 or lower. This represents an 85%+ reduction in capacity compared to a healthy pair of kidneys with a GFR of 100, and we no longer can use hyperfiltration to temporarily increase kidney filtering capacity. When GFRs are in the teens, it's very hard, if not impossible, to lower the workload enough to get back to a small amount of excess capacity.

However, if your GFR is between 30 and 70, you have a much better chance of achieving this.[5] For instance, let's assume your GFR is 50 today. If your diet sends a workload to your kidneys in excess of the current capacity of 50, then your numbers will start to go outside of the normal ranges, your symptoms will increase, and your kidney and heart disease progression will become accelerated. That's because a workload of 100 with a capacity of 50 results in excess waste products in your blood, acidosis, cramps, nausea, and so on. This excess workload is what causes your symptoms. Eating more than your capacity is the root of all your symptoms. It also has the power to greatly accelerate your disease.

That's the trick.

You can dramatically reduce or dramatically increase the workload on your kidneys with your diet choices.[6] What if we did the work for our kidneys by choosing foods wisely? What if our kidneys never had to filter out large amount of waste products? What if our kidneys never had to produce ammonia to offset a high-acid diet? What if our kidneys didn't have any oxidative stress or inflammation?

It's very simple:

Your kidneys cannot fully process your current diet when they are damaged. If they could, you would not have the symptoms you have. It's that simple. Don't overthink it. If your body could process your current diet, your numbers would be in the normal range. You have black and white information to answer your question. This is important, so I will say it again: If your kidneys can fully process your diet, your numbers will go back to normal. Your kidneys are handling the workload just like normal kidneys. This can be done through diet in many cases.

Now let's assume your GFR is the same 50, but you send a workload equivalent to a GFR of only 35 to your kidneys. Your kidneys have excess capacity now. When you do this over a long period of time, things start to change. Your body will think your kidneys are back to normal and everything will start to normalize. High cholesterol will start to drop, cramps and nausea will go away, vitamin D will get better, and so on. Your whole body will start working better.

For my part, by trial and error and thanks to research, I learned to reduce the workload to below my current GFR. I did the work for my kidneys with diet selection and supplements. The biggest surprise for me was that as soon as my metabolic numbers started getting back in the normal range, my body stopped attacking my kidneys. My incurable autoimmune disease finally stopped progressing. Something happened that strong drugs and the best hospitals and doctors in the country could not do. When I get off the diet for a few months (I am only human; I have given in to cravings and stress more times than I can count), my GFR starts to drop and the swelling slowly returns. This is when I know I am sending too much workload to my kidneys. You might say I am in voluntary remission. If I go off the dietary wagon, my disease may return at any time.

Before your disease, your kidneys could keep everything in the normal range despite a very high workload. You had no symptoms, and your blood and urine tests were in the normal range. You had no symptoms because your kidneys could handle the workload. If you trick your body into thinking everything is normal again, then your body may go back to normal. I think this is the secret to going into partial remission. My body stopped attacking my kidneys when everything looked and felt normal. My body no longer saw my kidneys as a defective part of my body. This happened only by dramatically reducing the workload for my kidneys and curing or managing every factor driving my disease. Every time you wrestle a blood test back into the normal range, your odds get better.

My turn for the better only happened with a certain combination of diet and supplements. I treated every aspect of kidney function I could find, including:

> Renal acid load or pH management

> Protein wastes or uremia

> Antioxidants

> Inflammation

> AGE's

I didn't just manage symptoms like you do with normal kidney diets. I did the work for my kidneys in many ways.

My current nephrologist argues that, even though my improved blood and urine tests exactly track with my change in diet and supplements, I could have gone into remission for several reasons. From a scientific point of view, he is 100% correct[7]. However, he is wrong in other ways. My other diet combinations did not change my blood and urine tests; as my other diets progressed, my blood and urine work barely changed. This time was different. It didn't happen overnight, but everything kept getting better the longer I stayed on the diet and plan. I could feel and see the difference. My ankles, hands, and face were not swollen anymore; in fact my wedding ring kept falling off because my hands were no longer swollen. I no longer had cramps nor nausea. Acidosis went away, cholesterol dropped, and so on.

One theory Dr. Walser expressed was that our kidneys were not designed to handle such a high workload for extended periods of time.[8] The diet and eating habits of most people in the United States today sends our kidneys and other internal organs more work than they were ever designed to handle.[9] Another theory is our kidneys are literally worked to death producing ammonia (an alkaline compound) to offset today's high-acid diets.[10]

If you doubt this idea, think about lifespans dropping for the first time in two hundred years. We might be eating ourselves to death.

Another way to look at the concept of kidney workload is caloric restriction. Caloric restriction is a term used to describe diets that are very low in calories but meet all nutritional requirements. Caloric restriction has been proven to extend lifespan in animal studies. Human studies are still ongoing.[11]

Kidney disease progression and related symptoms have been effectively slowed in animal models using restricted caloric diets. We also know that kidney disease rates are much higher in obese patients.[12] Walser writes[8]:

> *"Caloric restriction without protein restriction markedly retarded the development of glomerulosclerosis."*

Every calorie you eat increases the workload on your kidneys.

None of these theories are proven yet, but all point to one conclusion: Excessive workload is literally killing our kidneys — and might be killing us in the process. Reducing the workload by diet changes or by caloric restriction has the potential to slow or stop disease progression.

Think about what we know:

Increasing the workload on a damaged kidney accelerates a decline in kidney function. Taking the workload off slows kidney disease progression.

Once I made this realization, I made a determination, and now I share it with you. We are going all out to try for partial remission or dramatically slowing the progression of our disease. You can call it hardcore, extreme, the full-court press, damn the torpedoes, or whatever you want, but do whatever it takes to stop the progression of your disease. Remember, our disease is considered incurable at this point. The best doctors and hospitals have thrown in the towel. Going halfway isn't going work. We are going to treat our kidneys and all aspects of our disease—not just the protein part.

When I have been asked to talk to other patients, I get a lot of pushback initially regarding diet. We act like eating a diet for healthy kidneys is a form of punishment or going to an extreme. But how is eating healthy for your kidneys more extreme than letting a machine filter your blood for eighteen to twenty hours a week? Or having surgery to put someone else's kidney inside you? How is taking drugs that increase the rate of cancer 300% to 400% and come with some very nasty side effects somehow considered normal, but a kidney diet is extreme?

Extreme is praying that they will find a transplant match for you and you won't be one of the thirteen patients dying everyday waiting on a transplant. Extreme is not knowing if you will be alive next year. Extreme is not knowing if you will ever see your kids or grandkids. Extreme is leaving your wife with three kids when you were their sole support. Extreme is thinking about your parents burying you.

Trust me, the diet and treatment plan are absolutely nothing compared to any of the real-life alternatives. Diets seem extreme only because we are not used to them. They require change and a little willpower. I promise the so-called "extreme" diets are not extreme at all when you consider the alternatives. In fact, dietary treatment is the lowest risk option, and it is also the cheapest option. We can't forget that we have a deadly disease that may kill us thirty years prematurely and our last decade or so of life won't be a cakewalk.[13] It is extreme to allow this to happen and keep insisting on maintaining the lifestyle that may have caused the disease in the first place. It's extreme to choose cheeseburgers over your family, health, and life. It's extreme to choose five minutes of dietary pleasure over your spouse, kids, grandkids, and family.

So, I set out to devise a new diet plan. My first step was to identify all foods, food groups, or supplements that could accelerate my disease or create a large workload for my kidneys. Next, I identified all of the things I could do to slow my disease. The combination of these factors was going to save me, I thought.

After that, I set some parameters. I looked for foods that could put a very small load on my kidneys, or even protect them. The diet must reduce the workload on our kidneys, leave us well-nourished, and not break the bank account with special foods. Ideally, we want to be able to buy all the foods in any local grocery store and spend less per month than we spend today.

The next chapters consist of food or health issues that accelerate our disease. I was driving 100 mph toward kidney failure and never knew it. I could call these foods "accelerants," as they make our disease progress at a faster rate. Eliminating these foods is the first step to stop causing damage to our kidney and bodies so we can slow or stop disease progression. Remember, the part of the Hippocratic oath "First, do no harm."

Each chapter has research and data behind it. We don't want to guess; we want to know for sure what causes our disease to progress faster.

As I will show you, it's not impossible, and it's definitely not extreme. It's based on science as of 2019, not the 1950s like most kidney diet books or advice. The most current diet advice is based on managing sodium, potassium, and phosphorus. These need to be managed, but doing so does nothing or very little to slow the progression of our disease over the long term as you will see. As patients with a deadly disease, we deserve better than symptom management. We deserve a cure, we deserve a life. The focus on managing only symptoms and not slowing or trying to stop our disease is absolutely wrong. I get a little angry at the advice given to us by people who don't have the disease. I don't mean to imply they are bad people. However, it's easy to give advice based on old or bad research when you don't have to worry about dying young and when you stand to make a few bucks. This is how I feel about most (not all) renal or kidney diet books.

Our motivation is very different. The most well-meaning researchers or authors don't have the same motivation as someone with the disease. Therefore, I think the best non-drug research, diets, and treatments will come from us, people with kidney disease. Patient-to-patient may need to be the new model. We have to do for ourselves because, from what I have seen and experienced, no one is doing anything for us.

You will see the idea of patient-to-patient frequently. Collectively, we are a big group, spread all over the world. We have power together. An example of this is that people with kidney disease created a product for patients that is 60% lower in price, higher quality, made from more expensive ingredients, tailored to different stages of kidney disease, and manufactured to the highest standards. This is pretty earthshaking when you think about it, considering the price was reduced by over 60% and it's a much better product than previous options. Patients have a different motivation than corporations. We can put the needs of patients first instead of profits. I feel the traditional model is failing us, so we need a new model. Patient-to-patient allows for the cheapest costs and fastest research into new therapies, diets, supplements, and drugs. You will be hearing more about this later. I will be asking for your help.

Ok, enough ranting on my part.

The upcoming chapters are on foods or conditions that accelerate kidney disease. I have tried to summarize the most relevant research in each chapter. It was important for me, as a kidney patient, to understand the science behind the diet or condition. I needed understanding and education to stay on the diet. I think this is the first step in acquiring a little diet and treatment plan discipline. If you understand why you are doing something, you are more likely to stay with the plan.

The next chapters will summarize the research and data about foods and/or conditions that accelerate kidney disease progression. We need to start by doing no harm by stopping the drivers of kidney disease progression.

I don't expect you to read every study, but please read the text in the chapter to get an idea of how these factors accelerate kidney disease

References

1. Yang Q, Liu T, Kuklina EV, et al. Sodium and potassium intake and mortality among US adults: prospective data from the Third National Health and Nutrition Examination Survey. *Archives of internal medicine.* 2011;171(13):1183-1191.

2. Kasiske BL, Lakatua J, Ma JZ, Louis TA. A meta-analysis of the effects of dietary protein restriction on the rate of decline in renal function. *American Journal of Kidney Diseases.* 1998;31(6):954961.

3. Fouque D, Aparicio M. Eleven reasons to control the protein intake of patients with chronic kidney disease. *Nature clinical practice Nephrology.* 2007;3(7):383-392.

4. Coresh J, Astor BC, Greene T, Eknoyan G, Levey AS. Prevalence of chronic kidney disease and decreased kidney function in the adult US population: Third National Health and Nutrition Examination Survey. *American journal of kidney diseases.* 2003;41(1):1-12.

5. de Jong PE, Halbesma N, Gansevoort RT. Screening for early chronic kidney disease—what method fits best? *Nephrology Dialysis Transplantation.* 2006;21(9):2358-2361.

6. Beto JA. Which diet for which renal failure: Making sense of the options. *Journal of the American Dietetic Association.* 1995;95(8):898-903.

7. Ruggenenti P, Schieppati A, Remuzzi G. Progression, remission, regression of chronic renal diseases. *The Lancet.* 2001;357(9268):1601-1608.

8. Walser M, Thorpe B. *Coping with kidney disease: A 12-step treatment program to help you avoid dialysis.* John Wiley & Sons; 2010.

9. Frazão E. *High Costs of Poor Eating Patterns in the United States.* Food and Rural Economics Division, Washington: US Department of Agriculture, Economic Research Service;1999.

10. Hoffman JR, Falvo MJ. Protein–which is best? *Journal of Sports Science & Medicine.* 2004;3(3):118-130.

11. Roth LW, Polotsky AJ. Can we live longer by eating less? A review of caloric restriction and longevity. *Maturitas.* 2012;71(4):315-319.

12. Wickman C, Kramer H. Obesity and kidney disease: potential mechanisms. Paper presented at: Seminars in nephrology2013.

13. Neild GH. Life expectancy with chronic kidney disease: an educational review. *Pediatric Nephrology.* 2017;32(2):243–248.

Intro to the "Factors" That Contribute to the Speed of Kidney Disease Progression

The following chapters contain "Factors" that contribute to kidney disease progression and in most cases heart disease progression as well.

I am sure more "Factors" exist and we will add to this list in the future. What you need to understand is the more of these "Factors" you have the faster your disease will progress. Mortality rates start to rise dramatically when you have more than two of these "Factors" or comorbid conditions.

As you will see later in the treatment plan, one of our primary goals is to reduce the number of "Factors" contributing to the speed of kidney disease progression. I always use the analogy "Driving 100 mph toward kidney failure." The more "Factors" you have the faster you are driving towards kidney failure.

Another section will contain "Factors" I consider to be neutral or unknown, and another section on the "Factors" that slow or put the brakes on kidney disease progression.

I know it's a lot of research and technical jargon, but understanding how your kidney works and how these "Factors" affect your disease is the key to slowing or maybe even stopping your disease. Understand how your daily choices affect your kidneys and kidney disease progression is the first step.

CHAPTER 4

Low Albumin levels/Hypoalbuminemia

(The most important chapter in this book)

I am starting this section with albumin because the failure to treat low albumin levels is costing thousands of lives a year. If the needless death of thousands of patients is not enough to move you, then think about this: Low albumin is treatable in many cases. If these two facts are not enough to make you angry, maybe this fact will: The most proven and kidney-friendly treatment for raising albumin levels in people with kidney disease is not allowed in the U.S., but is allowed in over forty countries.

I believe not treating low-albumin levels is the biggest mistake made in kidney disease treatment/management today. I have been working for two years to bring a product to the U.S. that is safe, effective, and affordable, so we can start treating low-albumin levels.

This will be a long chapter, but don't skip it. Instead, read it two or three times instead. Our albumin level is tied lockstep to our disease and our future odds of survival. Let's say it again! Our albumin level is tied to our future odds of survival. Albumin levels may be one of the most accurate predictors of mortality and morbidity.[1] This is why this is the most important chapter in the entire book.

Albumin makes up 60% to 70% of the protein in our bloodstream. It is the most prevalent protein in our bloodstream. Albumin is made by the liver. Albumin levels drop due to a combination of proteinuria, inflammation, oxidative stress, acidosis, uremia, and reduced synthesis.

Prealbumin is a short-term measure of protein nutrition, and albumin is a longer-term measure. Albumin has a half-life of fifteen to twenty days. This means new albumin produced by the liver decays over fifteen to twenty days. Normally, the liver produces about 5% of our needed albumin each day. If, over the next fifteen or twenty days, a portion of our albumin escapes in urine (proteinuria) or is reduced by inflammation, oxidation, acidosis, or uremia, we end up with hypoalbuminemia even if our liver is producing normal amounts of albumin.

Production of albumin in our liver can drop for several reasons, such as liver disease/injury, a low-protein diet without protein supplementation, and insufficient calorie intake.

Albumin is debated as a nutrition factor. Some research suggests that low serum albumin is a marker for illness and not protein nutrition. The feeling is low serum albumin should be considered as an indicator of systemic illness instead of protein nutrition. Both are right. Albumin is an indicator of our body's ability to produce and successfully manage albumin. If production and management of albumin is failing, we have multiple problems.

The normal range for serum albumin is 3.5 to 5.5 g/dl (grams per deciliter) also expressed as 35 to 55 g/L. (grams per liter) In the U.S., albumin is normally expressed as grams per deciliter or g/dl. Albumin, like phosphorus, is another case where "normal" is bad for us.[2]

Why is albumin so important? Let us count the ways:

As you can see, albumin has a lot of jobs, but let's dig a little deeper.

FIGURE 4.1: **Physiological Effects of Exogenous Albumin**

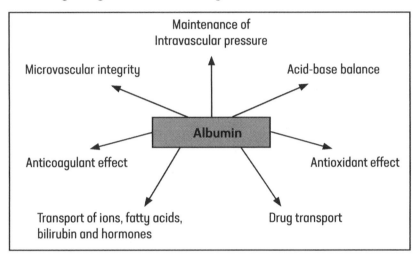

1. Albumin is an antioxidant that we need.[3]

2. Albumin regulates intravascular or oncotic pressure, which is related to edema/swelling.[4]

3. Albumin improves blood vessel strength or microvascular integrity, which reduces heart attack and stroke risk.[5]

4. Albumin acts as a buffer to smooth out acid-base balance, which is related to acidosis.[6]

5. Many drug molecules are transported by albumin in the bloodstream. Low albumin levels can interfere with proper drug dosage and delivery.[7]

6. Albumin transports and helps regulate things like calcium and magnesium. Low albumin equals reduced ability to control these levels.[8]

7. Albumin acts as carrier for anticoagulative enzymes like antithrombin and heparin.[9]

Albumin is a true workhorse in our bloodstream. This is probably why low albumin levels can be so deadly.

How deadly?

FIGURE 4.2: **30-day Mortality Rates Based on Albumin Levels**

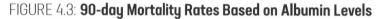

30-day mortality rates based on albumin levels. You can see mortality rates drop dramatically until you get to around 4.0 mg/dl or 40 g/L. 5.0 mg/dl + or 50 g/L + is even better. For someone to say albumin doesn't matter (which a nephrologist said to me) is wrong, crazy wrong.

How about those on dialysis?

FIGURE 4.3: **90-day Mortality Rates Based on Albumin Levels**

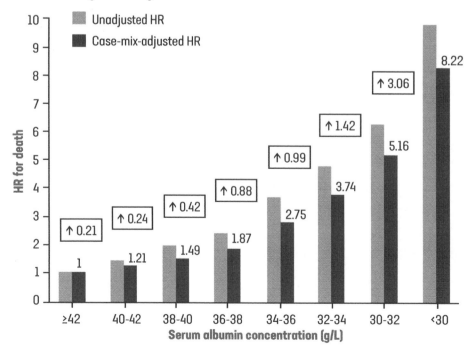

HR in this graph stands for hazard ratio. Hazard ratio is another word for death. I would say death is a pretty big hazard. The hazard of dying goes up as albumin drops. As your albumin (x-axis) gets higher, your odds get better even over periods of ninety-days (like in the chart above).

If these charts don't convince you that albumin is important, maybe this study will.

Study 4.1   **Preoperative Serum Albumin Level as a Predictor of Operative Mortality and Morbidity Results from the National VA Surgical Risk Study.[10]**

RESULTS:

A decrease in serum albumin from concentrations greater than 46 g/L to less than 21 g/L was associated with an exponential increase in mortality rates from less than 1% to 29% and in morbidity rates from 10% to 65%. In the regression models, albumin level was the strongest predictor of mortality and morbidity for surgery as a whole and within several subspecialties selected for further analysis. Albumin level was a better predictor of some types of morbidity, particularly sepsis and major infections, than other types.

CONCLUSIONS:

Serum albumin concentration is a better predictor of surgical outcomes than many other preoperative patient characteristics. It is a relatively low-cost test that should be used more frequently as a prognostic tool to detect malnutrition and risk of adverse surgical outcomes, particularly in populations in whom comorbid conditions are relatively frequent.

Serum albumin as a predictor of surgical outcomes is a big deal for us. Think about this for a second; as we age or our health declines, we are more likely to have some form of surgery or hospital stay. The reasons could be anything from a car wreck, to an accident around the house, a hernia, a burst appendix, or heart disease. If we don't get albumin under control, a normal hospital visit or a small surgical procedure can suddenly can become life-threatening.

I care about albumin because it is such a strong mortality indicator. Is it going to kill me and, if so, what can I do about it? This is what convinced me I had to improve my albumin levels or I was not going to get better.

Why is albumin so important? Albumin is a multifactorial indicator of how sick or healthy we are. That's what you and I need to focus on. Forget about the academic debates. Albumin is an indicator of protein nutrition and an indicator of how well our bodies are working to maintain that nutrition. If we have high oxidative stress, lots of inflammation, and so on, we may have low albumin levels. If our albumin levels are rising, we must be getting better. Commit this to memory: rising albumin good, falling albumin bad.

Let's look at additional research on people with kidney disease:

Study 4.2 Early changes in serum albumin: impact on 2-year mortality in incident hemodialysis patients.[11]

CONCLUSIONS:

Early sAlb (serum albumin) changes demonstrated a significant predictive power on mortality at two years in incident hemodialysis patients. Those with low initial sAlb may have a better prognosis if their sAlb rises. In contrast, patients with satisfactory initial levels can have a worsening of their prognosis in the case of an early reduction in sAlb.

*If you can raise your albumin levels, your odds improve. If albumin is dropping, your odds get worse.

Study 4.3 Precedent fluctuation of serum hs-CRP to albumin ratios and mortality risk of clinically stable hemodialysis patients.[12]

CONCLUSIONS:

Clinically stable HD patients with a fluctuating variation of hs-CRP/Alb are characterized by old age, and more co-morbidity and they tend to have longer subsequent hospitalization stay and higher mortality risk.

*Your ratio of CRP (aka inflammation) to albumin is a strong predictor of mortality. This further confirms we need to increase albumin and reduce inflammation at the same time.

Study 4.4 Serum oxidized albumin and cardiovascular mortality in normoalbuminemic hemodialysis patients: a cohort study.[13]

CONCLUSIONS:

Serum HNA (human serum albumin) level is a positive predictor of mortality in normoalbuminemic HD patients, especially among those with pre-existing CVD. Increased oxidative stress resulting from biological changes in serum albumin levels could contribute to accelerated atherosclerosis and the development of cardiovascular disease in HD patients.

Note: Oxidized albumin is what happens if your body is overwhelmed by oxidative stress. Instead of albumin acting as a mild antioxidant, the oxidized albumin now contributes to heart disease instead.

Study 4.5   **A lower level of reduced albumin induces serious cardiovascular incidence among peritoneal dialysis patients.**[14]

CONCLUSIONS:

Lower HMA (human serum albumin) level, which might be caused by chronic inflammation, anemia and accumulation of dialyzable uremic toxin(s), is closely related to serious CVD incidence among PD patients.

   *Uremia is also a factor, along with inflammation and anemia.

Study 4.6   **Revisiting mortality predictability of serum albumin in the dialysis population: time dependency, longitudinal changes, and population-attributable fraction.**[15]

Time-varying hypoalbuminemia predicts all-cause and CV death differently from fixed measures of serum albumin in MHD patients. An increase in serum albumin over time is associated with better survival independent of baseline serum albumin or other MICS surrogates. If this association is causal, an intervention that could increase serum albumin >3.8 g/dl might reduce the number of MHD deaths in the USA by approximately 10,000 annually. Nutritional interventions examining benefits of increasing serum albumin in MHD patients are urgently needed.

   Reducing deaths by 10,000 annually! Why aren't we working on this night and day? How many people could we save?

Study 4.7   **Association between serum albumin and mortality in dialysis patients is partly explained by inflammation, and not by malnutrition.**[16]

CONCLUSIONS:

In dialysis patients, a 1-g/dL decrease in serum albumin was associated with an increased mortality risk of 47% in HD patients and 38% in PD patients. These mortality risks were in part explained by the inflammatory pathway. The mortality risks associated with serum albumin were not a consequence of malnutrition, as measured with SGA [subjective global assessment] and nPNA. These findings imply that nutritional status cannot be assessed with precision by the measurement of serum albumin in dialysis patients.

   Note: A 1-gram decrease in albumin increased mortality risk by 47% and 38%. Again, these are big numbers. This study also confirms inflammation is partly responsible for low albumin.

Study 4.8   Serum Albumin Level and Risk for Mortality and Hospitalization in Adolescents on Hemodialysis.[17]

CONCLUSIONS:

This study demonstrates decreased mortality and hospitalization risk with albumin ≥3.5/3.2 g/dl and suggests that adolescent hemodialysis patients who can achieve serum albumin ≥4.0/3.7 g/dl may have the lowest mortality risk.

Note: Again, mortality risk drops even for adolescents with kidney disease if albumin can be raised.

Study 4.9   Relationship between trajectories of serum albumin levels and technique failure according to diabetic status in peritoneal dialysis patients: A joint modeling approach.[18]

RESULTS:

Using joint modeling approach, a relationship between trajectories of serum albumin with hazard of transfer to hemodialysis was estimated as -0.720 (95% confidence interval [CI], -0.971 to -0.472) for diabetic and -0.784 (95% CI, -0.963 to -0.587) for non-diabetic patients. From our findings, it was showed that predictors of low serum albumin over time were time on peritoneal dialysis for diabetic patients and increase in age and time on peritoneal dialysis, history of previous hemodialysis, and lower body mass index in non-diabetic patients.

CONCLUSIONS:

The results of the current study showed that controlling serum albumin over time in non-diabetic and diabetic patients undergoing continuous ambulatory peritoneal dialysis treatment can decrease the risk of adverse outcomes during the peritoneal dialysis period.

Study 4.10   Hypoalbuminemia in Renal Failure: Pathogenesis and Therapeutic Considerations.[19]

ABSTRACT:

Hypoalbuminemia is common in patients with end-stage renal disease (ESRD). It is caused by a combination of a reduced synthesis and an increased degradation of albumin. The altered albumin homeostasis in ESRD patients is caused by a systemic inflammatory state which correlates closely with mortality. Hypoalbuminemia is a strong predictor of an adverse prognosis, but it is not a pathogenic factor in itself. In critically ill patients in intensive care units, the intravenous administration of human serum albumin generally does not improve prognosis. In contrast, in hypoalbuminemic dialysis patients with volume overload and a reduced effective arterial volume the administration of albumin is based on the pathophysiological concept of increasing intravascular oncotic pressure to transfer extravascular fluid into the intravascular compartment for ultrafiltration to mobilize edema fluid.

| **Study 4.11** | Hypoalbuminemia, cardiac morbidity, and mortality in end-stage renal disease.[20] |

ABSTRACT:

A cohort of 432 ESRD (261 hemodialysis and 171 peritoneal dialyses) patients were followed up prospectively for an average of 41 months. Baseline and annual demographic, clinical, and echocardiographic assessments were performed, as well as serial clinical and laboratory tests measured, monthly, while patients were on dialysis therapy. Among hemodialysis patients, after adjustment was made for age, diabetes, and ischemic heart disease, as well as hemoglobin and blood pressure levels measured serially, a 10-g/L fall in mean serum albumin level was independently associated with the development of de novo (relative risk [RR], 2.22; $P = 0.001$) and recurrent cardiac failure (RR, 3.84; $P = 0.003$), de novo (RR, 5.29; $P = 0.001$) with recurrent ischemic heart disease (RR, 4.24; $P = 0.005$), cardiac mortality (RR, 5.60; $P = 0.001$), and overall mortality (RR, 4.33; $P < 0.001$). Among peritoneal dialysis patients, a 10-g/L fall in mean serum albumin level was independently associated with the progression of left ventricular dilation as seen on follow-up echocardiography (beta, 13.4 mL/m2; $P = 0.014$. The development of de novo cardiac failure (RR, 4.16; $P = 0.003$), and overall mortality (RR, 2.06; $P <0.001$). Hypoalbuminemia, a major adverse prognostic factor in dialysis patients, is strongly associated with cardiac disease.

I could go on, but you get the point. Albumin is a big deal. However, it's not just a big deal for us. Let's look at the data for other groups. Maybe albumin is important only to people with kidney disease?

| **Study 4.12** | Hypoalbuminemia Is a Strong Predictor of 30-Day All-Cause Mortality in Acutely Admitted Medical Patients: A Prospective, Observational, Cohort Study.[21] |

RESULTS:

We included 5,894 patients, and albumin was available in 5,451 (92.5%). A total of 332 (5.6%) patients died within 30 days of admission. Median plasma albumin was 40 g/L (IQR 37–43). Crude 30-day mortality in patients with low albumin was 16.3% compared to 4.3% among patients with normal albumin (p<0.0001). Patients with low albumin were older and admitted for a lon-ger period than patients with a normal albumin, while patients with high albumin had a lower 30-day mortality, were younger and were admitted for a shorter period. Multivariable logistic regression analyses confirmed the association of hypoalbuminemia with mortality (OR: 1.95 (95% CI: 1.31– 2.90)). Discriminatory power was good (AUROC 0.73 (95% CI, 0.70–0.77)) and calibration acceptable.

CONCLUSIONS:

We found hypoalbuminemia to be associated with 30-day all-cause mortality in acutely admitted medical patients. Used as a predictive tool for mortality, plasma albumin had acceptable discriminatory power and good calibration.

Study 4.13   Serum Albumin and Cerebro-cardiovascular Mortality During a 15-year Study in a Community based Cohort in Tanushimaru, a Cohort of the Seven Countries Study.[22]

CONCLUSIONS:

The serum albumin level was thus found to be a predictor of all-cause and cerebro-cardiovascular death in a general population.

Study 4.14   Decreased admission serum albumin level (SAL)is an independent predictor of long-term mortality in hospital survivors of acute myocardial infarction. Soroka Acute Myocardial Infarction II (SAMI-II) project.[23]

Out of 12,535 patients, 8750 were included. Patients with reduced SAL were older, a higher rate of women, with an increased prevalence of severe left ventricular dysfunction, chronic renal failure, diabetes mellitus and ST-elevation AMI, 3-vessel coronary artery disease, and in-hospital complications. While the prevalence of chronic ischemic coronary disease, dyslipidemia, smokers, and obesity, was lower. Mortality rates throughout the follow-up period increased as SAL decreased with 17.6%, 24%, 28.5%, 38.6%, and 57.5% for SAL of >4.1, 3.9-4.1, 3.7-3.9, 3.4-3.7 and <3.4g/dL respectively (p-for-trend <0.001). Using the SAL category of >4.1g/dL as the reference group, Adjusted Hazard Ratio values were 1.14 (p=0.107), 1.23 (p=0.007), 1.39 (p<0.001) and 1.70 (p<0.001) for the SAL categories of 3.9-4.1, 3.7-3.9, 3.4-3.7 and <3.4g/dL respectively.

CONCLUSIONS:

Decreased SAL (Serum albumin levels) on admission, including levels within "normal" clinical range, is significantly associated with long-term all-cause mortality in hospital survivors of AMI with a "dose-response" type association.

Study 4.15   Albumin correlates with all-cause mortality in elderly patients undergoing transcatheter aortic valve implantation.[24]

METHODS AND RESULTS:

A total of 150 patients (mean age 81±6 years) undergoing TAVI were included in the study. Patients with preprocedural albumin >4 g/dl (>40 g/L) (n=71) were compared to those >4 g/dl (>40 g/L) (n=79). The cut-off value of 4 g/ dl (40 g/L) was based on the mean value of albumin in the patients included in the study. During a mean follow-up of 2.1 years, the survival rate was 72%. Patients in both groups had similar baseline characteristics. The 2.1-year mortality was higher in the low albumin group compared with the normal albumin group (35% vs. 19%, p=0.01). Multivariate analysis indicated that low preprocedural albumin was independently associated with a more than twofold increase in 2.1-year all-cause mortality (p=0.01, HR=2.28; 95% CI: 1.17-4.44). Low post-procedural serum albumin remained a strong parameter correlated with all- cause mortality (HR=2.47; 95% CI: 1.28-4.78; p<0.01).

CONCLUSIONS:

Baseline albumin can be used as a simple tool that correlates with survival after TAVI. Low albumin is an important parameter associated with all-cause mortality after the procedure.

Study 4.16   **Lower Serum Albumin Shortly After Admission Predicts Prolonged Hospital Stay in Younger Burn Patients.[25]**

A composite score was created for the ≤40 years age group using ABSI and albumin levels to predict an increased length of stay. Thirty-eight of 198 (19.2%) patients had a stay >3 weeks. The AUCs for albumin level, total BSA [bovine serum albumin], and ABSI alone in younger patients were 0.97, 0.97, and 0.96, respectively. Among patients older than 40, the AUC values were substantially lower indicating lower predictive value. The probability of prolonged stay for patients with albumin level ≥2.4 g/dl was low (.8%) compared with those with albumin level <2.4 g/dl (96.5%). Adding ABSI to this model increased predictive accuracy.

Albumin level obtained within 72 hours of admission was an effective predictor of prolonged hospital stay in adult burn patients ≤40 years.

Study 4.17   **Lower serum albumin concentration and change in muscle mass: the Health, Aging and Body Composition Study.[26]**

CONCLUSIONS:

Lower albumin concentrations, even above the clinical cutoff of 38 g/L, are associated with future loss of ASMM (appendicular skeletal muscle mass) in older persons. Low albumin concentration may be a risk factor for sarcopenia.

Study 4.18   **Association Between Decreased Serum Albumin With Risk of Venous Thromboembolism(VTE) and Mortality in Cancer Patients.[27]**

RESULTS:

Patients (630 males [58.9%] and 440 females [41.1%]) were observed for a median of 723 days. During follow-up, 90 VTE events (8.4%) and 396 deaths (37.0%) occurred. The median albumin was 41.3 g/L (25th–75th percentile, 37.6–44.2). Patients with albumin levels below the 75th percentile had a 2.2-fold increased risk of VTE (95% confidence interval [CI] 1.09–4.32), as well as a 2.3-fold increased risk of death (95% CI 1.68–3.20) compared with patients with albumin above the 75th percentile.

CONCLUSIONS:

Decreased serum albumin levels in cancer patients were significantly associated with increased risk of VTE and mortality. Serum albumin, a marker of a cancer patient's overall prognosis, could be considered for risk assessment of important clinical outcomes such as VTE and mortality.

Ok, so albumin levels clearly matter to everyone regardless of health, illness, or disease. Burn patients, heart patients, older patients, pre- and postoperative cancer patients. No one can escape the importance of albumin levels.

My personal and very strong opinion is albumin is the closest thing to a perfect indicator for people with kidney disease. Albumin is a great indicator of the war going on in our bodies. If we are winning the war, our albumin levels are increasing. We might be winning the war on nutrition and uremia, but losing the battle on oxidative stress and inflammation. Albumin gives a composite view of the battle. Are we winning or losing? Albumin levels will continue to decline, or at least stay flat, if we are not addressing all the right issues.

Getting albumin levels to start rising is step one and the next step is to get your albumin level above 4.0 g/l and ideally up to the 4.5 g/l

Let's look at what must happen for albumin levels to rise:

1. Protein nutrition must be adequate. If we are not getting enough protein nutrition, albumin will not rise.

2. Calorie intake must be adequate.

3. Inflammation must be decreasing. If inflammation is rising, albumin levels may not increase, and may even fall.

4. Oxidative stress must be decreasing. If oxidative stress is increasing, albumin levels will be flat or falling.

5. Uremia must be decreasing. We don't fully understand how uremia decreases albumin, but it does. If uremia is increasing, albumin may not rise.

6. Acidosis must be decreasing. Acidosis decreases albumin synthesis. If albumin is rising, acidosis may be decreasing.

7. Proteinuria, or protein in our urine, is decreasing if albumin levels rise.

Think about it for a minute: tests like creatine clearance and blood urea nitrogen (BUN) tell you how well your kidneys are filtering waste products from your bloodstream today or over the recent days. These tests help determine GFR and uremia. Albumin in our urine tells us the severity of protein loss. However, these tests tell us very little, if anything, about protein nutrition, inflammation, oxidative stress and the impact these factors are having on our bodies.

We get lots of benefits that we don't see from increasing albumin.

Fetuin-A is a protein produced by the liver. Fetuin-A is the primary defense against vascular calcification. Remember vascular calcification is the number one killer of people with kidney disease. Fetuin-A is our body's main defense against heart disease. Low fetuin-A levels accelerate heart disease and increase mortality rates. Guess what increased albumin does to fetuin-A? If albumin is rising, so if fetuin-A. The same conditions that set the stage for albumin to increase also increase fetuin-A. Again, fetuin-A is strong mortality indicator, just like albumin. Increasing albumin, which in turn increases fetuin-A, lowers our risk of heart disease and vascular calcification.

Study 4.19   Associations of serum fetuin-A with malnutrition, inflammation, atherosclerosis and valvular calcification syndrome and outcome in peritoneal dialysis patients.[28]

CONCLUSIONS:

<u>Serum fetuin-A showed important associations with valvular calcification, atherosclerosis, malnutrition, and inflammation, and was linked to mortality and cardiovascular events in PD patients via its close relationships with the MIAC (Malnutrition, inflammation, atherosclerosis, and calcification) syndrome.</u>

The same conditions that allow albumin to rise also increase other proteins and hormones like fetuin-A. Here is a partial list of proteins/hormones produced by the liver:

Albumin

Fetuin-A

A-fetoprotein

Fibronectin

C-reactive protein

Ceruloplasmin

Transcortin

Haptoglobin

Hemopexin

IGF binding protein

Retinol-binding protein

Sex hormone binding globulin

Thyroxine-binding globulin

Transthyretin

Transferrin

Vitamin D binding protein

Insulin growth factor 1

Thrombopoietin

Hepcidin

Angiotensinogen

Polyprotein

The same conditions that allow albumin to increase may also allow many of these proteins and hormones to revert to normal levels. You don't need to know what these proteins and hormones do to see that albumin is a proxy for what is going on in our bodies. If albumin is rising, we are probably getting an increase in all kinds of other proteins, hormones, and so on. The good ones will be going up, and the bad ones will be going down if albumin is rising.

Some of these proteins are leading indicators of dropping serum albumin.

Study 4.20 **Increased urinary angiotensinogen (UAGT) precedes the onset of albuminuria in normotensive type 2 diabetic patients.[29]**

Based on these findings, the present study was performed to test the hypothesis that UAGT levels are increasing even before the development of DN in type 2 diabetic patients without hypertension. 102 patients with type 2 diabetes mellitus (T2DM) and 18 healthy volunteers were studied cross-sectionally. Clinical data were collected and morning spot urine samples were obtained from all participants. UAGT levels were detected by an enzyme-linked immunosorbent assay (ELISA). As a result, UAGT to creatinine ratio (UAGT/Cr) was significantly enhanced in T2DM patients before the appearance of urinary albumin (UALB) and further increased to a greater degree in albuminuric patients. UAGT/Cr levels were positively correlated with Log (UALB to creatinine ratio) and diastolic blood pressure, but negatively correlated with estimated glomerular filtration rate. These data indicate that elevated UAGT levels precede the onset of albuminuria in normotensive T2DM patients. UAGT might potentially serve as an early marker to determine intrarenal RAS [renal artery stenosis] activity and predict progressive kidney disease in T2DM patients without hypertension.

These studies suggest that other proteins produced in our livers are affected before albumin starts showing up in our urine. Oxidative stress, inflammation, etc., have been affecting us for some time before we start leaking protein in our urine.

Another example is edema, the swelling that we all know so well, which is caused by low oncotic pressure. Oncotic pressure is the pressure proteins in our blood (primarily albumin) that maintain pressure. This pressure helps to pull water out of our bloodstream. Increasing albumin decreases edema and swelling. Another unexpected benefit. Low serum albumin, salt, and edema go hand in hand.

I want to make this point repeatedly: The conditions that set the stage for albumin to rise help us in many ways. Almost too many to count. In fact, an entire book could be written on the factors that are affected by albumin levels. You get the idea; albumin is very important.

Studies show overwhelmingly that if our albumin is rising, our risk of death is decreasing. We want to increase our odds, right? Increasing our albumin levels is one of the best things we can do. To focus on raising your albumin levels, you will have to address several issues.

We can take separate measures of acidosis, uremia, inflammation, oxidative stress, and nutrition and the data would certainly be meaningful and helpful. Two of these measures could be better and three worse at any one time. Trust me; I have been there. It's confusing and frustrating to see some numbers get worse and others get better month after month. This is especially depressing when you are working for months to make a diet and treatment plan work. It's like getting punched in the gut. Fear and doubt creep in. You wonder if you are doing the right thing and it can drive you crazy. I came to fear my blood test results for a while. I just couldn't take more bad news.

If you focus on albumin over three-month periods, you will know if you are getting better or not. Albumin and many tests can be noisy on a monthly basis. It's better to look at longer time-frames and not just one-month tests. If albumin is increasing, you are winning the war overall. You can bet a lot of things other than albumin are getting better as well. If your albumin has gone up, many other proteins/hormones that we don't measure have gotten better as well. Not every issue or indicator will improve every month or every three months, but overall the good will start to outweigh the bad.

The other issue is how to increase albumin production. Low-protein or very low-protein diets reduce albumin production unless supplemented with a source of protein nutrition like keto acids or amino acids. Low-calorie diets may also decrease albumin production.

Increased intake of branched-chain amino acids or keto acids may also increase albumin production, but the increased albumin may be lost unless you treat all the factors: inflammation, oxidative stress, acidosis, proteinuria, and so on.

Eating more dietary protein from animal products makes the situation worse. It causes increasing inflammation, oxidative stress, uremia, acidosis, and so on. We need to address protein nutrition without increasing the very factors that make our kidneys fail faster. We have to increase nutrition with a foot on the brake and not on the gas.

I know there are exceptions to every rule and that many different types of kidney disease exist, but I would bet a large sum of money that no one has ever gone into partial remission without getting albumin levels under control. I don't see how it could be possible. Albumin is involved in too many body functions.

Screaming Again

Now, picture me jumping up and down, screaming, spitting, cussing, and red-faced for a minute. The reason I am so upset is hypoalbuminemia is treatable in most cases. I can't say this is true for everyone, but I can say the vast majority of us can increase our albumin levels by a measurable amount. Again, if we are increasing albumin, we are increasing our odds.

Remember the study that showed 10,000 patients could be saved each year if albumin could be treated? I am screaming because it can and should be treated in every kidney patient with albumin levels below 4 g/dl. Take a look at your last blood test to see where you are at.

When I stopped trying to cure my disease by just lowering protein intake and tried to improve my albumin as comorbid condition, that is when I started getting better. I tied together eating below my GFR and treating low albumin levels at the same time. The reason is the same conditions that set the stage for improving albumin numbers also set the stage for slowing or stopping kidney disease.

My personal experience in raising albumin was the key to getting better. I didn't get better until my albumin started rising. I had to take double the normal dosage of a protein supplement and later tried a keto acid supplement, which was better. We need healthy albumin levels for survival, no matter who we are.

Treating inflammation, uremia, oxidative stress, proteinuria, and acidosis also slows kidney disease progression. These same conditions are what led to our disease in many cases. This makes perfect sense when you think about it. Before, I was focused only on lowering protein, salt, and phosphorus. No one told me this might work for kidney disease. Low-protein diets are a one-factor approach. Protein is only part of the solution.

Summary

Increasing albumin should be the goal of every kidney patient. Any increase should be considered a win because your odds are getting better.

How to treat albumin is part of the treatment plan and diet in this book. A low-protein diet high in antioxidants and anti-inflammatory foods that don't cause uremia or acidosis is needed. A supplement is also needed to provide adequate protein nutrition without increasing acidosis, oxidative stress, inflammation, and uremia. In 2018, for the first time in history, a new product is available the U.S. that accomplishes all of these goals. We ended up with a patent pending on a product just for people with kidney disease (and others) to safely raise albumin levels. The website is www.albutrix.com.

I hope you can now see that albumin is a window into the war going on inside your body. Rising albumin means we are winning the war and increasing our odds of survival. Albumin may not be the perfect indicator, but it is as close to perfect as we have today. Focus on raising your albumin at all costs. It is key to living longer and living better.

Commit it to memory: Rising albumin good, falling albumin bad.

References

1. Phillips A, Shaper AG, Whincup P. Association between serum albumin and mortality from cardiovascular disease, cancer, and other causes. *The Lancet.* 1989;334(8677):1434-1436.

2. Nicholson J, Wolmarans M, Park G. The role of albumin in critical illness. *British Journal of Anaesthesia.* 2000;85(4):599-610.

3. Taverna M, Marie A-L, Mira J-P, Guidet B. Specific antioxidant properties of human serum albumin. *Annals of Intensive Care.* 2013;3(1):4.

4. Caironi P, Gattinoni L. The clinical use of albumin: the point of view of a specialist in intensive care. *Blood Transfusion.* 2009;7(4):259-267.

5. Gillum R. Assessment of serum albumin concentration as a risk factor for stroke and coronary disease in African Americans and whites. *Journal of the National Medical Association.* 2000;92(1):3.

6. Figge J, Rossing T, Fencl V. The role of serum proteins in acid-base equilibria. *The Journal of laboratory and clinical medicine.* 1991;117(6):453-467.

7. Larsen MT, Kuhlmann M, Hvam ML, Howard KA. Albumin-based drug delivery: harnessing nature to cure disease. Molecular and *Cellular Therapies.* 2016;4(1):3.

8. Blaine J, Chonchol M, Levi M. Renal control of calcium, phosphate, and magnesium homeostasis. *Clinical Journal of the American Society of Nephrology.* 2014:CJN. 09750913.

9. Finotti P, Pagetta A. Heparin-Induced Structural Modifications and Oxidative Cleavage of Human Serum Albumin in the Absence and Presence of Glucose. *The FEBS Journal.* 1997;247(3):1000-1008.

10. Gibbs J, Cull W, Henderson W, Daley J, Hur K, Khuri SF. Preoperative serum albumin level as a predictor of operative mortality and morbidity: results from the National VA Surgical Risk Study. *Archives of Surgery.* 1999;134(1):36-42.

11. Pereira GRM, Strogoff-de-Matos JP, Ruzany F, et al. Early changes in serum albumin: impact on 2-year mortality in incident hemodialysis patients. *Jornal Brasileiro de Nefrologia.* 2015;37(2):198-205.

12. Hwang J-C, Jiang M-Y, Lu Y-H, Wang C-T. Precedent fluctuation of serum hs-CRP to albumin ratios and mortality risk of clinically stable hemodialysis patients. *PloS One.* 2015;10(3):e0120266.

13. Lim PS, Jeng Y, Wu MY, et al. Serum oxidized albumin and cardiovascular mortality in normoalbuminemic hemodialysis patients: a cohort study. *PloS One.* 2013;8(7):e70822.

14. Terawaki H, Matsuyama Y, Matsuo N, et al. A lower level of reduced albumin induces serious cardiovascular incidence among peritoneal dialysis patients. *Clinical and Experimental Nephrology.* 2012;16(4):629-635.

15. Kalantar-Zadeh K, Kilpatrick RD, Kuwae N, et al. Revisiting mortality predictability of serum albumin in the dialysis population: time dependency, longitudinal changes, and a population-attributable fraction. *Nephrology Dialysis Transplantation.* 2005;20(9):1880-1888.

16. de Mutsert R, Grootendorst DC, Indemans F, et al. Association between serum albumin and mortality in dialysis patients is partly explained by inflammation, and not by malnutrition. *Journal of Renal Nutrition.* 2009;19(2):127-135.

17. Amaral S, Hwang W, Fivush B, Neu A, Frankenfield D, Furth S. Serum albumin level and risk for mortality and hospitalization in adolescents on hemodialysis. *Clinical Journal of the American Society of Nephrology.* 2008;3(3):759-767.

18. Khoshhali M, Kazemi I, Hosseini SM, Seirafian S. Relationship between trajectories of serum albumin levels and technique failure according to diabetic status in peritoneal dialysis patients: A joint modeling approach. *Kidney Research and Clinical Practice.* 2017;36(2):182.

19. Haller C. Hypoalbuminemia in renal failure: pathogenesis and therapeutic considerations. *Kidney & Blood Pressure Research.* 2005;28(5-6):307.

20. Foley RN, Parfrey PS, Harnett JD, Kent GM, Murray DC, Barre PE. Hypoalbuminemia, cardiac morbidity, and mortality in end-stage renal disease. *Journal of the American Society of Nephrology.* 1996;7(5):728-736.

21. Jellinge ME, Henriksen DP, Hallas P, Brabrand M. Hypoalbuminemia is a strong predictor of 30-day all-cause mortality in acutely admitted medical patients: a prospective, observational, cohort study. *PLoS One.* 2014;9(8):e105983.

22. Umeki Y, Adachi H, Enomoto M, et al. Serum Albumin and Cerebro-cardiovascular Mortality During a 15-year Study in a Community-based Cohort in Tanushimaru, a Cohort of the Seven Countries Study. *Internal Medicine.* 2016;55(20):2917-2925.

23. Plakht Y, Gilutz H, Shiyovich A. Decreased admission serum albumin level is an independent predictor of long-term mortality in hospital survivors of acute myocardial infarction. Soroka Acute Myocardial Infarction II (SAMI-II) project. *International Journal of Cardiology.* 2016;219:20-24.

24. Bogdan A, Barbash IM, Segev A, et al. Albumin correlates with all-cause mortality in elderly patients undergoing transcatheter aortic valve implantation. *EuroIntervention: journal of EuroPCR in collaboration with the Working Group on Interventional Cardiology of the European Society of Cardiology.* 2016;12(8):e1057-e1064.

25. Amavizca K, Yang S, Idicula A, Mata A, Dissanaike S. Lower Serum Albumin Shortly After Admission Predicts Prolonged Hospital Stay in Younger Burn Patients. *Journal of Burn Care & Research.* 2016;37(2):e145-e153.

26. Visser M, Kritchevsky SB, Newman AB, et al. Lower serum albumin concentration and change in muscle mass: the Health, Aging, and Body Composition Study. *The American Journal of Clinical Nutrition.* 2005;82(3):531-537.

27. Königsbrügge O, Posch F, Riedl J, et al. Association between decreased serum albumin with risk of venous thromboembolism and mortality in cancer patients. *The Oncologist.* 2016;21(2):252-257.

28. Wang AY-M, Woo J, Lam CW-K, et al. Associations of serum fetuin-A with malnutrition, inflammation, atherosclerosis and valvular calcification syndrome and outcome in peritoneal dialysis patients. *Nephrology Dialysis Transplantation.* 2005;20(8):1676-1685.

29. Zhuang Z, Bai Q, Lata A, Liang Y, Zheng D, Wang Y. Increased urinary angiotensinogen precedes the onset of albuminuria in normotensive type 2 diabetic patients. *International Journal of Clinical and Experimental Pathology.* 2015;8(9):11464.

CHAPTER 5

Potential Renal Acid Load (PRAL)

In my research, the most black-and-white issue was potential renal acid load (PRAL), which was initially surprising, as it is not covered in any kidney diet guidelines or books. Yet the evidence of its importance is overwhelming. My personal opinion is PRAL is at least as important as protein restriction and may even be more important, although I didn't come to this point of view until I started managing PRAL myself. I believe you need to be intimately familiar with the subject.

Let's begin with an explanation of what potential renal acid load is. According to Dr. David Collison at the Huntly Centre in Australia, PRAL is a calculated value of certain nutrients in food that have the most significant indication of changing the acidity or alkalinity–the pH–of the body.[1]

Your kidneys maintain the pH of your blood, working 24/7 to preserve a narrow pH range of 7.35 to 7.45. Above or below these numbers, bad things start to happen. Low numbers are acidic, and high numbers are alkaline, or base, or basic.[2]

Let's stop here for a key lesson: Your body only works well in only a very narrow range of values. This is true for many conditions, not just pH. By doing the work for your kidneys, you make it easy for your kidneys to maintain the narrow range. Back to acid load.

Your kidneys produce ammonia with a pH of 11 to offset acids; when you eat a largely acidic diet, your kidneys must work overtime to keep your body's pH in the normal range. Here is how it works:

Acid is produced from the metabolism of sulfur in certain dietary proteins, including meats, eggs, dairy, and many grains. Salts (not sodium, there is a difference) found primarily in fruits and veggies are absorbed in the gastrointestinal tract and produce bicarbonate (alkali). The difference between the acid and alkali is the dietary acid load, known as the net endogenous acid production (NEAP), which must be excreted by the kidney to maintain acid-base balance.[3] Our kidneys retain or excrete the appropriate amount of bicarbonate to maintain a balanced pH. If we have enough bicarbonate in our system, our kidneys don't have to produce ammonia to offset high levels of acid. Put another way, eating foods high in bicarbonate and restricting high acidic food equals no or very little ammonia production by the kidneys.

But as our kidney function declines, so does our ability to effectively manage bicarbonate levels, and our ability to produce ammonia declines as well. Remember, you have to treat every factor, not just protein. Renal acid load is a great example. Our kidneys have a lot of functions besides protein waste handling.

When we send more acid to our kidneys to process than can be balanced by the bicarbonate present in our system and the ammonia produced by our kidneys, we get acidosis. Acidosis, also called metabolic acidosis, occurs when the kidneys fail to maintain the slightly alkaline pH of the blood and fluids between cells. Even mild metabolic acidosis speeds up the rate at which your kidneys fail. It is a mortality indicator as early as stage 3 kidney disease.4 Remember how we talked about bad things happening earlier in kidney disease than everyone thought? Acidosis is an example. It is normally treated with sodium bicarbonate (yes, the same chemical as the baking soda you have in the kitchen cabinet). However, doctors will not treat acidosis if severe edema problems are present because sodium bicarbonate is a form of salt, and salt is restricted for patients with kidney disease. You will see a theme in this book about one condition leading to other conditions. Unmanaged acidosis leads to treatment with sodium bicarbonate which increases sodium intake leading to higher blood pressure, greater edema and more inflammation to name a few. Treating acidosis with diets stops this cascade of events that may increase the progression of your disease.

The Effects of High Dietary Acid Load on Chronic Kidney Disease

When I got to this stage of my research, I began to wonder whether lowering the workload on the kidneys might allow the body to maintain the proper pH when the kidneys are compromised. I became curious about whether anyone had studied or looked at the correlation between dietary acid load (DAL) or PRAL and chronic kidney disease (CKD)? Here are some excerpts from the conclusions of several studies that I found:

Study 5.1 High dietary acid load (DAL) predicts ESRD [end-stage renal disease] among adults with CKD.[5]

In conclusion, high DAL (dietary acid load) in persons with CKD (Chronic kidney disease) is independently associated with increased risk of ESRD (end-stage renal disease) in a nationally representative population.

Study 5.2 Dietary acid intake and kidney disease progression in the elderly.[6]

In elderly CKD patients, our findings suggest that high net endogenous acid production (NEAP) is independently associated with CKD progression. The decrease in NEAP may be an effective kidney-protective therapy.

Study 5.3 Dietary acid load and incident chronic kidney disease: results from the ARIC study.[7]

Dietary acid load is associated with incident CKD in a population-based sample. These data suggest a potential avenue for CKD risk reduction through diet.

Study 5.4 Dietary acid load and chronic kidney disease among adults in the United States.[8]

Higher NAE(es) is associated with albuminuria and low eGFR, and sociodemographic risk factors for CKD are associated with higher levels of NAE(es). DAL may be an important target for future interventions in populations at high risk for CKD.

Study 5.5   **Dietary acid-base load and risk of chronic kidney disease in adults: Tehran lipid and glucose study.[9]**

In the final model, after additional adjustment for dietary intake of total fat, carbohydrate, dietary fiber, fructose, sodium, diabetes mellitus, and hypertension, the risk of CKD in the highest dietary PRAL category, compared to the lowest, increased by 42%. After adjusting for possible confounding factors, we found that higher PRAL (more acidic diet) was associated with higher prevalent CKD.

If you were looking for a smoking gun in kidney disease, acid load is as close as you can get. High-acid diets are extremely bad for people with kidney disease. As for why this is so, it's a guess at this stage.

Ammonia toxicity could be a cause. From an evolutionary point of view, maybe our kidneys were never meant to produce ammonia 24 hours a day. Maybe our diets in the past were almost always alkaline, and our kidneys had to produce ammonia only in rare situations. From an autoimmune perspective, are our bodies attacking our kidneys because they are producing ammonia 24/7? Again, this is conjecture at this stage. But some research supports this theory.

We have focused on protein for so long when perhaps we should have been looking at acid loads instead, as the researchers did in this very large study completed in 2016, which points to the acid load being more important or as important as protein:

Study 5.6   **The association between renal hyperfiltration and the sources of habitual protein intake and dietary acid load in a general population with preserved renal function: the KoGES study[10]**

The odds for RHF (renal hyperfiltration) increased as the percentile rank of eNEAP increased until about the 50th percentile and then leveled off. The positive association between eNEAP [estimated net endogenous acid production] and RHF [renal hyperfiltration] was significant in both sexes and age groups. Dietary acid load was associated with RHF regardless of sex and age and rather than the amount of the total or the individual sources of habitual dietary protein may be a better target for the dietary intervention of chronic kidney disease.

Maybe like the tuna and bean curd study, it was the acid load, not the protein. Soybeans have a predicted renal acid load of -3.10, which is considered alkaline. Tuna has a predicted renal acid load of 7 to 10, which is highly acidic. The tuna and bean curd study leads us to believe acid load is the issue, not protein. Maybe the amount of protein was never the issue; it was the kind of protein.

How Alkali Can Help Chronic Kidney Disease

Some studies suggest that adding bicarbonate to your diet may be renoprotective. In other words, treating acidosis by increasing alkali may help slow the progression of your chronic kidney disease (CKD). By adding alkaline foods and/or increasing the natural bicarbonate found in your body, you are decreasing the amount of work your kidneys have to do.

Study 5.7 Metabolic acidosis and kidney disease: does bicarbonate therapy slow the progression of CKD?[11]

Metabolic acidosis is a risk factor for progressive CKD, possibly through various mechanisms that involve renal adaptation to chronic acidemia and that could cause renal injury when persistently activated. The administration of alkali to patients with early-to-advanced stages of CKD in small single-center clinical trials has been proved to be renoprotective. Larger clinical trials are awaited to better define treatment targets and therapeutic regimens that are applicable to a broad range of patients with CKD. For the time being it is advised to administer alkali therapy to patients with serum bicarbonate.

Study 5.8 Daily oral sodium bicarbonate preserves glomerular filtration rate by slowing its decline in early hypertensive nephropathy.[12]

After 5 years, the rate of eGFR [estimated glomerular filtration rate] decline, estimated using plasma cystatin C, was slower and eGFR was higher in patients given sodium bicarbonate than in those given placebo or sodium chloride. Thus, our study shows that in hypertensive nephropathy, daily sodium bicarbonate is an effective kidney protective adjunct to blood pressure control along with angiotensin-converting enzyme inhibition.

Study 5.9 Chronic kidney disease: Oral bicarbonate: renoprotective in CKD?[13]

Metabolic acidosis, a common complication of chronic kidney disease (CKD), can lead to the development and worsening of various serious conditions and might further deteriorate kidney function. Now, de Brito-Ashurst and colleagues report that administration of sodium bicarbonate to patients with metabolic acidosis in the context of non-dialysis-dependent CKD slows the decline in creatinine clearance and decreases the risk of developing end-stage renal disease (ESRD).

Not all studies have shown clear benefits with bicarbonate supplementation. Larger human trials are needed to determine the real effect. However, the studies lean towards bicarbonate supplementation. If eating an alkaline diet or a diet that has a negative acid load, you won't have to supplement with bicarbonate in most cases. This is very valuable, as sodium bicarbonate increase sodium intake which increases blood pressure, edema, and inflammation.

The chart below shows some data to support this. It comes from a study called "Ketoanalogue-Supplemented Vegetarian Very Low-Protein Diet and CKD Progression"[14] and it compares results of a conventional low-protein (higher-acid) diet (LPD) to a vegan, low-protein (more alkaline) diet (KD) in CKD patients. As you can see, the low-protein diet did not change serum bicarbonate levels. However, the vegan diet did raise serum bicarbonate (alkaline) to normal levels of 22-29 after 12 to 15 months. It didn't happen overnight, but continuous progress was made.

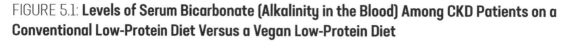

FIGURE 5.1: **Levels of Serum Bicarbonate (Alkalinity in the Blood) Among CKD Patients on a Conventional Low-Protein Diet Versus a Vegan Low-Protein Diet**

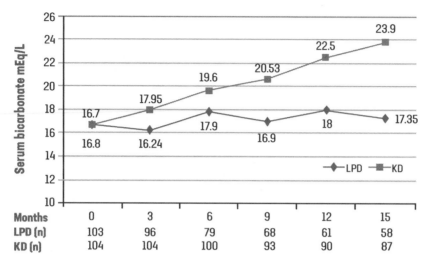

This chart has a lot of clues for us.

1. The conventional low-protein diet did not slow progression of the disease as well as the vegan diet.

2. Eating high-acid foods while on a low-protein diet did not help patients. Very low protein alone did not change bicarbonate levels.

3. The bicarbonate levels were still rising after 15 months. In other words, CKD patients' ability to deal with acid loads was still increasing after a year. This is a big key. Doing something for a few weeks isn't going to do much for us. If our kidneys are damaged, we may not respond to diets as quickly as a healthy person. The lower your kidney function, the longer it may take for you to realize the full benefits of any dietary modifications.

4. Depending on the severity of acidosis, it may be completely cured by diet alone. Remember, acidosis speeds the decline in our kidney function, but it is easily ignored, and many times it is left untreated. This is a huge mistake. You have every right to talk to your doctor about options. Diet should be your first treatment. This could eliminate the need for sodium bicarbonate to increase pH, which many doctors avoid recommending because it can also increase swelling, blood pressure, and edema. Fruits and veggies are alkaline. The bottom line is the higher the acid level or case of acidosis, the faster your kidney will fail and the less likely you are to stop or slow your disease.

5. Keto acids were used to reduce kidney workload further and provide protein nutrition. An alkaline diet with keto acids, which also reduce the amount of acid your body produces, was the best combination. Keto acids produce less of an acid load than amino acids. We will talk more about keto acids.

Another study supports the idea that the secret to halting the progression of CKD might be fruits and vegetables or bicarbonate supplements:

| Study 5.10 | Treatment of metabolic acidosis in patients with stage 3 chronic kidney disease with fruits and vegetables or oral bicarbonate reduces urine angiotensinogen and preserves glomerular filtration rate.[15] |

Alkali therapy of metabolic acidosis in patients with chronic kidney disease (CKD) with plasma total CO_2 (TCO_2) below 22mmol/l per KDOQI guidelines appears to preserve estimated glomerular filtration rate (eGFR). By contrast, urine excretion of angiotensinogen, an index of kidney angiotensin II, increased in Usual Care but decreased with bicarbonate or fruits and vegetables. Creatinine-calculated and cystatin C–calculated eGFR decreased in all groups, but the loss was less at 3 years with bicarbonate or fruits and vegetables than Usual Care. Thus, dietary alkali treatment of metabolic acidosis in CKD that is less severe than that for which KDOQI recommends therapy reduces kidney angiotensin II activity and preserves eGFR.

In regular English, this study shows that eating alkaline fruits and veggies or adding a daily dose of an alkalizing agent like bicarbonate slowed disease progress better than traditional care or recommendations. Again, we are treating early in stage 3 and not waiting until ESRD.

The study demonstrates another important benefit: Angiotensin II, a hormone that increases blood pressure, is reduced by an alkaline diet or supplementation. A decrease in angiotensin II is a big benefit for us because high blood pressure is also a kidney killer.

The Problem of Acidosis

Acidosis has other effects as well. A direct correlation exists between bicarbonate levels and the amino acid valine in muscle tissue in people with kidney disease. Acidosis appears to interfere with normal amino acid metabolism. Another direct correlation exists between bicarbonate and albumin or blood protein levels. Again, in some way, acidosis interferes with normal protein metabolism resulting in lower albumin levels. Albumin is the most abundant protein in your blood. Acidosis may also have a detrimental effect on vitamin D syntheses and bone health as well. Remember, we want to treat every factor of our kidney workload, not just the protein component. Kidney disease is a multifactorial disease.

The evidence from my point of view is overwhelming that low-acid or alkaline diets may be the most important factor in stopping or slowing your kidney disease. This is as close to an open-and-shut case as you can get from a dietary point of view. This evidence might also explain why I didn't do as well on the low-protein diet. It was because I was still eating foods with a high acid load. As people with kidney disease, we should absolutely limit the acid load in our diets and go as alkaline as possible. We will talk more about this later in Chapter 32. In the meantime, the following chart will give you an idea of which foods increase the workload on your kidneys (those with a higher PRAL) and which foods can greatly decrease the workload on your kidneys (those with a lower PRAL). The table is helpful because, while dietary acid load is highly correlated to protein content, this is not always the case.

Potential Renal Acid Loads

The following chart is an estimate of dietary effects on pH balance. Foods with a negative value (milliequivalents per 100g) are alkaline or "basic" foods. Foods with a positive value are considered acidic. The more acid in your diet, the harder your kidneys must work to maintain your body's narrow pH range. We need to eat foods with negative numbers. The higher the number, the higher the acid load.

Beverages

FOOD	PRAL
Beer, draft	−0.2
Beer, pale	0.9
Beer, stout, bottled	−0.1
Coca-Cola	0.4
Cocoa, made with semi-skimmed milk	−0.4
Coffee, infusion, 5 minutes	−1.4
Mineral water	−1.8
Mineral water (Volvic)	−0.1
Red wine	−2.4
Tea, Indian, infusion	−0.3
White wine, dry	−1.2

Fats and oils

FOOD	PRAL
Butter	0.6
Margarine	−0.5
Olive oil	0.0
Sunflower seed oil	0.0

Fish

FOOD	PRAL
Cod, fillets	7.1
Haddock	6.8
Herring	7.0
Trout, brown, steamed	10.8

Fruits, nuts, and fruit juices

FOOD	PRAL
Apple juice, unsweetened	-2.2
Apples, 15 varieties, flesh and skin, average	-2.2
Apricots	-4.8
Bananas	-5.5
Black currants	-6.5
Cherries	-3.6
Grape juice, unsweetened	-1.0
Hazelnuts	-2.8
Kiwi fruit	-4.1
Lemon juice	-2.5
Orange juice, unsweetened	-2.9
Oranges	-2.7
Peaches	-2.4
Peanuts, plain	8.3
Pears, 3 varieties, flesh and skin, average	-2.9
Pineapple	-2.7
Raisins	-21.0
Strawberries	-2.2
Walnuts	6.8
Watermelon	-1.9

Vegetables

FOOD	PRAL
Asparagus	-0.4
Broccoli	-1.2
Carrots, young	-4.9
Cauliflower	-4.0
Celery	-5.2
Chicory, Endive	-2.0
Cucumber	-0.8
Eggplant	-3.4
Leeks	-1.8
Lettuce, average of 4 varieties	-2.5
Lettuce, iceberg	-1.6
Mushrooms, common	-1.4
Onions	-1.5
Peppers, green bell	-1.4
Potatoes, gold	-4.0
Radish, red	-3.7
Spinach	-14.0
Tomato juice	-2.8
Tomatoes	-3.1
Zucchini	-4.6

Grain products

FOOD	PRAL
Bread, rye flour, mixed	4.0
Bread, rye flour	4.1
Bread, wheat flour, mixed	3.8
Bread, wheat flour, whole meal	1.8
Bread, white wheat	3.7
Cornflakes	6.0
Crispbread, rye	3.3

Grain products continued

FOOD	PRAL
Noodles, egg	6.4
Oat flakes, rolled oats	10.7
Rice, brown	12.5
Rice, white, easy cook	4.6
Rice, white, easy cook, boiled	1.7
Rye flour, whole	5.9
Spaghetti, white	6.5
Spaghetti, whole wheat	7.3
Wheat flour, white, plain	6.9

Legumes

FOOD	PRAL
Beans, green/French beans	-3.1
Lentils, green and brown, whole, dried	3.5
Peas	1.2

Meat and meat products

FOOD	PRAL
Beef, lean only	7.8
Chicken, meat only, no skin	8.7
Corned beef, canned	13.2
Frankfurters, hot dogs	6.7
Liver sausage	10.6
Luncheon meat (deli meats like salami, ham)	10.2
Pork, lean only	7.9
Rump steak, lean and fat	8.8
Salami	11.6
Turkey, meat only	9.9
Veal, fillet	9.0

Milk, dairy products, and eggs

FOOD	PRAL
Buttermilk	0.5
Cheese, Camembert	14.6
Cheese, Cheddar-type, reduced fat	26.4
Cheese, Gouda	18.6
Cottage cheese, plain	8.7
Creams, fresh, sour	1.2
Eggs, whole	8.2
Eggs, whites	1.1
Eggs, yolk	23.4
Full-fat soft cheese, aka cream cheese	4.3
Hard cheese, average of 4 types	19.2
Ice cream, dairy, vanilla	0.6
Milk, whole, evaporated	1.1
Milk, whole, pasteurized and sterilized	0.7
Cheese, Parmesan	34.2
Processed cheese, plain	28.7
Yogurt, whole milk, fruit	1.2
Yogurt, whole milk, plain	1.5

Sugar, preserves, and sweets

FOOD	PRAL
Chocolate, milk	2.4
Honey	−0.3
Marmalade, jam	-1.5
Sugar, white	-0.1

It's never too early to start managing your disease. The following study shows that as early as stage 2, kidney disease can be slowed by lowering your acid load. This is tragic, as most patients wait until too much kidney function has been lost before trying to aggressively manage their diets to slow or stop their disease.

The Key to Halting Progression of CKD Might Be in the Produce Market, Not in the Pharmacy

The current study by Goraya et al. tests the hypothesis that, as the daily acid load is primarily dependent on the type of food ingested, increasing the daily intake of fruits and vegetables might have effects similar to those of alkali therapy in preserving renal function.[15] Indeed, the study showed similar effects of oral $NaHCO_3$ and a diet rich in fruits and vegetables (calculated to reduce acid load by 50%) in patients with stage 2 CKD, although no effects were noted in stage 1 CKD patients.

<u>Moreover, a diet rich in fruits and vegetables could potentially slow down renal disease progression by several effects independent of decreasing acid load; for example, the relative increase of potassium over sodium intake, decreased phosphorus load, and increased intake of fibers, antioxidants, vitamins, and chemicals such as sulforaphane.</u>

Gray *et al.* recognize that a significant effect of the fruit-and-vegetable-rich diet is decreasing blood pressure, a factor known to slow loss of kidney function. Regardless of mechanisms, a fruit-and-vegetable-rich diet has so many potential beneficial effects that it could be easily accepted for implementation. This study is also important because it illustrates a very simple and safe way to treat metabolic acidosis, an intervention to slow CKD progression that has not received enough attention.

Reducing dietary acid load is a win on every level. Heart health, antioxidants, fiber, blood pressure, and the list goes on.

A Word on High-Acid Foods

I do understand that many people, including myself, do not want to stop eating meat. I love the taste of a good steak, fried chicken, and blackened snapper. I like it all. One of the biggest obstacles for me was giving up meat. Giving up meat is usually the biggest obstacle to slowing kidney disease progression. If you can't or won't give it up, your chances of slowing your disease or going into remission are very low.

My experience could be described as losing a bad habit. Many of us are used to eating meals based around meats. Breakfast may be the exception, but most lunches and dinners are often based around meat as the main component. It is a habit we have had for many decades, maybe fifty or more years.

The benefits of giving up meat (high-acid) foods and sticking to the diet are too numerous to mention here, but I can tell you with 100% confidence the following:

1. You will look better.

2. You will feel better.

3. Your health will be better.

4. Your future prognosis will be better.

5. You might even put a deadly disease into remission or slow its progression to a snail's pace.

You just have to change the habit of expecting to eat meat at every meal. You will get five huge benefits if you can change one habit. What is more important, a cheeseburger or steak or spending more very high-quality years with your family? It's easy when you think about it this way. In addition, a large amount of research supports this approach to preventing or stopping heart disease progression.

Here is what I can say with complete certainty based on the science as of 2019:

"The more high-acid foods you eat like beef, chicken, fish, egg, dairy, and grains the faster your kidney disease will progress. It will also be much harder to manage your metabolic numbers and to manage the day-to-day symptoms of your disease."

As you can see, what started out as something relatively simple got complicated very quickly. This is the nature of kidney disease. But here's a good summation of the valuable data I found while reviewing the studies specified in this chapter, as well as others:

1. High-acid diets are associated with heart disease, which is the last thing we need.

2. Alkaline diets may have a renoprotective effect, slowing the decline in our kidneys.

3. No data suggests that low-acid diets are bad for us.

4. No data suggests that high-acid diets are good for us.

5. Acidosis, even mild acidosis, accelerates a decline in kidney function.

6. Acidosis is associated with bone and muscle loss.

7. Acidosis increases our odds of death and is a mortality indicator as early as stage 3.

8. Acidosis reduces our absorption of amino acids, especially valine, leucine, and isoleucine.

9. A direct correlation exists between bicarbonate levels and albumin levels.

10. Acidosis may also reduce vitamin D synthesis.

11. Blood pressure may be reduced by an alkaline diet.

Simply put, your life with kidney disease will be harder and likely shorter if you continue to abuse your kidneys with a high-acid diet.

The weight of scientific research overwhelmingly supports a low-acid or alkaline diet to slow the progression of kidney disease. Furthermore, it may eliminate metabolic acidosis in many cases with no known harmful side effects. Alkaline diets may even protect your kidneys.

If you pick up a kidney or renal diet book that says you should be eating meat or most grains, throw it away. This is advice from the 1950s. Do you own research if you don't believe me; PubMed and Google Scholar are good places to start.

In Summary

Potential renal acid load maybe one of the biggest factors driving our disease progression. Considering its impact on your health, it is underappreciated.

Reducing high-acid foods and increasing alkaline foods decreases the amount of ammonia your kidney has to produce to offset a high-acid diet.

Not one study can be found suggesting a diet high in acid is good for people with kidney disease. All available research says just the opposite.

The data is overwhelming on this issue; it's not up for debate anymore.

References

1. Collison D. PRAL - Potential Renal Acid Load: A Measure of the Effect of Foods on the pH of the Body. 2010; http://www. huntlycentre.com.au/updates/posts/view/118. Accessed May 12th, 2017.

2. Frassetto LA, Morris RC, Sebastian A. Effect of age on blood acid-base composition in adult humans: role of age-related renal functional decline. *American Journal of Physiology-Renal Physiology.* 1996;271(6):F1114-F1122.

3. Scialla JJ, Anderson CA. Dietary acid load: a novel nutritional target in chronic kidney disease? *Advances in chronic kidney disease.* 2013;20(2):141-149.

4. Navaneethan SD, Schold JD, Arrigain S, et al. Serum bicarbonate and mortality in stage 3 and stage 4 chronic kidney disease. *Clinical Journal of the American Society of Nephrology.* 2011;6(10):2395-2402.

5. Banerjee T, Crews DC, Wesson DE, et al. High dietary acid load predicts ESRD among adults with CKD. *Journal of the American Society of Nephrology.* 2015;26(7):1693-1700.

6. Kanda E, Ai M, Kuriyama R, Yoshida M, Shiigai T. Dietary acid intake and kidney disease progression in the elderly. *American journal of nephrology.* 2014;39(2):145-152.

7. Rebholz CM, Coresh J, Grams ME, et al. Dietary acid load and incident chronic kidney disease: results from the ARIC study. *American journal of nephrology.* 2015;42(6):427-435.

8. Banerjee T, Crews DC, Wesson DE, et al. Dietary acid load and chronic kidney disease among adults in the United States. *BMC nephrology.* 2014;15(1):137.

9. Mirmiran P, Yuzbashian E, Bahadoran Z, Asghari G, Azizi F. Dietary Acid-Base Load and Risk of Chronic Kidney Disease in Adults. *Iranian Journal of Kidney Diseases.* 2016;10(3):119-125.

10. So R, Song S, Lee JE, Yoon H-J. The Association between Renal Hyperfiltration and the Sources of Habitual Protein Intake and Dietary Acid Load in a General Population with Preserved Renal Function: The KoGES Study. *PloS one.* 2016;11(11):e0166495.

11. Kovesdy CP. Metabolic acidosis and kidney disease: does bicarbonate therapy slow the progression of CKD? *Nephrology Dialysis Transplantation.* 2012;27(8):3056-3062.

12. Mahajan A, Simoni J, Sheather SJ, Broglio KR, Rajab M, Wesson DE. Daily oral sodium bicarbonate preserves glomerular filtration rate by slowing its decline in early hypertensive nephropathy. *Kidney international.* 2010;78(3):303-309.

13. Kovesdy CP, Kalantar-Zadeh K. Chronic kidney disease: Oral bicarbonate: renoprotective in CKD? *Nature Reviews Nephrology.* 2010;6(1):15-17.

14. Garneata L, Stancu A, Dragomir D, Stefan G, Mircescu G. Ketoanalogue-Supplemented Vegetarian Very Low–Protein Diet and CKD Progression. *Journal of the American Society of Nephrology.* 2016;27:2164-2176.

15. Goraya N, Simoni J, Jo C-H, Wesson DE. Treatment of metabolic acidosis in patients with stage 3 chronic kidney disease with fruits and vegetables or oral bicarbonate reduces urine angiotensinogen and preserves glomerular filtration rate. *Kidney international.* 2014;86(5):1031-1038.

CHAPTER 6

The Protein Debate

As we saw in the previous chapter, the benefit of a diet with a low potential renal acid load (PRAL) is an open-and-shut case. Protein and protein load, on the other hand, are not as clear-cut and require a little more research. We'll begin with what we know: Renal acid load and protein are closely related; high-acid foods are normally high-protein foods. We are aware high-protein/high-acid food is bad for us but is it the protein load, the acid load, or the combination that is the culprit? In most cases, we don't know. Like many issues in kidney disease, everything is related in some way, and untangling these issues can be hard. We are not always sure of the causes and outcomes.

The good news is we don't have to know every possible issue; we just need to know which foods are good and which are bad for our kidneys. We need to know which foods accelerate the progression of our disease, and which ones are protective in some way.

One of the first questions we need to deal with is how much protein we truly need. Many of us—and our well-meaning families and friends—assume we are experts on protein. I know from personal experience that the comments can get wild if you say you are on a very low-protein diet.

These are some things well-meaning friends and family have told me:

"How can you live without eating protein? Aren't you going to die?"

"Oh, but don't you know this is good protein? It's okay to eat chicken."

"Your doctor has given you horrible advice. The reason you are sick is not eating enough protein."

"I would seek a second opinion. Clearly, your doctor has no understanding of how the body really works."

"What? You're not eating protein? Do you feel dizzy or sick? Have you sought medical help?"

We are protein-obsessed as a nation. I, too, fell into this group and had no real understanding before my experience at Johns Hopkins. Conventional wisdom is that large amounts of protein are good for us, and, further, we are all probably protein deficient. So many food labels claim to be high in protein as a selling point. But are we getting *too much* protein in our diets?

A little protein education is needed. Remember, our bodies work in only a narrow range. Too much or too little of anything can be bad for us; it can put an extra workload on our bodies. As we discovered with alkali and bicarbonate in Chapter 4, we keep what we need and get rid of the rest—and protein is no different. Our bodies have robust mechanisms to conserve what is necessary and get rid of what is excessive. Once our bodies have enough protein, we excrete the excess protein.

The standard recommendation of protein is usually 0.8 grams per kg of body weight,[1] so a 75 kg (165 pound) person would need to consume 60 grams of protein a day, which can be obtained from just one chicken breast and a glass of milk. This means that the full recommended daily allowance can be obtained very easily. However, protein is in almost everything we eat. One stalk of broccoli contains four or five grams of protein.[2]

Low-protein diets (LPD) traditionally aim for 0.6 grams per kg of body weight, or 45 grams per day for a 75 kg (165 pound) person. Very low-protein diets (VLPD) recommend 0.3 grams per kg, or 22.5 grams a day for our 75-kg person. These diets include a special supplement of special amino acids or keto acids to ensure protein nutrition is always provided.[3]

During my decade of trying different diets, I went as low as 0.45 grams per kg of body weight a day for six months with no protein supplements. My blood tests looked great, and I had no problems. When you are on these diets, especially the VLPD, you find out protein is in everything. I was very uneducated on this issue before the Johns Hopkins/Walser diet. I never realized how hard it was to eat only 22.5 grams of protein a day. Check out these examples:

Protein rich foods	Grams of protein
One chicken breast	43
1 cup soybeans	68
4 cups cooked brown rice	20
1 cup cheese	33
1 cup scrambled eggs	22
3 cups milk	24

You can see that it is very easy to get to 60 grams of protein. Many of us are getting 60 grams or more *per meal*. The average male consumes 102 grams of protein per day,[4] almost twice the recommended daily intake. And many people I know take additional protein supplements or favor foods with high protein.

Could it be that the giant increase in kidney disease has something to do with eating 200% to 400% more protein than required?

Protein Workload and Nitrogen Waste

To understand the problem here, we first need to understand the workload protein puts on our kidneys. As our bodies digest (break down) proteins, the by-products of this process are nitrogen-based waste products called urea. Creatinine is another waste product that's produced by your muscle metabolism and, to a smaller extent, by eating protein. Healthy kidneys filter urea and creatinine and excrete them in your urine. Uremia is the diagnosis when your kidneys cannot remove end products like urea and creatinine from the blood fast enough.[5]

Albumin is the most abundant protein in the human body. Serum albumin is the blood test for albumin levels. Your serum albumin test levels from a blood test will give your insight into your level of protein nutrition and inflammation. Low albumin levels are a strong mortality predictor. Our main problem is we can't eat enough protein to raise our albumin levels in many cases. Impaired amino acid metabolism, inflammation, and leaking protein in your urine cause low albumin levels despite adequate levels of protein consumption. Eating higher amounts of protein to solve low albumin levels leads to accelerated kidney and heart disease and doesn't work either. The fact that people with kidney disease have low albumin to start with tells us that eating more dietary protein won't solve the problem.[6] Later, we will talk about bypassing normal amino acid metabolism to avoid this issue.

Animal proteins have all the essential amino acids we need, but a few essential amino acids may be bad for us at higher levels. Methionine, an essential amino acid, has been implicated in aging and can be toxic in high levels. Methionine also happens to be the amino acid most associated with acidosis due to its high sulfur content. Methionine-restricted diets improve epithelial barrier function in cell-to-cell junctions. Impairments to these junctions have been described in several neurological disorders including multiple sclerosis, stroke, Alzheimer's disease, Parkinson's disease, and epilepsy. Methionine is also a precursor to homocysteine, another amino acid. Homocysteine is related to several diseases, including heart disease. Data is mixed on whether high methionine intake promotes high homocysteine levels.[7]

Methionine restriction may also be the reason caloric restriction works, but more on this later.

Tryptophan, another essential amino acid, generates uremic toxins during the digestion process. These compounds are considered cardio- and nephrotoxic and accelerate kidney disease progression.[8] We will cover this in Chapter 8.

It's All About the Nitrogen

Blood Urea Nitrogen (BUN) is the blood test normally used to monitor the amount of waste products in your bloodstream. High BUN levels are related to decreased survival rates for people with heart and kidney disease. BUN levels are directly correlated with how much nitrogen we consume.[9] So when we talk about protein, we are really talking about nitrogen. Amino acids contain nitrogen, but so do other food components. Components like purines, pyrimidines, creatine, creatinine, and other free amino acids, as well as amino sugars and vitamins, can all contribute to the total nitrogen content. That said, as a rule, high-nitrogen foods are foods high in amino acids or high in protein.

Different kinds of proteins have different nitrogen levels despite having similar protein or amino acid content.

Here is the nitrogen content of different proteins:

Food	Nitrogen content of 100 grams of dry food (about 3 oz)
Soybeans	8.19
Beef	15.71
Pork	15.53
Chicken	15.64
Fish	15.21

And the percentage of nitrogen content:[10]

Food	Nitrogen content percentage
Cheese	4.96%
Cured Ham	4.41%
Mixed nuts	4.18%
Soy Cutlet (processed soybean food)	2.48%
Veggie burger	0.65%

As you can see, soybeans have almost half the amount of nitrogen as meats. The same is true for a veggie burger, which has a much lower nitrogen content than cheese or ham. A fifty percent reduction in waste workload for our kidneys for a similar protein intake is a big deal for us.

You may wonder why soybeans are so high in protein but low in nitrogen. The reason is that soybeans do not have many of the extras that add to nitrogen content. Creatine and creatinine are in meats, but not soybeans. An equal serving of chicken breast has a purine content that's 300% higher than soybeans.[11] You get the idea. Meats have all the essential amino acids and so are considered a higher quality of protein. Plant proteins rarely contain all the essential amino acids, and therefore are thought of as a low-quality protein by the public. But for our purposes, it is reversed. We want protein nutrition with the lowest possible nitrogen load on our kidneys. High-quality protein for us is low-acid, or alkaline, and as low in nitrogen as we can get. Traditional dietary guidelines do not apply to us anymore.

My point is that eating a diet high in nitrogen, aka protein, may come with more baggage than our kidneys can carry. As people with kidney disease, we need to be a little smarter about the foods we eat and how we get our protein. Amino acids are essential for our survival, but data suggests we want to consume the minimum amount required to avoid protein malnutrition and maintain our blood albumin levels.

BUN levels are managed in kidney disease patients because high BUN levels lead to uremia, which will kill you if left untreated. Without dialysis or other intervention, uremia will progress to cause coma, stupor, and then death.[12]

The possible effects of uremia can be seen in GFR levels.[13]

GFR and their effects

GFR (mL/min)	Effects
100-120	Normal GFR
‹60	Uremic symptoms may be present, reduced well-being
30-60	Cognitive impairment
55	Fatigue and reduced stamina
‹50	Insulin resistance
‹30	Possibly lead to coma
≤15	Kidney failure

Symptoms can start as early as stage 2 kidney disease. The same is true for renal acid load (see Chapter 4). Therefore, low-protein diets were initially designed to reduce BUN levels and reduce the odds of uremia. Treating uremia is necessary, but in many cases we are still treating the symptom, not the cause. The symptom is high BUN levels, but the cause is eating more nitrogen-rich foods than your kidney can process.

Using the kidney workload concept, we need to eat below our current GFR. Sending a BUN workload of 100 to kidneys with a GFR of 50 will cause BUN levels to rise.

In the previous chart, we saw that ham had 7 times more nitrogen than a veggie burger.

If we send a workload of 35 to our kidneys and have a GFR of 50, then our BUN levels will start to drop slowly over the following weeks and months. Our kidneys can handle the workload with a little left in reserve.

It's that simple. What is less simple is managing your diet so the amount of nitrogen waste products you produce is as small as possible. Protein is in everything we eat, so limiting nitrogen/amino acid intake can be tricky.

Let's look at what the research says about high-protein diets:

Study 6.1   Associations of diet with albuminuria and kidney function decline.[14]

Results did not vary by diabetes status for microalbuminuria and eGFR outcomes or in those without hypertension at baseline for eGFR decline. No significant associations were seen for other types of protein, fat, vitamins, folate, fructose, or potassium.

Study 6.2   Withdrawal of red meat from the usual diet reduces albuminuria and improves serum fatty acid profile in type 2 diabetes patients with microalbuminuria.[15]

In macroalbuminuric patients with type 2 diabetes, withdrawing red meat from the diet reduces the urinary albumin excretion rate (UAER).

Study 6.3   The Western-style diet: a major risk factor for impaired kidney function and chronic kidney disease.[16]

(This study has so much information I am posting several parts of the study instead of just the conclusion.)

Study 6.4   A High-Fat Diet as a Risk Factor for CKD

The Western-style diet is high in animal fat with elevated levels of saturated fats and trans-fatty acids. A cross sectional study (Reasons for Geographic and Racial Differences in Stroke Study; REGARDS), including more than 19,000 adults >45 yr. of age, found a significant association between saturated fat intake and hyper albuminuria (95). Other subtypes of fat such as PUFAs [polyunsaturated fatty acids] and trans-fatty acids were associated neither with hyper albuminuria nor with estimated glomerular filtration rate.

Study 6.5   A Protein-Rich Diet and Impaired Kidney Function

However, convincing evidence indicates that reduced protein intake favorably affects disease progression in patients with stage 3–4 CKD and delays the time to renal death.[17] Reduced blood urea levels and proteinuria in CKD patients on low- and very low-protein diets delay kidney function decline; however, a close monitoring of these patients including supplementation of certain nutrients is required. Reduced kidney function is found in ~40% of diabetic patients.[18] Thus high intakes of red meat represent a risk for further deterioration of kidney function in this patient population.[19]

Moreover, consumption of high amounts of animal proteins leads to a marked acid load to the kidney and has been associated with the development of kidney stones.[20] High meat protein intakes result in increased dietary acid loads and compensatory increases in renal acid excretion and ammonia production, leading to metabolic acidosis with a higher risk for tubulointerstitial injury.[21] Restricted protein intake is therefore recommended for the prevention of recurrent kidney stones and the progression of kidney function decline.[22]

CONCLUSION:

A chronic nutrient overload causes various tissue-specific and systemic metabolic dysfunctions that increase the risk of kidney damage and promote CKD. Especially, the combination of high amounts of saturated fat, fructose, and salt promotes dyslipidemia, hormonal disturbances, oxidative stress, inflammation, and fibrosis with impaired glomerular function and hypertension.

Study 6.6 | **Low carbohydrate-high protein diet and incidence of cardiovascular diseases in Swedish women: prospective cohort study.[23]**

Low carbohydrate-high protein diets, used on a regular basis and without consideration of the nature of carbohydrates or the source of proteins, are associated with increased risk of cardiovascular disease.

Study 6.7 | **Low-carbohydrate-high-protein diet and long-term survival in a general population cohort.[24]**

Prolonged consumption of diets low in carbohydrates and high in protein is associated with an increase in total mortality.

Study 6.8 | **Low-carbohydrate diets and all-cause mortality: a systematic review and meta-analysis of observational studies.[25]**

Low-carbohydrate diets were associated with a significantly higher risk of all-cause mortality, and they were not significantly associated with a risk of CVD [cardiovascular disease] mortality and incidence. However, this analysis is based on limited observational studies, and large-scale trials on the complex interactions between low-carbohydrate diets and long-term outcomes are needed.

The National Kidney Foundation has an excellent summary page on dietary protein intake.[26] Following are some highlights.

Study 6.9 | **Low-protein diets[26]**

Based on 2 meta-analyses, low-protein diets reduced risks of loss of kidney function (GFR or creatinine-based measurements) and/or increased albuminuria (measured as urinary excretion of either albumin or total protein), with more pronounced benefits in DKD than in non-DKD (Fig 21).[27,28] More recently, even a modest limitation of dietary protein (0.89 versus 1.02 g/kg body weight per day) substantially reduced the risk of CKD stage 5 or death (RR, 0.23; 95% CI, 0.07 to 0.72; P = 0.04) in people with type 1 diabetes and CKD stage 2 (inferred based on levels of albuminuria and GFR; Fig 22). These patients (85% to 89% during the course of the study) also received ACE [angiotensin-converting enzyme] inhibitors and had similar control of blood pressure and other risk factors irrespective of diet group assignment, indicating that reducing dietary protein provided benefits beyond established medical therapies.[29] Benefits of limiting dietary protein intake are more evident in type 1 than type 2 diabetes, but fewer studies have been done in the latter population. Based on the available evidence (Table 37 and Table 38), the Work Group concluded that limiting dietary protein will slow the decrease in kidney function and progression of albuminuria, and it may prevent CKD stage 5.

Study 6.10   High-protein diets[26]

At the other end of the spectrum, high-protein diets are a particular concern in patients with diabetes because they increase albuminuria and may accelerate the loss of kidney function. Glomerular hyperfiltration and increased intraglomerular pressure are well-recognized mechanisms of kidney damage induced by excess dietary protein. <u>Based on both human studies and experimental mod-els, higher protein intake appears to have more pronounced effects on kidney hemodynamics and kidney damage in diabetes.</u>[30-32] Emerging epidemiological evidence indicates that higher protein intake (≥20% versus 10% of total daily calories) is associated with loss of kidney function in women with mild kidney insufficiency (defined as estimated GFR < 80 and > 55 mL/min/1.73 m2) and development of microalbuminuria in people with diabetes and hypertension.[33,34] <u>Therefore, in the opinion of the Work Group, people with diabetes and CKD should avoid high-protein diets (≥20% of total daily calories). Some common fad diets that recommend high protein are Atkins°, Protein Power, the Zone, South Beach°, and Sugar Busters°.</u>

Study 6.11   Low-protein diets for chronic kidney disease in nondiabetic adults.[35]

<u>Reducing protein intake in patients with chronic kidney disease reduces the occurrence of renal death by 32% as compared with higher or unrestricted protein intake.</u> The optimal level of protein intake cannot be confirmed by these studies.

A reduction in renal death by 32% is a pretty strong statement when ten studies and 2,000 patients are analyzed.

As you can see, science strongly suggests that high-protein diets are bad for all of us as people with kidney disease. Protein-restricted diets have been around for a very long time to slow or stop the progression of kidney disease. The main goal of low-protein diets had simply been to reduce uremia.

Mentioning low-protein diets to a nephrologist will get dismissive gestures in many cases.

The main reason low-protein diets are not recommended in the United States is a study called "Modification of Diet in Renal Disease (MDRD)." This study took place from 1989 to 1993 and was inconclusive, with some patients doing well and others showing no improvements. Years later, the MDRD study was reanalyzed, and the result changed to "some benefit," but it's far from the conclusive evidence that we would like.[36]

What if our protein sources didn't have saturated fats or a put a large acid load on our bodies? Would that make a difference? I wanted to dig a little deeper. Vegetable sources of protein like soybeans, lentils, and other beans are high protein. This includes soybean foods like tofu and tempeh. (Seitan is another source of vegetable protein, but it's made from wheat protein or wheat gluten. We know grains have a high renal acid load, so seitan is excluded from our consideration.) Here's what I found:

Study 6.12 — Effects of soy protein containing isoflavones in patients with chronic kidney disease: A systematic review and meta-analysis.[37]

Soy protein containing isoflavones intake significantly decreased serum creatinine, serum phosphorus, CRP and proteinuria in predialysis patients, while no significant change was found in creatinine clearance and glomerular filtration rate. We also found that soy protein intake could maintain the nutritional status in dialysis patients, though no significant change in CRP, BUN, and serum phosphorus was detected. Future large, long-term RCTs are still needed to clarify the effects of soy protein intake in patients with CKD.

Study 6.13 — The effects of soy protein on chronic kidney disease: a meta-analysis of randomized controlled trials[38]

The meta-analysis suggested a protective effect of soy protein consumption on SCR and serum phosphorus concentrations in pre-dialysis CKD patients. It may also have a significant effect on lowering serum TG concentrations. However, nonsignificant effects on TC and Ca were observed. Evidence was limited because of the relatively small number of available trials and subjects.

Study 6.14 — Renal, metabolic and hormonal responses to ingestion of animal and vegetable proteins.[39]

No differences were found in plasma amino acid levels following the two protein loads. Thus, independently of the quantity of protein, vegetable protein has significantly different renal effects from animal protein in normal humans which could be partly explained by differences in glucagon and renal vasodilatory prostaglandin secretion.

The type of protein ingested is therefore crucial to the pattern and magnitude of the renal response elicited. Vegetable proteins seem to induce renal changes comparable to those obtained by reducing the total amount of protein in the diet and prevent the vasodilatory and proteinuric effects of meat. These effects appear to be mediated by hormonal changes involving glucagon secretion and renal prostaglandin production. Protein modified, rather than protein restricted, diets may prove advantageous in the long-term treatment of chronic renal failure.

The results of this research surprised me since I was taught all protein was dangerous for people with kidney disease regardless of source. In the Johns Hopkins program, every source protein was off limits. But now we were getting somewhere. A direct comparison on what happens in our kidneys when we eat different kinds of proteins shows us that kidney workload is much higher when we eat animal proteins as opposed to soy-based proteins. And here's a study from 2016 that sheds more light on the issue, suggesting that we don't have to limit ourselves to protein from vegetable sources—only protein from meats, eggs, fish, dairy, and grains.

Study 6.15 — The Associations of Plant Protein Intake with All-Cause Mortality in CKD.[40]

A diet with a higher proportion of protein from plant sources is associated with lower mortality in those with eGFR<60mL/min/1.73m (2). Future studies are warranted to determine the causal role of plant protein intake in reducing mortality in those with eGFR<60mL/ min/1.73m (2).

The study analyzed health information from 14,866 participants in the National Health and Nutrition Examination Survey III (NHANES III). Of those participants, 1,065 were classified as having CKD (eGFR <60). Dietary information was gathered through 24-hour dietary recall interviews. The death rate in the participants without CKD was 11.1% over an average follow-up of 8.6 years, while the death rate in the CKD population was 59.4% over an average follow-up period of 6.2 years.

After adjusting for age, gender, race, tobacco use, alcohol use, comorbid conditions, body mass index, physical inactivity, and total protein and calorie intake, with each 33% increase in the ratio of plant to total protein in the diet, there was a significantly lower risk of death (HR 0.77, 95% CI 0.61 to 0.96) in the CKD group.

"We were surprised to see such an impressive association. Every 33 percent plant of total protein ratio increase was associated with a 23% lower risk of mortality in those with CKD," said co-author Xiaorui Chen, MS, of University of Utah School of Medicine. "However, this health-preserving benefit was not seen in 'normal' individuals with an eGFR ≥ 60."

Two facts need to be repeated:

> Every 33% increase in plant protein was associated with a 23% lower risk of mortality.

> Health-preserving benefits were found in individuals with GFRs over 60.

That the health-preserving effect happened only in those with GFRs lower than 60 is kind of earth-shattering. Finally, we are starting to explain a few things. Eating plant protein did not affect mortality rates unless the subjects had kidney disease (GFR below 60)! Lowering the workload on the kidney by reducing meat consumption reduced mortality rates for kidney disease patients. The more plant protein consumed, the lower the risk of mortality. This confirms data from the tuna and bean curd study. A GFR of 60 was the tipping point in terms of our kidneys being able to handle protein loads. This also goes hand in hand with the tuna/bean curd study. Two different study point to a GFR around 60 being the tipping point.

In other words, a healthy kidney can handle any workload you throw at it, so no benefit was seen in healthy patients. However, an impaired kidney cannot process the same amount of protein (with its corresponding increased workload) as a healthy kidney. Giving the kidneys a break reduced mortality rates.

This is exactly what we have been talking about with kidney workload. For a little more proof, we can look at a more recent study comparing a low-protein diet and a very low-protein vegetarian diet. This is the study[41] I mentioned in Chapter 4 that compares results of a conventional low-protein (higher-acid) diet (LPD) to a vegan, low-protein (more alkaline) diet (KD) on CKD patients with a GFR of 18.

FIGURE 6.1: **Median Changes in eGFR (Estimated Glomerular Filtration Rate) Between Study Moments**

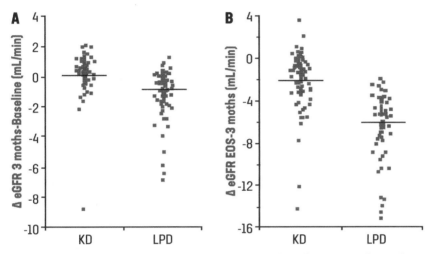

Median changes in eGFR (95% CI) between study moments (Δ implies statistically significant differences between the two groups). EOS, end of study. (A) In the first 3 months after randomization, eGFR significantly increased in KD arm and decreased in LPD. (B) The decrease in eGFR was lower in KD when considering the interval between 3 months after randomization and the end of study.

The following chart shows the same information in a more dramatic fashion. The KD group, the vegetarian low-protein group using keto acids, had a much better outcome and slowed progression dramatically compared to the regular LPD group using a traditional or conventional low-protein diet.

FIGURE 6.2: **Adjusted event-free survival rates of patients assigned to the KD or the LPD**

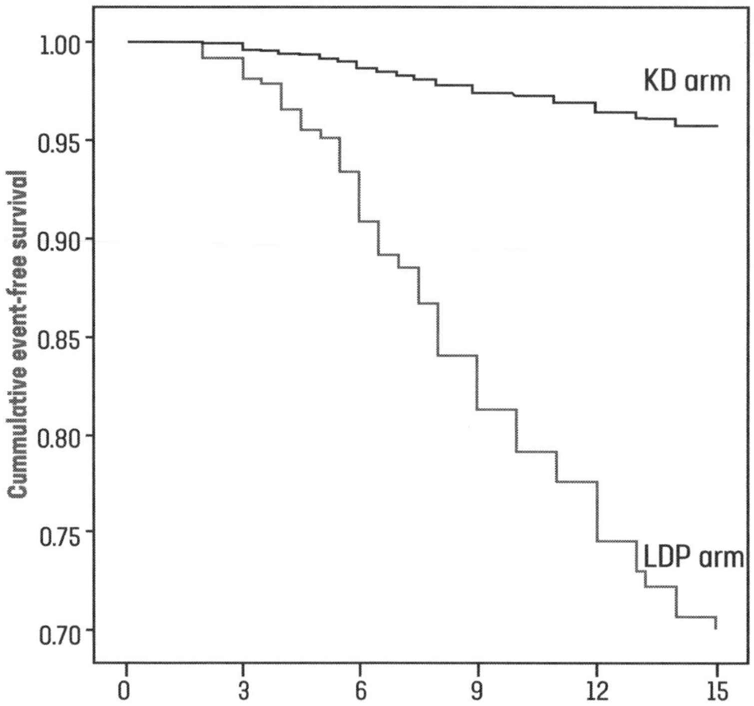

Adjusted event-free survival rates of patients assigned to the KD or the LPD. The probability to reach the end-point was even lower in KD group when adjusted for the other significant predictors of outcome in a Cox proportional hazard model.

On the table, KD stands for the vegetarian group, which consumed 0.3 grams of vegetarian protein per kg of body weight. LPD was the group on a low-protein diet, consuming 0.6 grams of protein per kg body weight, with no restrictions on the source of protein. So, three things are going on with this study: a lower amount of protein, a vegetarian diet, and the use of a protein supplement (keto acids again).

Comparing the KD group between tables A and B, we see that eGFR barely dropped for the group average over 15 months. By comparison, the LPD group dropped dramatically.

Was it the increased protein restriction, or the vegetarian diet, or a combination? We don't know the exact reason. Remember, the GFRs of all patients in this study were 18 at the start of the study. These patients are almost on dialysis, yet the KD group still benefited.

Other data from the same study is excerpted in this table:

Nitrogen waste productSerum urea (mg/dl)	KD	LPD
Baseline	187 (164 to 225)	213 (183 to 248)
End of Study	122 (114 to 127)	226 (191 to 252)

Urea dropped 34% in the vegetarian KD group, despite having a GFR around 18, while urea increased 5% in the LPD group. So, decreasing any-source protein by a moderate amount (0.6 grams per kg per day, or 45 grams for a 75 kg person) did nothing to help deal with uremia; it was still too much for the kidneys to process. However, 22.5 grams a day of vegetable proteins influenced slowing disease progression.

Back to the workload model, we can say that a GFR of 18 is too low to handle 45 grams of protein a day, but it could handle 22.5 grams of alkaline protein sources (fruits and veggies). The workload must be very low to reap the benefits. Remember, moderation kills.

Another factor from this study is that calcium and phosphorus rates improved in the KD group, but not in the LPD group, another clue that reducing the workload allows our bodies to work towards self-correction.

The bottom line is that the amount of protein and the type of protein matter. You can dramatically change the workload on your kidneys with your protein or protein supplement selection. In fact, if you've been told to eat a low or very low-protein diet, the fact is that if you focus only on vegetable proteins, you may be able to eat more protein than you thought. With vegetable proteins, we get amino acids, but we don't get all the extras that raise the nitrogen content. On average, about 15% to 20% of meat consists of the essential amino acids we need for nutrition. The other 80% are things we don't need, and many are considered bad for us.

Summary

The weight of the scientific evidence is apparent. There is no evidence that eating eggs, dairy, chicken, beef, or fish helps our kidney disease. In fact, all evidence points to high-protein diets accelerating disease progression and creating uremic conditions faster than plant-based protein diets. On the other hand, no evidence exists to suggest that vegetarian sources of protein are bad for us. All the available evidence suggests that plant proteins are good for people with kidney disease and may even be protective.

One is proven to accelerate our disease, and the other is proven to slow disease progression or protect our kidneys. Which one should you be eating? Once you have been diagnosed with kidney disease, meats, eggs, dairy, and fish products have no place in your diet.

Uremia and or uremic malnutrition are mortality indicators for us. High-protein and high acid foods must go if we want to slow or maybe even stop kidney disease progression.

As I said in the last chapter, advocating that people with kidney disease should be eating meats or other animal products is 1950s diet advice

References

1. Chernoff R. Protein and older adults. *Journal of the American College of Nutrition.* 2004;23(sup6):627S-630S.

2. FDA. Raw Vegetables Poster (Text / Accessible Version). 2015; https://www.fda.gov/food/ingredientspackaginglabeling/ labelingnutrition/ucm114222.htm. Accessed 20th May, 2017.

3. Piccoli GB, Capizzi I, Vigotti FN, et al. Low protein diets in patients with chronic kidney disease: a bridge between mainstream and complementary-alternative medicines? *BMC Nephrology.* 2016;17(1):76.

4. Ulmer G. How Much Protein is Needed Daily for the Ideal Protein Diet? 2015; http://www.livestrong.com/article/369551how-much-protein-is-needed-daily-for-the-ideal-protein-diet/. Accessed 24th May, 2017.

5. Witko-Sarsat V, Friedlander M, Capeillère-Blandin C, et al. Advanced oxidation protein products as a novel marker of oxidative stress in uremia. *Kidney international.* 1996;49(5):1304-1313.

6. Kaysen GA, Dubin JA, Müller HG, Rosales LM, Levin NW. The acute-phase response varies with time and predicts serum albumin levels in hemodialysis patients. *Kidney international.* 2000;58(1):346-352.

7. Lee BC, Kaya A, Gladyshev VN. Methionine restriction and lifespan control. *Annals of the New York Academy of Sciences.* 2016;1363(1):116-124.

8. Vitetta L, Linnane AW, Gobe GC. From the gastrointestinal tract (GIT) to the kidneys: live bacterial cultures (probiotics) mediating reductions of uremic toxin levels via free radical signaling. *Toxins.* 2013;5(11):2042-2057.

9. Wu BU, Johannes RS, Sun X, Conwell DL, Banks PA. Early changes in blood urea nitrogen predict mortality in acute pancreatitis. *Gastroenterology.* 2009;137(1):129-135.

10. Krotz L, Leone F, Giazzi G. *Nitrogen/Protein Determination in Food and Animal Feed by Combustion Method (Dumas) using the Thermo Scientific FlashSmart Elemental Analyzer.* Milan, Italy: Thermo Fisher Scientific;2016.

11. Kaneko K, Aoyagi Y, Fukuuchi T, Inazawa K, Yamaoka N. Total purine and purine base content of common foodstuffs for facilitating nutritional therapy for gout and hyperuricemia. *Biological and Pharmaceutical Bulletin.* 2014;37(5):709-721.

12. Ahmad S, Blagg CR. Neurologic and psychiatric disorders in renal failure. *Therapy of renal diseases and related disorders:* Springer; 1991:719-732.

13. Meyer TW, Hostetter TH. Uremia. *New England Journal of Medicine.* 2007;357(13):1316-1325.

14. Lin J, Hu FB, Curhan GC. Associations of diet with albuminuria and kidney function decline. *Clinical Journal of the American Society of Nephrology.* 2010;5(5):836-843.

15. de Mello VD, Zelmanovitz T, Perassolo MS, Azevedo MJ, Gross JL. Withdrawal of red meat from the usual diet reduces albuminuria and improves the serum fatty acid profile in type 2 diabetes patients with macroalbuminuria. *The American Journal of Clinical Nutrition.* 2006;83(5):1032-1038.

16. Odermatt A. The Western-style diet: a major risk factor for impaired kidney function and chronic kidney disease. *American Journal of Physiology-Renal Physiology.* 2011;301(5):F919-F931.

17. Chauveau P, Aparicio M. Benefits in nutritional interventions in patients with CKD stage 3-4. *Journal of Renal Nutrition.* 2011;21(1):20-22.

18. Coresh J, Astor BC, Greene T, Eknoyan G, Levey AS. Prevalence of chronic kidney disease and decreased kidney function in the adult US population: Third National Health and Nutrition Examination Survey. *American Journal of Kidney Diseases.* 2003;41(1):1-12.

19. American-Diabetes-Association. Evidence-based nutrition principles and recommendations for the treatment and prevention of diabetes and related complications. *Diabetes Care.* 2002;25(1):202-212.

20. Reddy ST, Wang C-Y, Sakhaee K, Brinkley L, Pak CY. Effect of low-carbohydrate high-protein diets on acid-base balance, stone-forming propensity, and calcium metabolism. *American Journal of Kidney Diseases.* 2002;40(2):265-274.

21. van den Berg E, Hospers FA, Navis G, et al. Dietary acid load and rapid progression to end-stage renal disease of diabetic nephropathy in Westernized South Asian people. *Journal of Nephrology.* 2011;24(1):11-17. 22. Goldfarb DS, Coe FL. Prevention of recurrent nephrolithiasis.

22. *American Family Physician.* 1999;60(8):2269-2276.

23. Lagiou P, Sandin S, Lof M, Trichopoulos D, Adami H-O, Weiderpass E. Low carbohydrate-high protein diet and incidence of cardiovascular diseases in Swedish women: prospective cohort study. *BMJ.* 2012;344:e4026.

24. Trichopoulou A, Psaltopoulou T, Orfanos P, Hsieh C, Trichopoulos D. Low-carbohydrate-high-protein diet and long-term survival in a general population cohort. *European Journal of Clinical Nutrition.* 2007;61(5):575.

25. Noto H, Goto A, Tsujimoto T, Noda M. Low-carbohydrate diets and all-cause mortality: a systematic review and meta-analysis of observational studies. *PLoS One.* 2013;8(1):e55030.

26. National-Kidney-Foundation-Inc. NFK KDOQI Guidelines: Guideline 5: Nutritional Management in Diabetes and Chronic Kidney Disease. 2007; https://www2.kidney.org/ professionals/ KDOQI/guideline_diabetes/guide5.htm#tab37. Accessed 29th May, 2017.

27. Kasiske BL, Lakatua J, Ma JZ, Louis TA. A meta-analysis of the effects of dietary protein restriction on the rate of decline in renal function. *American Journal of Kidney Diseases.* 1998;31(6):954-961.

28. Pedrini MT, Levey AS, Lau J, Chalmers TC, Wang PH. The Effect of Dietary Protein Restriction on the Progression of Diabetic and Nondiabetic Renal Diseases A Meta-Analysis. *Annals of internal medicine.* 1996;124(7):627-632.

29. Hansen HP, Tauber-Lassen E, Jensen BR, Parving H-H. Effect of dietary protein restriction on prognosis in patients with diabetic nephropathy. *Kidney International.* 2002;62(1):220-228.

30. Brenner BM, Meyer TW, Hostetter TH. Dietary protein intake and the progressive nature of kidney disease: the role of hemodynamically mediated glomerular injury in the pathogenesis of progressive glomerular sclerosis in aging, renal ablation, and intrinsic renal disease. *New England Journal of Medicine.* 1982;307(11):652-659.

31. Tuttle KR, Johnson EC, Cooney SK, et al. Amino acids injure mesangial cells by advanced glycation end products, oxidative stress, and protein kinase C. *Kidney international.* 2005;67(3):953-968.

32. Vora J, Thomas D, Peters J, Coles G, Williams J. Preservation of Renal Haemodynamic Response to an Oral Protein Load in Non-insulin-dependent Diabetes Mellitus. *Diabetic medicine.* 1993;10(8):715-719.

33. Knight EL, Stampfer MJ, Hankinson SE, Spiegelman D, Curhan GC. The impact of protein intake on renal function decline in women with normal renal function or mild renal insufficiency. *Annals of internal medicine.* 2003;138(6):460-467.

34. Wrone EM, Carnethon MR, Palaniappan L, Fortmann SP. Association of dietary protein intake and microalbuminuria in healthy adults: Third National Health and Nutrition Examination Survey. *American Journal of Kidney Diseases.* 2003;41(3):580-587.

35. Fouque D, Laville M. Low protein diets for chronic kidney disease in non-diabetic adults. *Cochrane Database of Systemic Reviews.* 2009(3).

36. Koulouridis E, Koulouridis I. Is the dietary protein restriction achievable in chronic kidney disease? The impact upon quality of life and the dialysis delay. *Hippokratia.* 2011;15(Suppl 1):3.

37. Jing Z, Wei-Jie Y. Effects of soy protein containing isoflavones in patients with chronic kidney disease: A systematic review and meta-analysis. *Clinical Nutrition.* 2016;35(1):117-124.

38. Zhang J, Liu J, Su J, Tian F. The effects of soy protein on chronic kidney disease: a meta-analysis of randomized controlled trials. *European Journal of Clinical Nutrition.* 2014;68(9):987-993.

39. Kontessis P, Jones S, Dodds R, et al. Renal, metabolic and hormonal responses to ingestion of animal and vegetable proteins. *Kidney International.* 1990;38(1):136-144.

40. Chen X, Wei G, Jalili T, et al. The associations of plant protein intake with all-cause mortality in CKD. *American Journal of Kidney Diseases.* 2016;67(3):423-430.

41. Garneata L, Stancu A, Dragomir D, Stefan G, Mircescu G. Ketoanalogue-Supplemented Vegetarian Very Low–Protein Diet and CKD Progression. *Journal of the American Society of Nephrology.* 2016;27:2164-2176.

CHAPTER 7

Proteinuria/Albuminuria/Microalbuminuria/ Nephrotic Syndrome

As you might guess, albumin, inflammation, and albuminuria are all closely related. Albumin levels are directly correlated to the severity of proteinuria.[1]

Proteinuria is correlated to the severity of inflammation.[2] The three amigos of kidney disease.

Let's start with some definitions. Three terms are used to describe the similar conditions. The difference is the severity of protein leakage.

Microalbuminuria is the presence of albumin in urine. Albumin is the smallest protein in our bloodstream, so it is the first to leak from our kidneys. 30 to 300 mg of albumin leakage in a 24-hour period is the usual definition of microalbuminuria. Microalbuminuria is considered an early indicator of kidney and heart disease.[3,4]

Albuminuria and proteinuria are used interchangeably in some cases. Albuminuria and proteinuria can be considered 300 mg or more of albumin leakage in a 24-hour period. For most of us, protein leakage is measured in grams, not milligrams.

Nephrotic syndrome is the combination of protein leakage of 3 grams a day or more and low serum albumin. Edema may also be part of the diagnosis. In many cases nephrotic syndrome is the result of prolonged, or more severe, albuminuria.[5]

Albuminuria is protein in our urine. Albuminemia is low albumin in our blood.

For our purposes, we will stick with albuminuria to describe all forms of protein leakage into the urine.

If we can attain a partial remission, we will still have albuminuria in most cases. In my case, I still have the champagne of urine with lots of bubbly, but my disease progression stopped. Our disease may have stopped its progression, but part of our kidneys are still permanently damaged. The severity of protein leakage is a mortality indicator. The ability to slow or stop protein leakage is also a mortality indicator.

The cause of albuminuria starts with the smallest parts of our kidneys which are designed to hold the good stuff in (like albumin) and let urea and other waste products pass to be excreted through our urine. The proper name is "kidney filtration barrier," which allows the right things to pass through into the urine. Imagine a colander or strainer working like normal for decades. Now imagine the small holes in the colander/strainer have slowly enlarged over the years. You might think of albuminuria the same way. The part of our kidneys that lets waste products out of our bloodstream has enlarged enough to allow albumin to escape into our urine.

There are several ways that the small holes can be enlarged. High blood pressure, diabetes, lupus, inflammation, and kidney diseases are the top causes of proteinuria. In the case of high blood pressure, imagine running water at high pressure through these small holes. Over time the pressure would slowly enlarge those holes.

Inflammation is a little different. The theory is that these small holes become inflamed, which causes the tissue to swell, enlarging the holes. The difference between inflammation and blood pressure damage is inflammation might be reversible. Damage from high blood pressure is not. If inflammation is stopped or lessened, 90% of the time the albuminuria symptoms will lessen. My personal experience is the amount of albumin in my urine was directly correlated to the amount of inflammation revealed by my blood tests. This is not an absolute, but it is a pretty good rule of thumb. If the markers of inflammation are dropping, then albuminuria should be improving.

For diabetics, strict control of blood glucose reduces proteinuria. High blood glucose levels increase inflammation. The improvement in proteinuria may come from reducing inflammation caused by high blood glucose levels.

I made a strong statement in the next chapter: Inflammation is killing us. Let's look at how proteinuria impacts our future prognosis.

FIGURE 7.1: **Effect of Proteinuria on Mortality**

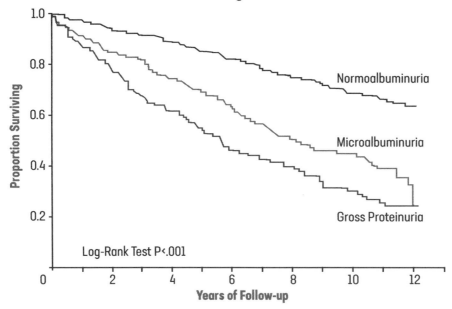

This chart[6] shows how the severity of albumin loss affects our future odds. This chart is based on a study using older-onset diabetes. What is interesting to me about this chart is that micro-albuminuria is almost as bad as proteinuria (albuminuria) over the long-term. The reason is that microalbuminuria turned into albuminuria over time in many cases. This was a one-time measurement at the beginning of the study, which turned out to be predictive over the next ten years.

Study 7.1   **Summary from this study[6]:**

CONCLUSION:

Results from our population-based study strongly suggest that both microalbuminuria and gross proteinuria are significantly associated with subsequent mortality from all causes, and from cardiovascular, cerebrovascular, and coronary heart diseases. These associations were independent of known cardiovascular risk factors and diabetes-related variables.

Another study on the relationship of myocardial infarctions (heart attacks) and proteinuria.

FIGURE 7.2: **Reltionship Between Proteinuria and Myocardial Infractions**

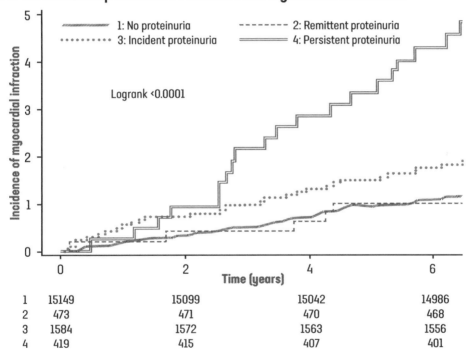

1	15149	15099	15042	14986
2	473	471	470	468
3	1584	1572	1563	1556
4	419	415	407	401

As you can see, if proteinuria can be halted, our prognosis is pretty good (dashed line --------).

However, the double line (══════)shows proteinuria that cannot be slowed or stopped. Study information is below.

Study 7.2 Changes in proteinuria and the risk of myocardial infarction in people with diabetes or pre-diabetes: a prospective cohort study.[7]

CONCLUSION:

Persistent proteinuria is an independent risk factor for the incidence of MI in the pre-diabetic and diabetic population. These findings may help clinicians to interpret proteinuria changes in the outpatient setting and provide possible preventive approaches for those with pre-diabetes or diabetes.

The reason that heart attacks are related to persistent proteinuria is that inflammation is still out of control. Proteinuria that has been cured may mean inflammation has been controlled or reduced. Other reasons exist, but we know inflammation is correlated with the severity of proteinuria.

In Chapter 14, we discuss inflammation. Proteinuria is linked to inflammation, but to a more specific inflammatory protein. Tumor necrosis factor (TNF), also called tumor necrosis factor alpha (TNF-A), sounds ominous, and it is when it comes to proteinuria. TNF is another inflammatory protein produced by macrophages just like C-reactive protein.

TNF seems to be more associated with proteinuria when compared to other inflammatory proteins.

Study 7.3 Not all inflammatory markers are linked to kidney function: results from a population-based study.[8]

CONCLUSION:

We did not confirm a significant association between renal function and IL-6, IL-1β, and hsCRP in the general population. However, our results demonstrate a significant association between TNF-α and renal function, suggesting a potential link between inflammation and the development of CKD. This data also confirms the association between MAU (Microalbuminuria) and inflammation.

Study 7.4 TNF-α and microalbuminuria in patients with type 2 diabetes mellitus.[9]

CONCLUSION:

In patients with type 2 DM, urinary, but not serum, TNF-α levels are associated with the presence and severity of microalbuminuria.

Study 7.5 Correlation Between Tumor Necrosis Factor Alpha and Proteinuria in Type-2 Diabetic Patients.[10]

RESULTS:

Levels of the three inflammatory parameters were significantly higher in diabetic patients when compared to control subjects, and they were positively correlated to urinary protein excretion.

<u>There was a significant positive correlation between serum and urine TNF-α and duration of diabetes, as well as between serum TNF-α and glycemic control.</u> Serum and urine TNF-α remained as independent predictors of urine protein excretion in diabetic patients with overt proteinuria after forward, stepwise multiple regression analysis.

CONCLUSION:

<u>Serum and urine TNF-α and CRP levels are</u> <u>significantly elevated in this group of diabetic patients, and</u> <u>correlate positively with the severity of proteinuria.</u> This suggests a significant role for TNF-α in the pathogenesis and progression of renal injury in diabetes mellitus.

> We can see that TNF has something to with the severity of proteinuria. I tried to fact-check this by looking at studies that blocked TNF. I found one study on TNF and albumin that focused on blocking TNF.

Study 7.6   **Effect of TNF-alpha inhibition on urinary albumin excretion in experimental diabetic rats.[11]**

ABSTRACT:

The objective is to assess the effect of TNF-alpha inhibition on urinary albumin excretion in experimental diabetic rats. Male Wistar rats, 8-week-old, were categorized into four groups, which were the control (n = 9), diabetes (n = 9), infliximab-treated diabetes (n = 10), and FR167653-treated diabetes (n = 9) groups. Diabetes was induced by intraperitoneal injection of STZ (40 mg/kg). Thereafter, infliximab was injected intraperitoneally once a month (5.5 mg/kg), and FR167653 was administered orally by mixing with the rat chow (0.08%). The effects of infliximab and FR167653 on urinary albumin excretion was observed for 12 weeks. Body weight, blood sugar, 24-h urinary TNFalpha, and 24-h urinary albumin/creatinine ratio (Ualb/ Ucr) levels were determined at 1, 4, 8, and 12 weeks after the STZ-injection. Treatment of rats with STZ caused a significant loss of body weight, as well as polyuria and hyperglycemia within 1 week, while the urinary excretions of albumin and TNF-alpha were increased. Neither infliximab nor FR167653 affected body weight or blood sugar levels, <u>whereas both decreased urinary albumin excretion, together with a modest decrease in the urinary excretion of TNF-alpha. These results suggest a role of TNF-alpha in the pathogenesis of diabetic nephropathy and show that TNF-alpha inhibition is a potential therapeutic strategy.</u>

> In rats, when TNF is inhibited, proteinuria improved. Proteinuria was not cured but lessened by reducing the amount of TNF.

> TNF is not the only cause of inflammation; other inflammatory agents are involved. The point I want to make again is that inflammation is the real issue. The most likely reason microalbuminuria is predictive of our future prognosis is because it is an indicator of inflammation. It could also be an indicator of malnutrition due to low albumin levels. Early inflammation that is not corrected leads to greater inflammation over time.

If high blood pressure, a drug reaction, or another kidney injury did not cause proteinuria, then it is very likely inflammation. Higher inflammation equals higher rates of protein in our urine and lower serum albumin levels in our blood.

Other research points us in the direction of oxidative stress. Oxidative stress causes our kidney filters to become more permeable, allowing albumin to pass into our urine.

Study 7.7 **Development of albuminuria and enhancement of oxidative stress during chronic renin-angiotensin system suppression.**[12]

CONCLUSION:

We conclude that albuminuria is accompanied by an amplified oxidative damage in patients in early stages of chronic kidney disease. These results indicate that chronic RAS [renal artery stenosis] protection must be directed to avoid development of albuminuria and oxidative damage.

In Chapter 14, we will discuss about the stress response and inflammation. What about proteinuria?

Study 7.8 **Assessment of stress & related albuminuria in caregivers of severely mentally ill persons.**[13]

INTERPRETATION & CONCLUSIONS:

The study demonstrated depression, anxiety, and albuminuria amongst primary caregivers of patients with mental illness. Increase in the caregivers' burden, depression, and anxiety resulted in an increase in the urinary albumin: creatinine ratio. This indicates that psychological stress is one of the determinants of albumin excretion rate in otherwise healthy subjects.

As a parent of an autistic child and a caregiver for an elderly family member, I'm really bothered by these kinds of studies.

Stress may also be a factor in albuminuria due to the inflammation response.

I could not find one study that tied albuminuria to normal inflammation markers. In other words, I could not find a study that proved albuminuria was common in patients without inflammation. It seems that albuminuria only exists when inflammation is present.

This concept is big news for us. We can treat inflammation and possibly lower the amount of protein in our urine. Looking back on the Walser study and other low-protein diets, I see that inflammation and oxidative stress are not treated. I believe, therefore, the results were inconclusive. Kidney disease treatment must take all possible factors into account, not just one.

What Lowers TNF?

First, let's start with drug therapies.

In addition to healthy eating and living, the standard treatment for almost all people with kidney disease is blood pressure medication or angiotensin-converting enzyme inhibitors known as ACE inhibitors.

Most of us will be on blood pressure medication for life. The reason is that lowering blood pressure overall lowers blood pressure in the kidneys as well. Remember the colander/strainer example? We want to control pressure so we don't do any more damage.

However, blood pressure does not entirely explain how these drugs slow kidney disease progression. These drugs work better than they should at slowing kidney disease based on blood pressure reduction alone.

The real reason why ACE inhibitors perform better than expected may be related to TNF. The combination of low blood pressure and lower TNF may be the true cause of slowed disease progression.

Study 7.9   Do ACE-inhibitors suppress tumor necrosis factor alpha (TNF) production in advanced chronic renal failure?[15]

CONCLUSION:

The present data suggests that the use of ACE-inhibitors is associated with lower plasma TNF-alpha and CRP levels as well as a lower prevalence of malnutrition in patients with advanced CRF. Further studies are needed to establish if there is a causal relationship between these findings and, if so, the molecular mechanism(s).

Study 7.10   Angiotensin-converting enzyme inhibitors suppress production of tumor necrosis factor-alpha in vitro and in vivo.[16]

ABSTRACT:

It has been reported that angiotensin-converting enzyme (ACE) inhibitors have beneficial effects on insulin resistance and congestive heart failure, in which elevations of serum tumor necrosis factor-alpha (TNFalpha) level have been indicated. Therefore, in this study, we examined the effect of ACE inhibitors on TNF-alpha production both in vitro and in vivo by using human blood mononuclear cells and mice, respectively. LPS (20 micrograms/ml)-induced in vitro TNF-alpha production, measured by bioassay and enzyme-linked immunosorbent assay, was significantly inhibited with captopril, delapril, and cilazapril in a concentration of 10(-3) mol/l. A single, oral administration of captopril, delapril, and cilazapril at more than 10-fold doses of common clinical use in man significantly inhibited LPS (2 mg/kg)-induced serum TNFalpha activity in Balb/c mice. These results indicate that ACE inhibitors such as captopril, delapril, and cilazapril have an inhibitory effect on TNF-alpha production not only in vitro as previously reported but also in vivo, although relatively high concentrations and large doses were required in this study.

Study 7.11   Angiotensin-converting-enzyme inhibitors suppress synthesis of tumor necrosis factor and interleukin 1 by human peripheral blood mononuclear cells.[17]

ABSTRACT:

Administration of angiotensin-converting-enzyme (ACE) inhibitors reduces vascular proliferation following endothelial injury, as well as the progression of renal disease in various animal models. These effects might be due to interference with cytokines such as interleukin 1 (IL-1) or tumor necrosis factor alpha (TNF) since they have been implicated in regulating the effects of vascular cell growth factors such as fibroblast- and platelet-derived growth factors. We investigated the in vitro synthesis of IL-1 and TNF from human peripheral blood mononuclear cells (PBMC) in the presence of various ACE-inhibitors. Captopril dose-dependently suppressed the IL-1 betainduced synthesis of TNF by 74% (P < 0.01) and the IL-1 beta-induced synthesis of IL-1 alpha by 60% (P < 0.01). Cytokine synthesis, induced by lipopolysaccharide, was less affected. At concentrations suppressing TNF and IL-1, captopril did not reduce the synthesis of complement C3 in the same cells. Enalapril and cilazapril also suppressed cytokine-induced cytokine synthesis. Ramipril, lisinopril, perindopril, and spirapril had no significant effect on TNF synthesis suggesting that the effect was not related specifically to the inhibition of ACE. Accumulation of mRNA for IL-1 and TNF were not affected by captopril, suggesting a posttranscriptional effect. We conclude that certain ACE-inhibitors suppress IL-1 and TNF synthesis at a post-transcriptional level and might, therefore, influence cytokine-mediated cell growth.

ACE inhibitors are good for us for two main reasons: blood pressure control and inflammation control. We should all be taking an ACE inhibitor except in rare cases. If you are not on an ACE inhibitor, talk to your doctor about it.

Do we have other ways to reduce inflammatory agents like TNF?

We can lower inflammatory factors like TNF pretty easily. The same things that reduce inflammation work for lowering TNF as well. The same basic diet for heart disease, with some adjustments for protein, potassium, phosphorus, sodium, and acid load, works for lowering inflammatory proteins as well.

Study 7.12   Non-soya legume-based therapeutic lifestyle change diet reduces inflammatory status in diabetic patients: a randomized cross-over clinical trial.[18]

ABSTRACT:

The present, randomized, cross-over, clinical trial investigated the effects of two intervention diets (nonsoya legume-based therapeutic lifestyle change (TLC) diet v. isoenergetic legume-free TLC diet) on inflammatory biomarkers among type 2 diabetic patients. A group of thirty-one participants (twenty-four women and seven men: weight 74.5 (SD 7.0) kg; age 58.1 (SD 6.0) years) were randomly assigned to one of the two following intervention diets for 8 weeks: legume-free TLC diet or non-soya legume-based TLC diet. The latter diet was the same as the legume-free TLC diet, except that two servings of red meat were replaced with different types of cooked nonsoya legumes such as lentils, chickpeas, peas, and beans over a period of 3 days per week. The intervention period was followed by a washout period of 4 weeks, after which the groups followed the alternate treatment for 8 weeks. Concentrations of inflammatory markers were measured at baseline and after the intervention periods. Compared with the legume-free TLC diet, the non-soya legume-based TLC diet significantly decreased high-sensitivity C-reactive protein, IL-6, and TNF-α in overweight diabetic patients. The replacement of two servings of red meat by non-soya legumes in the isoenergetic TLC diet for a period of 3 days per week reduced the plasma concentrations of inflammatory markers among overweight diabetic patients, independent of weight change.

Note: Just three days a week of soy protein vs. red meat lowered inflammatory proteins. Soy protein includes beans and peas.

Study 7.13   Effects of Antioxidant Polyphenols on TNF-Alpha Related Diseases[19]

ABSTRACT:

Oxidative stress and inflammatory responses sustained for a long period of time, cause many diseases. A proinflammatory cytokine, tumor necrosis factor α (TNF-α), plays a pivotal role in the pathogenesis of chronic and autoimmune diseases. The present review, supplemented by hitherto unpublished data of the authors and their coworkers, shows that the intake of polyphenols contained in natural sources, such as hydroxytyrosol, tyrosol, oleuropein (olives), naringin, and hesperidin (citrus fruits), resveratrol, procyanidins or oligomeric procyanidin (grapes or grape seed extracts), (-)-epigallocatechin gallate (green tea) and quercetin (grapes, green tea) etc., are able to modulate chronic inflammatory diseases, such as type 2 diabetes, rheumatoid arthritis, inflammatory bowel disease, and affect the formation and interaction of advanced glycation end products with their respective receptors. Furthermore, potent activities of fermented grape marc, prepared as a fine lyophilized powder from fresh skin and seeds of a Japanese grape strain (Koshu) and then fermented with Lactobacillus Plantarum, are described. Finally, the bioavailability of representative polyphenols will be discussed.

Note: Antioxidants appear to reduce TNF.

Study 7.14   INHIBITION of TUMOR NECROSIS FACTOR α INDUCTION IN MACROPHAGES*

Chemoprotection by Phenolic Antioxidants[20]

The pivotal role of TNF-α in inflammation and the potent anti-inflammatory activity of phenolic antioxidants raises the question of whether the induction of TNF-α during inflammation serves as a target of anti-inflammation by phenolic antioxidants. In this study, we tested this hypothesis by examining the effect of phenolic antioxidants on the induction of TNF-α by LPS in macrophage cells. Our data reveal that phenolic antioxidants block LPS-induced expression of TNF-α both time- and dose-dependently; the inhibition occurs at a transcriptional level and involves inhibition of NF-κB activation, the major regulator of TNF-α transcription in macrophage cells. To our knowledge, this study is the first report of inhibition of signal-induced TNF-α production by phenolic chemicals. Our findings provide new insights into the mechanism of chemoprotection against inflammatory diseases by phenolic antioxidants.

Note: Phenols refers to polyphenols, an antioxidant found in many berries and fruits.

Study 7.15   Anti-inflammatory effect of white wine in CKD patients and healthy volunteers.[21]

CONCLUSION:

Plasma markers of chronic inflammation were significantly reduced in CKD patients during the combined consumption of white wine and olive oil, suggesting a possible anti-inflammatory effect of this nutritional intervention.

Note: Red wine may be better, but white wine works as well.

Study 7.16   Effect of flavonoids on circulating levels of TNF-α and IL-6 in humans: a systematic review and metaanalysis.[22]

ABSTRACT:

Epidemiological or in-vitro evidence suggests a potential role for flavonoids as anti-inflammatory agents. We investigated the effect of flavonoid-rich foods or supplements on tumor necrosis factor- alpha (TNF-α) and interleukin-6 (IL-6) in long-term placebo-controlled human intervention trials. From 110 human intervention studies selected, (MEDLINE, EMBASE, CHORANE, and FSTA databases), 32 long-term placebo-controlled trials were suitable for meta-analysis. After sensitivity analysis, seven studies imputed of bias were excluded, and 25 studies were analyzed (TNF-α, n = 2404; IL-6, n = 2174).

Levels of TNF-α decreased after flavonoid consumption in the fixed model only (mean difference (MD) (95% CI): -0.098 (-0.188, -0.009), p = 0.032), but meta-regression results showed that neither higher dose, nor a longer duration of intervention were associated with a greater effect size. Subgroup analysis did not reveal any significant effect for quercetin and soy, but other sources (red wine, pomegranate, and tea extracts) showed a significant effect size both in fixed (MD (95% CI): TNF-α -0.449 (-0.619, -0.280), p < 0.001; IL-6 -0.346 (-0.612, -0.079), p = 0.011) and random (MD (95% CI): TNF-α -0.783 (-1.476, -0.090), p = 0.027; IL-6, -0.556 (-1.062, -0.050), p = 0.031) effect models. High-quality placebo-controlled trials are needed to identify flavonoids as the active ingredients.

Note: Interesting that TNF reduction was more prevalent in wine, pomegranate, and tea compared with soy or apples.

Omega 3s

Study 7.17   Effect of marine-derived n-3 polyunsaturated fatty acids on C-reactive protein, interleukin 6 and tumor necrosis factor α: a meta-analysis.[23]

CONCLUSION:

Marine-derived n-3 PUFAs supplementation had a significant lowering effect on CRP, IL-6, and TNF-α level. The lowering effect was most effective in non-obese subjects, and consecutive long-term supplementation was recommended.

Exercise

Study 7.18   Moderate-intensity regular exercise decreases serum tumor necrosis factor-α and HbA1c levels in healthy women[24]

CONCLUSION:

Changes in serum TNF-α that occur with exercise may play an important role in improving glucose metabolism parameters.

Study 7.19   Inflammation and exercise: Inhibition of monocytic intracellular TNF production by acute exercise via β2-adrenergic activation.[25]

This inhibitory response in TNF production by exercise was mirrored by β-AR agonists in an agonist-specific and dose-dependent manner in vitro: similar isoproterenol (EC50=2.1-4.7×10-10M) and epinephrine (EC50=4.4-10×1010M) potency and higher norepinephrine concentrations (EC50=2.6-4.3×10-8M) needed for the effects. Importantly, epinephrine levels observed during acute exercise in vivo significantly inhibited TNF production in vitro. The inhibitory effect of the AR agonists was abolished by β2, but not by β1- or α-AR blockers. We conclude that the down-regulation of monocytic TNF production during acute exercise is mediated by elevated epinephrine levels through β2-ARs. <u>Decreased inflammatory responses during acute exercise may protect us against chronic conditions with low-grade inflammation.</u>

Note: In a part of the study that's not discussed in the summary, researchers found that twenty minutes of exercise was enough to reduce TNF levels by 5% or more.

Summary

As you can see, we have several options for reducing inflammation and reducing proteinuria. All the options sound like a healthy lifestyle except for ACE inhibitors. Let's look at our options:

Maintain a healthy diet rich in fruits and vegetables

Eat foods high in antioxidants, flavonoids, and polyphenols

Reduce or eliminate red meat or processed meat consumption

Enjoy a glass of wine every occasionally (no more than five glasses per week and only one per day)

Increase polyunsaturated fatty acid consumption, including omega-3 oil

Exercise twenty minutes or more every day

Reduce stress

My message is you can reduce albuminuria, but only by treating inflammation.

In my mind, inflammation and albuminuria are two sides of the same coin. They can't be separated. If you can successfully treat inflammation, you can reduce albuminuria.

References

1. Peterson PA, Evrin P-E, Berggård I. Differentiation of glomerular, tubular, and normal proteinuria: Determinations of urinary excretion of β2-microglobulin, albumin, and total protein. *Journal of Clinical Investigation*. 1969;48(7):1189.

2. Taslıpınar A, Yaman H, Yılmaz MI, et al. The relationship between inflammation, endothelial dysfunction, and proteinuria in patients with diabetic nephropathy. *Scandinavian Journal of Clinical and Laboratory Investigation*. 2011;71(7):606-612.

3. de Zeeuw D, Parving H-H, Henning RH. Microalbuminuria as an early marker for cardiovascular disease. *Journal of the American Society of Nephrology*. 2006;17(8):2100-2105.

4. Bigazzi R, Bianchi S, Baldari D, Sgherri G, Baldari G, Campese VM. Microalbuminuria in salt-sensitive patients. A marker for renal and cardiovascular risk factors. *Hypertension*. 1994;23(2):195-199.

5. Churg J, Habib R, White RR. Pathology of the nephrotic syndrome in children: a report for the International Study of Kidney Disease in Children. *The Lancet*. 1970;295(7660):12991302.

6. Valmadrid CT, Klein R, Moss SE, Klein BE. The risk of cardiovascular disease mortality associated with microalbuminuria and gross proteinuria in persons with older-onset diabetes mellitus. *Archives of Internal Medicine*. 2000;160(8):1093-1100.

7. Wang A, Sun Y, Liu X, et al. Changes in proteinuria and the risk of myocardial infarction in people with diabetes or pre-diabetes: a prospective cohort study. *Cardiovascular Diabetology*. 2017;16(1):104.

8. Pruijm M, Ponte B, Vollenweider P, et al. Not all inflammatory markers are linked to kidney function: results from a population-based study. *American Journal of Nephrology*. 2012;35(3):288294.

9. Lampropoulou I-T, Stangou M, Papagianni A, Didangelos T, Iliadis F, Efstratiadis G. TNF-α and microalbuminuria in patients with type 2 diabetes mellitus. *Journal of Diabetes Research*. 2014;2014(Article ID 394206):1-7.

10. Refat H, Mady GE, El Ghany MMA, et al. Correlation between tumor necrosis factor alpha and proteinuria in type-2 diabetic patients. *Arab Journal of Nephrology and Transplantation*. 2010;3(1):33-38.

11. Moriwaki Y, Inokuchi T, Yamamoto A, et al. Effect of TNF-α inhibition on urinary albumin excretion in experimental diabetic rats. *Acta Diabetologica*. 2007;44(4):215-218.

12. Ruiz-Hurtado G, Condezo-Hoyos L, Pulido-Olmo H, et al. Development of albuminuria and enhancement of oxidative stress during chronic renin-angiotensin system suppression. *Journal of Hypertension*. 2014;32(10):2082-2091.

13. Dalui A, Guha P, De A, Chakraborty S, Chakraborty I. Assessment of stress & related albuminuria in caregivers of severe mentally ill persons. *The Indian Journal of Medical Research.* 2014;139(1):174.

14. Schwedhelm C, Pischon T, Rohrmann S, Himmerich H, Linseisen J, Nimptsch K. Plasma Inflammation Markers of the TNF Pathway but not C-Reactive Protein Are Associated with Processed Meat and Unprocessed Red Meat Consumption in Bavarian Adults. *The Journal of Nutrition.* 2016;2016(jn237180):1-8.

15. Stenvinkel P, Andersson P, Wang T, et al. Do ACE-inhibitors suppress tumor necrosis factor-α production in advanced chronic renal failure? *Journal of Internal Medicine.* 1999;246(5):503-507.

16. Fukuzawa M, Satoh J, Sagara M, et al. Angiotensin converting enzyme inhibitors suppress production of tumor necrosis factor-α in vitro and in vivo. *Immunopharmacology.* 1997;36(1):49-55.

17. Schindler R, Dinarello CA, Koch K-M. Angiotensin-converting enzyme inhibitors suppress synthesis of tumor necrosis factor and interleukin 1 by human peripheral blood mononuclear cells. *Cytokine.* 1995;7(6):526-533.

18. Hosseinpour-Niazi S, Mirmiran P, Fallah-Ghohroudi A, Azizi F. Non-soya legume-based therapeutic lifestyle change diet reduces inflammatory status in diabetic patients: a randomised cross-over clinical trial. *British Journal of Nutrition.* 2015;114(2):213-219.

19. Kawaguchi K, Matsumoto T, Kumazawa Y. Effects of antioxidant polyphenols on TNF-alpha-related diseases. *Current Topics in Medicinal Chemistry.* 2011;11(14):1767-1779.

20. Ma Q, Kinneer K. Chemoprotection by Phenolic Antioxidants - Inhibition of tumor necrosis factor α induction in macrophages. *Journal of Biological Chemistry.* 2002;277(4):2477-2484.

21. Migliori M, Panichi V, de la Torre R, et al. Anti-inflammatory effect of white wine in CKD patients and healthy volunteers. *Blood Purification.* 2015;39(1-3):218-223.

22. Peluso I, Raguzzini A, Serafini M. Effect of flavonoids on circulating levels of TNF-α and IL-6 in humans: A systematic review and meta-analysis. *Molecular Nutrition & Food Research.* 2013;57(5):784-801.

23. Li K, Huang T, Zheng J, Wu K, Li D. Effect of marine-derived n-3 polyunsaturated fatty acids on C-reactive protein, interleukin 6 and tumor necrosis factor α: a meta-analysis. *PloS One.* 2014;9(2):e88103.

24. Tsukui S, Kanda T, Nara M, Nishino M, Kondo T, Kobayashi I. Moderate-intensity regular exercise decreases serum tumor necrosis factor-[alpha] and HbA1c levels in healthy women. *International Journal of Obesity.* 2000;24(9):1207.

20. Dimitrov S, Hulteng E, Hong S. Inflammation, and exercise: Inhibition of monocytic intracellular TNF production by acute exercise via β 2-adrenergic activation. *Brain, Behavior, and Immunity.* 2017;61(March):60-68.

CHAPTER 8

Inflammation

Let me start off with a strong statement: "Inflammation is killing us."

There is no other way to say it. The evidence is everywhere for us to see. Inflammation could have been number one on our list of disease-causing agents. Inflammation is the most likely cause of many diseases and, if not, inflammation can at least accelerate our disease.[1]

No standard exists to treat systemic inflammation or inflammation in our kidneys. This leaves us guessing on how to reduce inflammation.

If inflammation is not the cause of our disease, then it is at least a strong predictor of mortality and morbidity.[2] It is also very likely that inflammation was the first on the scene months or years before you showed symptoms. This chapter was overwhelming to write, adding up to more than 140 pages before I cut it down to size. The most unexpected part of this chapter will be the part on stress.

Stress can affect our immune system and convert anti-inflammatory cells to inflammatory cells.[3] I personally never equated work or social stress with inflammation.

Inflammation is currently treated by knocking down our immune system so that our bodies don't respond to the factors causing inflammation. Again, we treat the symptoms of inflammation and not the cause.[4]

You know the saying "Necessity is the mother of all invention"? Then "Inflammation is the mother of all diseases." Inflammation is a precursor to almost all serious diseases. The latest theory is inflammation could mark the beginning of all diseases. It's a kind of unified theory of disease.

Inflammation is supposed to protect our bodies. An increased blood flow allows more white blood cells into the affected area to fight infections or other insults. If you cut your finger or stub your toe, you can see and feel inflammation around the affected area within hours.

How Does Inflammation Go from Helping Us to Hurting Us?

Autoimmune diseases like FSGS, lupus, and others might be described as a runaway or overzealous response by our immune systems. Our bodies are attacking themselves in an effort to cure something our bodies thinks is harming us. Could it be that these diseases are trying to correct chronic inflammation? Our bodies are attacking something they perceives as a threat. Inflammation is a predictor of type 2 diabetes[6] and a predictor of how fast your kidney function will decline.[7] While reading this chapter, keep in mind the idea of runaway inflammation while reading this chapter.

When I look back to when my symptoms started, I know I was working 55 to 60 hours a week. I was eating fast food on the way to work, at lunch, and sometimes on the way home. I didn't get home until 7 or 8 p.m. I was back at work by 7 a.m. the next morning. I was in a job that was highly stressful and very competitive.

As a part of this book, I talked to a few others who had autoimmune diseases. I was looking for a common thread. I found that stress, combined with a faulty diet, was a possible common thread.

Two family members have psoriatic arthritis, an autoimmune disease. Both of these people experienced the first symptoms of psoriatic arthritis during a stressful period in their lives. Both describe this period as the most stressful they ever experienced.

I, too, was under tremendous stress when I was diagnosed. Two people with lupus, another autoimmune disease, tell a similar story. Again, both say the symptoms started during one of the most stressful periods of their lives. In their cases, one experienced a painful, unexpected divorce with small children involved, and the other was saving a family business, which employed many family members from bankruptcy.

While these personal stories are far from conclusive, we can let science answer the question of stress some of which are discussed below.

Are Autoimmune Diseases Caused or Triggered by Stress

Study 8.1   **Stress as a trigger of autoimmune disease.**[8]

ABSTRACT:

The etiology of autoimmune diseases is multifactorial: genetic, environmental, hormonal, and immunological factors are all considered important in their development. Nevertheless, the onset of at least 50% of autoimmune disorders has been attributed to "unknown trigger factors". Physical and psychological stress has been implicated in the development of autoimmune disease, since numerous animal and human studies demonstrated the effect of sundry stressors on immune function. Moreover, many retrospective studies found that a high proportion (up to 80%) of patients reported uncommon emotional stress before disease onset. Unfortunately, not only does stress cause disease, but the disease itself also causes significant stress in the patients, creating a vicious cycle. Recent reviews discuss the possible role of psychological stress, and of the major stress-related hormones, in the pathogenesis of autoimmune disease. It is presumed that the stress-triggered neuroendocrine hormones lead to immune dysregulation, which ultimately results in autoimmune disease, by altering or amplifying cytokine production. The treatment of autoimmune disease should thus include stress management and behavioral intervention to prevent stress-related immune imbalance. Different stress reactions should be discussed with autoimmune patients, and obligatory questionnaires about trigger factors should include psychological stress in addition to infection, trauma, and other common triggers.

Note: 50% of autoimmune diseases have been attributed to "unknown" factors. In my experience, the "unknown" factor has been stress.

Study 8.2   **The influence of stress on the development and severity of immune-mediated diseases.**[9]

ABSTRACT:

Evidence that psychological stress can increase inflammation and worsen the course of immune-mediated inflammatory disease (IMID) is steadily accumulating. The majority of data supporting this hypothesis come from studies in patients with inflammatory bowel disease (IBD). While there is no evidence to suggest that stress is a primary cause of IBD, many, although not all, studies have found that patients with IBD experience increased stress and stressful life events before disease exacerbations. Further, the disease itself can cause psychological stress, creating a vicious cycle. In addition to reviewing the epidemiological evidence supporting a stressed relationship, this article also briefly discusses how stress-related changes in neural, endocrine, and immune functioning may contribute to the pathogenesis of immune diseases, IBD in particular. The effects of different pharmacological and nonpharmacological interventions, including stress management and behavioral therapy, on stress, mood, quality of life (QOL), and activity of the underlying IMID are also summarized.

Note: A link exists between inflammatory bowel disease and stress.

Study 8.3   **Social stress up-regulates inflammatory gene expression in the leukocyte transcriptome via β-adrenergic induction of myelopoiesis**[10]

SIGNIFICANCE:

Chronic exposure to adverse social environments is associated with increased risk of disease, and stress related increases in the expression of proinflammatory genes appear to contribute to these effects. The present study identifies a biological mechanism of such effects in the ability of the sympathetic nervous system to up-regulate bone marrow production of immature, proinflammatory monocytes. These effects are mediated by β-adrenergic receptors and the myelopoietic growth factor GM-CSF, and suggest new targets for interventions to protect health in the context of chronic social stress.

Note: Stressful periods tell our bodies to produce inflammatory cells and not anti-inflammatory cells. This was the bombshell for me. In some crazy way, stress tells our bodies to increase inflammation.

Study 8.4 — Chronic stress, glucocorticoid receptor resistance, inflammation, and disease risk[11]

ABSTRACT:

We propose a model wherein chronic stress results in glucocorticoid receptor resistance (GCR) that, in turn, results in failure to down-regulate inflammatory response. Here we test the model in two viral-challenge studies. In study 1, we assessed stressful life events, GCR, and control variables including baseline antibody to the challenge virus, age, body mass index (BMI), season, race, sex, education, and virus type in 276 healthy adult volunteers. The volunteers were subsequently quarantined, exposed to one of two rhinoviruses, and followed for 5 d with nasal washes for viral isolation and assessment of signs/ symptoms of a common cold. In study 2, we assessed the same control variables and GCR in 79 subjects who were subsequently exposed to a rhinovirus and monitored at baseline and for 5 d after viral challenge for the production of local (in nasal secre-tions) proinflammatory cytokines (IL-1β, TNF-α, and IL-6). Study 1: After covarying the control variables, those with recent exposure to a longterm threatening stressful experience demonstrated GCR; and those with GCR were at higher risk of subsequently developing a cold. Study 2: With the same controls used in study 1, greater GCR predicted the production of more local proinflammatory cytokines among infected subjects. These data provide support for a model suggesting that prolonged stressors result in GCR, which, in turn, interferes with appropriate regulation of inflammation. Because inflammation plays an important role in the onset and progression of a wide range of diseases, this model may have broad implications for understanding the role of stress in health.

Note: We lose the ability to turn off inflammation during periods of high stress.

Study 8.5 — Type 2 diabetes mellitus and psychological stress - a modifiable risk factor.[12]

ABSTRACT:

Psychological stress is common in many physical illnesses and is increasingly recognized as a risk factor for disease onset and progression. An emerging body of literature suggests that stress has a role in the etiology of type 2 diabetes mellitus (T2DM) both as a predictor of new onset T2DM and as a prognostic factor in people with existing T2DM. Here, we review the evidence linking T2DM and psychological stress. We highlight the physiological responses to stress that are probably related to T2DM, drawing on evidence from animal work, large epidemiological studies and human laboratory trials. We discuss population and clinical studies linking psychological and social stress factors with T2DM, and give an overview of intervention studies that have attempted to modify psychological or social factors to improve outcomes in people with T2DM.

Note: Stress may predict type 2 diabetes onset.

Study 8.6   **Stress and type 2 diabetes: a review of how stress contributes to the development of type 2 diabetes.**[13]

ABSTRACT:

Current policy and research around type 2 diabetes (T2D) interventions largely invoke a behavioral model. We suggest that activation of the physiologic stress response (PSR) from chronic exposure to stressors, low socioeconomic status (SES), severe mental health problems, or aggressive behavior increases the risk of T2D. This article is a comprehensive review of the literature on the link between T2D and psychosocial factors focusing on prospective studies of the risk for developing diabetes. The review found an increased risk for T2D in people: exposed to stressful working conditions or traumatic events; with depression; with personality traits or mental health problems that put them in conflict with others; of low SES, either currently or in childhood; and in racial/ ethnic minority populations, independent of current SES. This review suggests that T2D prevention research would be more effective if (a) the PSR to psychosocial factors (especially social disparities) was recognized and (b) intervention programs evaluated reduction in social disparities as part of a comprehensive approach.

Note: This is another study showing increased risk of developing type 2 diabetes after a stressful period.

Study 8.7   **Stressful life events precede exacerbations of multiple sclerosis.**[14]

RESULTS:

Eighty-five percent of MS exacerbations were associated with stressful life events in the preceding 6 weeks. Stressful life events occurred an average of 14 days before MS exacerbations, compared with 33 days before a randomly selected control date (p < .0001). Survival analysis confirmed that an increase in frequency of life events was associated with greater likelihood of MS exacerbations (hazard ratio = 13.18, p < .05).

CONCLUSION:

These results are consistent with the hypothesis that stress is a potential trigger of disease activity in patients with relapsing-remitting MS.

Note: A stressful event preceded MS symptoms.

Study 8.8　　Stress and cardiovascular disease.[15]

ABSTRACT:

The physiological reaction to psychological stress, involving the hypothalamic-pituitary-adrenocortical and sympatho-adrenomedullary axes, is well characterized, but its link to cardiovascular disease risk is not well understood. Epidemiological data show that chronic stress predicts the occurrence of coronary heart disease (CHD). Employees who experience work-related stress and individuals who are socially isolated or lonely have an increased risk of a first CHD event. In addition, short-term emotional stress can act as a trigger of cardiac events among individuals with advanced atherosclerosis. A stress-specific coronary syndrome, known as transient left ventricular apical ballooning cardiomyopathy or stress (Takotsubo) cardiomyopathy, also exists. Among patients with CHD, acute psychological stress has been shown to induce transient myocardial ischemia and long-term stress can increase the risk of recurrent CHD events and mortality. Applications of the 'stress concept' (the understanding of stress as a risk factor and the use of stress management) in the clinical settings have been relatively limited, although the importance of stress management is highlighted in European guidelines for cardiovascular disease prevention.

Note: Stress is one of the most well-known causes of heart diseases.

Take your pick of autoimmune diseases like IBD, MS, FSGS, and others, and you will find evidence that stress plays a role in their development. These studies confirm what I have witnessed and experienced. However, I had no idea that our bodies could change the type of cells produced or change our genes when we are chronically stressed. We may lose the ability to regulate the normal inflammatory response. This is not true of every kind of kidney disease, but may be true for autoimmune diseases.

This chapter is about inflammation, and stress has the power to contribute greatly to inflammation. Stress is harder to correct in many ways. What most of us are going through is pretty stressful. Learning to control stress has got to be a part of the plan.

I looked for additional proof for the development of diseases caused when our bodies had lost the control over inflammatory processes. IL-18 is an inflammation-producing protein and IL-18BP is the anti-inflammatory version of the same protein. In healthy adults, IL-18BP is 20 times higher than IL-18. We normally have 20 times more anti-inflammatory protein than inflammatory protein. The 20:1 ratio assures us we can control any inflammatory response so that inflammation does not get out of hand.

Look at the following chart that shows different levels of IL-18 (inflammatory) vs IL-18BP (anti-inflammatory) to get an idea of what happens in our body[16]:

TABLE 8.1: **Levels of IL-18 and IL-18BP in Human Disease**

Disease	IL-18a	IL-18BPb	Free IL-18a	Reference
Sepsis	500–2,000	ND	ND	Emmanuilidis et al. [100]
Sepsis	250–10,000	22.5	250–3,000	Novick et al. [73]
Trauma	300–600	ND	ND	Mommsen et al. [101]
Schizophrenia	518	10	253	Palladino et al. [102]
Ulcerative colitis	274	ND	ND	Haas et al. [103]
Ulcerative colitis	393	4.7	250	Ludwiczek et al. [104]
Crohn's disease	387	ND	ND	Haas et al. [103]
Crohn's disease	546	5	340	Ludwiczek et al. [104]
Wegener's disease	240	14.5	84	Novick et al. [74]
Rheumatoid arthritis	230–400	ND	ND	Bokarewa and Hultgren [105]
SLEc	700	7.5	408	Favilli et al. [99]
SLEc	400	15	167	Novick et al. [75]
MASd	2,200	35	660	Mazodier et al. [32]
Systemic JIAe	1,600–78,000	ND	ND	Jelusic et al. [106]
Adult Still's disease	1,000–6,000	ND	ND	Kawashima et al. [107]
Myocardial infarction	238	ND	ND	Blankenberg et al. [108]
Myocardial infarction	355	ND	ND	Narins et al. [109]
Coronary artery disease	356	13.7	125	Thompson et al. [110]
Metabolic syndrome	380	ND	ND	Troseid et al. [111]
Acute kidney injuryf	500	ND	ND	Parikh et al. [112]
Acute kidney injuryf	2,000	ND	ND	Vaidya et al. [113]
Acute kidney injuryf	>360	ND	ND	Parikh et al. [114]
Acute kidney injuryf	884	ND	ND	Sirota et al. [115]

aLevels in picograms per milliliter, range, or mean.
bLevels in nanograms per milliliter, range, or mean.
cSystemic lupus erythematosus.
dMacrophage activation syndrome.
eSystemic juvenile idiopathic arthritis.
fUrine levels (mean in picograms per milliliter).

Take a look at the column labeled IL-18BP (ND stands for not detectable). Look at the number of diseases where IL-18BP is not detectable anymore. They include myocardial infarction (heart attack), acute kidney injury, metabolic syndrome, Crohn's disease, ulcerative colitis, arthritis, lupus, and so on.

Our bodies have lost the ability to stop a runaway inflammatory response. We have lost the power to control inflammation. This is when the body succumbs to inflammation and these diseases begin to develop or greatly accelerate.

How Important is the Power to Stop Inflammation

The following chart shows how accurate IL-18 was in predicting mortality over a two-year period.

FIGURE 8.1: **Accuracy of IL-18 in Predicting Mortality Over a Two-Year Period**

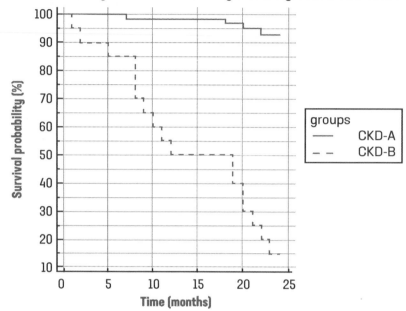

CKD-A includes the patients with serum concentration of IL-18 ≤ 1584.5 pg/mL, and CKD-B includes the patients with serum concentration of IL-18 > 1584.5 pg/mL.

The related study shows a 20-fold increase in fatalities by a single indicator for inflammation. Remember, this chart is about us, people with kidney disease. This is pretty shocking when you think about it.

Study 8.9   Usefulness of serum interleukin-18 in predicting cardiovascular mortality in patients with chronic kidney disease—systems and clinical approach.[24]

ABSTRACT:

It was found that an increase in serum concentration of IL-18 above the cut-off point (1584.5 pg/mL) was characterized by 20.63-fold higher risk of cardiovascular deaths among studied patients. IL-18 serum concentration was found to be superior to the well-known cardiovascular risk parameters, like high sensitivity C-reactive protein (hsCRP), carotid intima media thickness (CIMT), glomerular filtration rate, albumins, ferritin, N-terminal prohormone of brain natriuretic peptide (NT-proBNP) in prognosis of cardiovascular mortality. The best predictive for IL-18 were 4 variables, such as CIMT, NT-proBNP, albumins and hsCRP, as they predicted its concentration at 89.5%. Concluding, IL-18 seems to be important indicator and predictor of cardiovascular death in two-year followup among non-diabetic patients suffering from CKD, with history of AMI in the previous year. The importance of IL18 in the process of atherosclerotic plaque formation has been confirmed by systems analysis based on a formal model expressed in the language of Petri nets theory.

Note: A 20-fold higher risk of heart disease! Albumin was predicitve of IL-18 levels.

Survival probability drops to just 15% over two years vs 95% if inflammation is controlled. This may be another reason why heart disease is the number one killer of people with kidney disease. Inflammation is strongly correlated to the risk of heart attacks. If inflammation is controlled or stopped, our future prognosis can be pretty good. However, if we don't deal with inflammation effectively, our odds drop dramatically.

I will say it again for effect: Inflammation is killing us.

C-Reactive Protein and All-Cause Mortality in a Large Hospital-Based Cohort[25]

FIGURE 8.2: **Effect of C-Reactive Protein**

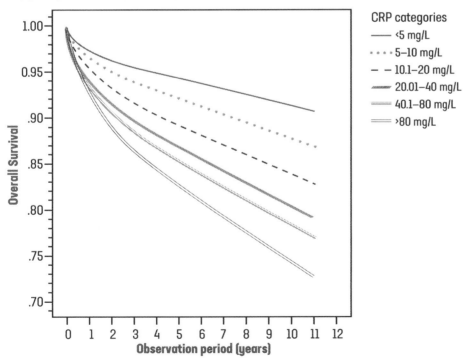

As you can see, with higher C-reactive protein, the odds of survival drop, lockstep with the severity of inflammation. We know which group we want to be in, and that is the group that has less than 5 mg per liter of CRP.

No matter how you look at the data, it's clear that inflammation may be the strongest driver for the progression of kidney diseases.

We can't say for sure how many cases of autoimmune diseases are triggered by stress. It is likely that many factors must come together at once to trigger an autoimmune disease.

While we can't tell if stress was the cause of our woes, we do have several ways to gauge inflammation. Blood tests can reveal systemic inflammation through the detection of the levels of C-reactive protein or "CRP." CRP is a protein produced by the liver in response to inflammation. CRP is considered a non-specific marker for inflammation. It is considered non-specific because we don't know the exact source of inflammation. We don't know which body part or parts are inflamed.

Other markers for inflammation, such as Interleukin 8 (IL-8), IL-18, and suPAR, are not as common. However, all inflammatory markers increase due to kidney diseases. We can use CRP levels as an indicator for inflammation. It's not a perfect indictor, but every doctor's office can do this test. Other, less common indicators may be better guides to gauge inflammation. But a CRP test can be done easily.

One of the most frustrating aspects of the kidney disease treatment is the lack of guidance once the drugs fail. But there are a few steps you can take to make things a little better. Kidney disease symptoms and, most importantly, the acceleration of kidney disease, starts as early as stage 2. Why aren't we treating inflammation in the early stages of this disease? If we wait until stage 3 or stage 4, we miss years (maybe a decade) of treating inflammation, thus missing a chance to slow the progression of heart and kidney diseases. It's a form of medical malpractice. The idea of "let's wait until you get really sick and run out of options before treatment" has got to go.

We know that heart diseases and related inflammation can be treated with diet to a large extent.[17] The bare minimum for kidney patients should be a heart-healthy diet. For most patients, we don't even do that. This might be the reason why we are still like a third world country when it comes to kidney outcomes. We wait until 80% of the kidney functions are affected before taking action. This has to stop. Ok, now back to inflammation.

What effect does inflammation have on kidney disease progression?

Study 8.10   C-reactive protein and long-term risk for Chronic kidney disease: a historical prospective study.[18]

CONCLUSION:

Elevated CRP level is an independent risk factor for CKD development. In patients with DM (Diabetes Mellitus) HTN (hypertension) or baseline eGFR between 60-90 ml\min\1.73 m (2) its predictive role is enhanced.

Note: When you add high CRP with one other condition, the risk for kidney diseases gets higher. We are stacking up comorbid conditions.

Study 8.11   Inflammation in chronic kidney disease: role in the progression of renal and cardiovascular disease.[19]

ABSTRACT:

Inflammation is the response of the vasculature or tissues to various stimuli. An acute and chronic proinflammatory state exists in patients with chronic kidney disease (CKD), contributing substantially to morbidity and mortality. There are many mediators of inflammation in adults with CKD and end-stage kidney disease (ESKD), including hypoalbuminemia/malnutrition, atherosclerosis, advanced oxidation protein products, the peroxisome proliferators-activated receptor, leptin, the thiobarbituric acid reactive system, asymmetric dimethyl arginine, iron, fetuin-A, and cytokines. Inflammation contributes to the progression of CKD by inducing the release of cytokines and the increased production and activity of adhesion molecules, which together contribute to T cell adhe-sion and migration into the interstitium, subsequently attract-ing pro-fibrotic factors. Inflammation in CKD also causes mortality from cardiovascular disease by contributing to the development of vascular calcifications and endothelial dysfunction. Similar to the situation in adults, cardiovascular disease in pediatric CKD is linked to inflammation: abnormal left ventricular wall geometry is positively associated with markers of inflammation. This review focuses on traditional and novel mediators of inflammation in CKD and ESKD, and the deleterious effect inflammation has on the progression of renal and cardiovascular disease.

Study 8.12   Biomarkers of inflammation and progression of chronic kidney disease.[20]

Higher CRP (C reactive protein) and sTNFrii (soluble tumor necrosis factor receptor II) are inde-pendently associated with faster rates of kidney function loss in chronic kidney disease. Pravas-tatin appears to prevent loss of kidney function to a greater extent in individuals with greater evidence of inflammation, although this was of borderline significance. These data suggest that inflammation may mediate the loss of kidney function among subjects with chronic kidney disease and concomitant coronary disease.

Note: As our kidney function declines, inflammation increases.

Study 8.13   Progressive Increase of Inflammatory Biomarkers in Chronic Kidney Disease and End-Stage Renal Disease.[21]

ABSTRACT:

Chronic kidney disease (CKD) has reached epidemic levels. It is a multisystem disease associ-ated with elevated systemic inflammatory and hypercoagulable states. Most concerning are the cardiovascular risks associated with all stages of kidney disease. It is difficult to assess kidney disease stage progression and cardiovascular risk with current indicators such as estimated glomerular filtration rate and conventional cardiovascular risk factors. However, the use of biomarkers to assess the underlying pathological disease state may bridge the gap. This study evaluated biomarkers of inflammation including C-reactive protein, D-dimer, neuron-specific enolase, neutrophil gelatinase–associated lipocalin, tumor necrosis factor receptor I, and thrombomodulin in 3 groups of patients: CKD stages 2-4, end-stage renal disease (ESRD), and age-matched controls. The study demon-strated a statistically significant progressive upregulation in mean concentration of all markers when comparing controls to CKD and ESRD. Therefore, biomarkers may be able to evaluate the inflammatory state in kidney disease and potentially predict the cardiovascular risk.

Note: Again, as our disease progresses, inflammation gets worse!

Study 8.14   **Serum IL-18 Is Closely Associated with Renal Tubulointerstitial Injury and Predicts Renal Prognosis in IgA Nephropathy[22]**

In conclusion, simple histopathologic measures of tubulo-interstitial injury and serum IL-18 may improve the identification of IgAN patients who are at high risk and have potential for progressive loss of kidney function. These results require confirmation and validation in an independent cohort of patients with biopsy-proven IgAN. We suggest that higher serum IL-18 may represent an ongoing inflammatory and fibrotic process in IgA nephropathy, which indicates for intensive therapy from onset.

Study 8.15   **Serum Interleukin-18 as a Biomarker of Tubular Kidney Damage in Patients with Chronic Glomerulonephritis[23]**

Results: according to the results of renal microscopy 88% patients had mesangial proliferative glomerulonephritis, 7%–membranous nephropathy, 5%–membranous proliferative glomerulonephritis. Patients with CGN and AH have more severe histological tubulo-interstitial lesion parameters than patients with CGN without AH. On the basis of rank correlation analysis, we proved that serum IL18 directly correlates with indicators of tubulo-interstitial kidney tissue lesion 186 Oleg Kraydaschenko et al. In patients with CGN, strong direct relationship was found between the level of serum IL-18 and dystrophic changes in epithelial tubules ($r = 0.81$, $p < 0.05$). Diagnostics of dystrophic changes in epithelial tubules by determining of the serum IL-18 level is a highly sensitive and specific method, with the efficiency of 96.6%.

Digging a Little Deeper

In mouse and bovine studies, disabling the inflammatory response stopped or dramatically reduced the progression of kidney disease. In humans, the immune-suppressing drugs are used to blunt the body's response to inflammation.

These facts confirm the idea that inflammation is the driving force of our disease. Yet, I rarely read that kidney disease is an inflammatory disease. Let me say it for the record:

Treating inflammation should be our highest priority, along with increasing albumin levels.

suPar (Soluble urokinase-type plasminogen activator receptor) is another pro-inflammatory substance circulating in our bloodstream, similar to CRP and IL18. suPAR was thought to be a factor in FSGS (Focal Segmental Glomerulosclerosis).

The reason suPAR was suspected to be the factor responsible for inflammation is that plasmapheresis seemed to help patients with FSGS. Plasmapheresis works like dialysis, but on our blood plasma, removing certain antibodies from the blood plasma. The idea behind this theory was that a "circulating factor" was present in the plasma that caused FSGS relapse in the patients who had undergone a kidney transplant.

FSGS has been estimated to reoccur in about 30% to 40% of transplant patients. This leads to the idea that the dysfunction was not in the kidneys. Removing suPAR from the plasma helped some patients when FSGS relapsed. After aggressive plasmapheresis treatment (3x per week), suPAR levels rebounded to 100% of the pre-plasmapheresis numbers in two weeks. It takes two weeks for the inflammation to go back to the same level as before.

These studies show that plasma exchange (plasmapheresis) can save the transplanted kidneys from developing FSGS.

Study 8.16   Plasma Exchange for the Recurrence of Primary Focal Segmental Glomerulosclerosis(rFSGS) in Adult Renal Transplant Recipients: A Meta-Analysis

CONCLUSION:

Not withstanding the inherent limitations of small, observational trials, <u>PLEX (Plasma exchange) appears to be effective for PR in rFSGS.</u> Additional research is needed to further elucidate its optimal use and impact on long-term allograft survival.

Study 8.17   The role of plasma exchange in treating post-transplant focal segmental glomerulosclerosis: A systematic review and meta-analysis of 77 case reports and case-series.

CONCLUSION:

<u>In this systematic review of patients with recurrent post-transplant FSGS, 71 % of patients achieved full or partial remission after treatment with plasma exchange;</u> however, extensive missing data and lack of a control group limit any conclusions on causality.

However, other studies show conflicting data. Treating FSGS with plasma exchange didn't work in all cases. These studies suggest something systemic is going on, but no one is sure exactly what it could be. I suspect suPAR is more of a symptom than a cause.

suPAR levels predict kidney diseases and albuminuria in diabetes, just like other inflammation indicators. We also know that inflammation comes before albuminuria. Inflammation markers start to rise before the proteins show up in your urine. Inflammation comes before kidney diseases or albuminuria.

It could be suPAR, IL-18, CRP, or any number of others related to inflammation that drive our diseases and predict our future outcomes. The actual name of the pro-inflammatory substance is not important. What is important is that when inflammation was stopped or the pro-inflammatory substance was blocked, the disease progression also stopped, as is evident in several studies.

These facts tell us that stopping inflammation should be the cornerstone of the kidney disease treatment and management plan.

When I say inflammation is everywhere, let me show you what I mean.

Inflammation and Albumin

Study 8.18   Serum albumin: relationship to inflammation and nutrition.[26]

ABSTRACT:

Hypoalbuminemia is the result of the combined effects of inflammation and inadequate protein and caloric intake in patients with chronic disease such as chronic renal failure. Inflammation and malnutrition both reduce albumin concentration by decreasing its rate of synthesis, while inflammation alone is associated with a greater fractional catabolic rate (FCR) and, when extreme, increased transfer of albumin out of the vascular compartment. A vicious cascade of events ensues in which inflammation induces anorexia and reduces the effective use of dietary protein and energy intake and augments catabolism of the key somatic protein, albumin. Hypoalbuminemia is a powerful predictor of mortality in patients with chronic renal failure, and the major cause of death in this population is due to cardiovascular events. Inflammation is associated with vascular disease and likely causes injury to the vascular endothelium, and hypoalbuminemia as two separate expressions of the inflammatory process. Albumin has a myriad of important physiologic effects that are essential for normal health. However, simply administering albumin to the critically ill patients with hypoalbuminemia has not been shown to improve survival or reduce morbidity. Thus, the inference from these clinical studies suggests that the cause of hypoalbuminemia, rather than low albumin levels specifically, is responsible for morbidity and mortality.

Note: This is why we have to treat inflammation at the same time we are treating the low albumin levels.

Study 8.19 Serum albumin level adjusted with C-reactive protein predicts hemodialysis patient survival[27]

CONCLUSION:

CRP-adjusted albumin was shown to be a better predictor of mortality among the HD patients. When assessing serum albumin values, inflammatory status should be taken into account. Malnutrition or wasting was shown to be associated with a poor outcome independent of inflammation.

What about Proteinuria and Inflammation

Study 8.20 Urinary cytokines after HCT (hematopoietic cell transplantation) evidence for renal inflammation in the pathogenesis of proteinuria and kidney disease.[28]

ABSTRACT:

We compared urinary levels of cytokines in patients with and without albuminuria, proteinuria and kidney disease (glomerular filtration rate<60 mL/min per 1.73 m(2)) after HCT. Plasma and urine were collected at baseline and weekly through day 100 and monthly through year 1, for measurement of IL-6, gp130, sIL6r, IL-10, IL15, MCP1 and urine albumin-to-creatinine ratios (ACRs). Coxproportional hazards modeling examined associations between urinary cytokine levels and development of these renal end points. The association of ACR with the hazard of overall mortality was assessed using Cox regression. Increasing urinary IL-6 and IL-15 were associated with an increased risk of developing proteinuria. Urinary MCP-1 during the first 100 days post HCT was associated with kidney disease at 1 year. The degree of albuminuria at any time point in the first 100 days post-transplant was related to the subsequent risk of death (for ACR 30-299, hazard ratio (HR)=1.91; 95% confidence interval (CI): 1.27-2.87; for ACR >300, HR=2.82; 95% CI: 1.60-4.98). After HCT, elevated urinary levels of pro-inflammatory cytokines are associated with development of albuminuria and proteinuria, suggesting early intra-renal inflammation as an important pathogenetic mechanism. Albuminuria and proteinuria within the first 100 days post HCT are associated with decreased overall survival.

Inflammation and Phosphorus

Study 8.21 High phosphate induces a pro-inflammatory response by vascular smooth muscle cells and modulation by vitamin D derivatives.[29]

ABSTRACT:

In chronic kidney disease patients, high phosphate (HP) levels are associated with cardiovascular disease, the major cause of morbidity and mortality. Since serum phosphate has been independently correlated with inflammation, the present study aimed to investigate an independent direct effect of HP as a pro-inflammatory factor in VSMCs. A possible modulatory effect of vitamin D (VitD) was also investigated. The study was performed in an in vitro model of human aortic smooth muscle cells (HASMCs). Incubation of cells in an HP (3.3 mM) medium caused an increased expression of the pro-inflammatory mediators intercellular adhesion molecule 1 (ICAM-1), interleukins (ILs) IL-1β, IL-6, IL-8 and tumour necrosis factor α (TNF-α) (not corroborated at the protein levels for ICAM-1), as well as an increase in reactive oxygen/ nitrogen species (ROS/ RNS) production.

Inflammation and Heart Disease Progression

Study 8.22 Vascular inflammation and media calcification are already present in early stages of chronic kidney disease.[30]

CONCLUSION:

Early stages of CKD are already associated with local up-regulation of proinflammatory and proteogenic molecules in the vascular wall and calcification of the aortic media. These findings point to the importance of local microinflammation in CKD.

Inflammation and Fat

Study 8.23 Increased production of proinflammatory cytokines in adipose tissue of patients with end-stage renal disease.[31]

CONCLUSION:

Subcutaneous and visceral adipose tissues in ESRD express higher amounts of proinflammatory cytokines and may play a role in the development of systemic inflammation.

It is absolute insanity that we don't treat inflammation from the first day of diagnosis. We do treat inflammation via immune-suppressing drugs. But, are these drugs treating the symptom or the cause? I don't think we know at this stage. Knocking down our immune system does reduce the the body's response to inflammation. However, it doesn't allow us to address why our body is attacking itself, or why inflammation is out of control. How did we lose control of inflammation? That is the question we should be asking.

My message is that we have to control and ideally stop inflammation at all costs. Every reduction in inflammation markers has the potential to add years to our lives or slow the disease progression. If we can't stop or slow inflammation, our odds of survival are greatly reduced. This is a fact we can't escape.

We know a few things:

1. Inflammation started well before you became aware of the symptoms.

2. Markers for inflammation start very early in kidney diseases, as early as stage 2.

3. As kidney disease progresses, inflammation increases.

4. Inflammation accelerates the progression of kidney diseases.

5. Inflammation accelerates the progression of heart diseases.

6. Dialysis does little to treat inflammation.

7. Excess fat or adipose tissue can worsen inflammation.

8. Diet is one of the primary drivers of inflammation, when infection, injury, or viruses are not present.

9. Stress likely plays a factor as a trigger for initiating the disease or in disease progression.

10. Inflammation is linked to many factors in kidney and heart diseases such as albumin and phosphorous in urine, proteinuria, and so on.

If these facts are correct (and they are), restoring the body's ability to properly regulate inflammation should be our goal. For most of us, our bodies did a pretty good job at controlling inflammation until we got sick.

Treating kidney diseases with a low-protein diet corrects only uremia. In my experience, eating a low-protein diet without treating inflammation has very little chance of success. I believe this is one of the reasons why other low-protein diets and/or protein supplements have a bad history. If we are not treating inflammation, we have little chance of achieving success. We have to treat everything, not just one part of the disease.

Turning Off Runaway Inflammation

Macrophages are two types of immune cells. The pro-inflammatory M1 macrophages produce the pro-inflammatory molecules that tell other cells to join the fight. M2 macrophages calm down the M1 macrophages by secreting anti-inflammatory substances.

Something called the "polarization" of M1 and M2 cells takes place when certain conditions are present. The cells are converted from being positive (anti-inflammatory) into being negative (pro-inflammatory). Our bodies can turn M2 anti-inflammatory cells into M1 inflammatory cells. The body sends M1 cells to fight, but the problem still exists.

Our bodies think we need more inflammatory cells to fight the perceived threat. It's a vicious cycle. Our bodies experience inflammation and create more inflammatory cells to fight the perceived threat. The number of M1 cells increase and the number of M2 cells start to drop. Runaway inflammation can take place when our bodies start producing more inflammatory cells than the anti-inflammatory cells.

C-reactive protein helps turn the good M2s into the bad M1s. The higher the inflammation, the higher the conversion rate.

Study 8.24   C-reactive protein polarizes human macrophages to an M1 phenotype and inhibits transformation to the M2 phenotype.[32]

CONCLUSION:

Collectively, these results further support a role for CRP in promoting differentiation of human monocytes toward a proinflammatory M1 phenotype.

Study 8.25   Macrophage polarization in kidney diseases[33]

ABSTRACT:

Macrophage accumulation associates closely with the degree of renal structural injury and renal dysfunction in human kidney diseases. Depletion of macrophages reduces while adoptive transfer of macrophages worsens inflammation in animal models of the renal injury. However, emerging evidence support that macrophage polarization plays a critical role in the progression of a number of kidney diseases including obstructive nephropathy, ischemia-reperfusion injury, glomerulonephritis, diabetic nephropathy, and other kidney diseases. In this minireview, we briefly summarize the macrophage infiltration and polarization in these inflammatory and fibrotic kidney diseases, discussing the results mostly from studies in animal models. In view of the critical role of macrophage in the progression of these diseases, manipulating macrophage phenotype may be a potential effective strategy to treat various kidney diseases.

Study 8.26   Enhanced M1 and Impaired M2 Macrophage Polarization and Reduced Mitochondrial Biogenesis via Inhibition of AMP Kinase in Chronic Kidney Disease[34]

RESULTS:

Our data showed that macrophages from RRM rats displayed enhanced M1 and impaired M2 polarization as revealed by increased M1 markers (tumor necrosis factor α, IL-6, IL-12p40, nitric oxide) and decreased M2 markers (IL-10, CD206, arginase activity) in response to LPS and IL-4 induction.

| Study 8.27 | Macrophage Polarization in Obesity and Type 2 Diabetes: Weighing Down Our Understanding of Macrophage Function?[35] |

Obesity and type 2 diabetes are now recognized as chronic pro-inflammatory diseases. In the last decade, the role of the macrophage in particular has become increasingly implicated in their pathogenesis. Abundant literature now establishes that monocytes get recruited to peripheral tissues (i.e., pancreas, liver, and adipose tissue) to become resident macrophages and contribute to local inflammation, development of insulin resistance, or even pancreatic dysfunction. Furthermore, an accumulation of evidence has established an important role for macrophage polarization in the development of metabolic diseases. The general view in obesity is that there is an imbalance in the ratio of M1/M2 macrophages, with M1 "pro-inflammatory" macrophages being enhanced compared with M2 "anti-inflammatory" macrophages being down-regulated, leading to chronic inflammation and the propagation of metabolic dysfunction.

As the body perceives that an injury or some other problem is not being healed by sending enough M1 cells, the body cranks up the production of more M1 cells, creating ever more inflammation. This cycle continues until the anti-inflammatory cells cannot control inflammation.

Once this cycle starts, it may be hard to turn off. We can't say that this scenario happens at all times and in all patients. But evidence points us in this direction. Oxidative stress, acidosis, uremia, etc. also play a role. We do know that the anti-inflammatory cells diminish when kidney diseases and inflammation are present.

This is a simplified version of a complex issue, but you get the idea.

The Good News

We can take steps to stop the runaway inflammation. The steps are easier than you may think. The different heart and cancer diets and research have showed us the right ways to do so. Heart diseases can be stopped and reversed, in part, by controlling or stopping inflammation.

Diet may be contributing to ongoing or systemic inflammation. One meal won't do it. It took years of tiny insults adding up to make the problem worse. Death by a thousand meals. We need to convince our bodies that everything is okay again. Our bodies can stop sending out the inflammatory troops and get back to normal. This is our primary goal. Our secondary goal is to slow the progression of the disease to a snail's pace. These goals overlap in many areas.

We know that diet can turn off certain genes. This is an emerging science. But the research tells us that our diet can at least partially control our genes. Micro RNA, or micro ribonucleic acid, can turn on and off genes. Micro RNA has recently been shown to change based on your diet.

Study 8.28 MicroRNA expression in relation to different dietary habits: a comparison in stool and plasma samples.[36]

ABSTRACT:

MicroRNAs (miRNAs), a class of small non-coding RNAs, are fundamental for the post-transcriptional regulation of gene expression. Altered expression of miRNAs has been detected in cancers, not only in primary tissue but also in easily obtainable specimens like plasma and stools. miRNA expression is known to be modulated by diet (micro and macronutrients, phytochemicals) and possibly by other lifestyle factors; however, such influence has not yet been exhaustively explored in humans. In the present study, we analysed the expression levels of a panel of seven human miRNAs in plasma and stool samples of a group of 24 healthy individuals characterised by different dietary habits (eight vegans, eight vegetarians and eight subjects with omnivorous diet, all groups with similar age and sex distribution). The dual aim of the study was to identify possible differences in miRNA expression due to diet (or other lifestyle factors recorded from questionnaires) and to compare results in both types of specimens. miR-92a was differentially expressed in both plasma and stool samples and with the same trend, among the three groups
with different diets (P = 0.0002 and P = 0.02, respectively, with expression levels of vegans> vegetarians>omnivores). miR-92a was also associated with low body mass index (P = 0.04 and P = 0.05, respectively) in both types of specimens, and with several dietary factors. Other analysed miRNAs (miR-16, miR-21, mir-34a and miR-222) were associated with dietary and lifestyle factors, but not consistently in both stool and plasma. Our pilot study provides the first evidence of miRNA modulation by diet and other factors, that can be detected consistently in both plasma and stools samples.

Study 8.29 Aberrant expression of microRNA induced by high-fructose diet: implications in the pathogenesis of hyperlipidemia and hepatic insulin resistance.[37]

ABSTRACT:

Fructose is a highly lipogenic sugar that can alter energy metabolism and trigger metabolic disorders. In the current study, microRNAs (miRNAs) altered by a high-fructose diet were comprehensively explored to elucidate their significance in the pathogenesis of chronic metabolic disorders. miRNA expression profiling using small noncoding RNA sequencing revealed that 19 miRNAs were significantly upregulated and 26 were downregulated in the livers of high-fructose-fed mice compared to chow-fed mice. Computational prediction and functional analysis identified 10 miRNAs, miR-19b-3p, miR-101a-3p, miR-30a-5p, miR-223-3p, miR-378a-3p, miR33-5p, miR-145a-3p, miR-128-3p, miR-125b-5p and miR582-3p, assembled as a regulatory network to potentially target key genes in lipid and lipoprotein metabolism and insulin signaling at multiple levels. qRT-PCR analysis of their potential target genes [IRS-1, FOXO1, SREBP-1c/2, ChREBP, insulin-induced gene-2 (Insig-2), microsomal triglyceride transfer protein (MTTP) and apolipoprotein B (apoB)] demonstrated that fructose-induced alterations of miRNAs were also reflected in mRNA expression profiles of their target genes. Moreover, the miRNA profile induced by high-fructose diet differed from that induced by high-fat diet, indicating that miRNAs mediate distinct pathogenic mechanisms in dietary-induced metabolic disorders. This study presents a comprehensive analysis of a new set of hepatic miRNAs, which were altered by high-fructose provides novel insights into the interaction between miRNAs and their target genes in the development of metabolic syndrome.

| Study 8.30 | A High-Fat Diet Promotes Mammary Gland Myofibroblast Differentiation through MicroRNA 140 Downregulation.[38] |

ABSTRACT:

Human breast adipose tissue is a heterogeneous cell population consisting of mature white adipocytes, multipotent mesenchymal stem cells, committed progenitor cells, fibroblasts, endothelial cells, and immune cells. Dependent on external stimulation, adipose-derived stem cells differentiate along diverse lineages into adipocytes, chondrocytes, osteoblasts, fibroblasts, and myofibroblasts. It is currently not fully understood how a high-fat diet reprograms adipose-derived stem cells into myofibroblasts. In our study, we used mouse models of a regular diet and of high-fat-diet-induced obesity to investigate the role of dietary fat on myofibroblast differentiation in the mammary stromal microenvironment. We found that a high-fat diet promotes myofibroblast differentiation by decreasing microRNA 140 (miR-140) expression in mammary adipose tissue through a novel negative-feedback loop. Increased transforming growth factor β1 (TGF-β1) in mammary adipose tissue in obese mice activates SMAD3 signaling, causing phospho-SMAD3 to bind to the miR-140 locus and inhibit miR-140 transcription. This prevents miR-140 from targeting SMAD3 for degradation, resulting in amplified TGF-β1/SMAD3 signaling and miR-140 downregulation-dependent myofibroblast differentiation. Using tissue and coculture models, we found that myofibroblasts and the fibrotic microenvironment created by myofibroblasts impact the stemness and proliferation of normal ductal epithelial cells and early-stage breast cancer invasion and stemness.

Many more studies exist coming to the same conclusion: The food we eat gives instructions to our cells. This is still an emerging science. But the bulk of the evidence all comes to the same conclusion: food tells our body what to do and how to behave.

High-fat diets, in particular, appear to promote the inflammatory cell development.

In 2012, Chinese researchers found the RNA from rice in human microRNA. This means the same microRNA found in rice has the ability to make it into our cells. I guess we really are what we eat. Plant microRNA can alter the gene expression (turn on and off certain genes) in humans.

In a study of breast cancer, the microRNA found in broccoli was higher in the healthy subjects than cancer patients. An inverse correlation existed. The higher the broccoli microRNA, the less severe the breast cancer appeared to be. For the first time, it was proven that the plant RNA can inhibit cancer growth in humans.

We can look at this issue from another viewpoint to try to confirm this theory. Telomeres are the caps on the ends of our chromosomes (DNA). Think of it like a cap end on a shoelace. Telomeres keep our chromosomes intact and prevent them from mixing with nearby chromosomes. Telomere length is a subject of research. The longer the telomere, the healthier or younger you are. A shorter or shortening telomere is associated with aging and disease.

Study 8.31 — The telomere/telomerase system in autoimmune and systemic immune-mediated diseases.

ABSTRACT:

Telomeres are specialized nucleoproteic structures that cap and protect the ends of chromosomes. They can be elongated by the telomerase enzyme, but in telomerase negative cells, telomeres shorten after each cellular division because of the end replicating problem. This phenomenon leads ultimately to cellular senescence, conferring to the telomeres a role of biological clock. Oxidative stress, inflammation and increased cell renewal are supplementary environmental factors that accelerate age-related telomere shortening. Similar to other types of DNA dam-age, very short/dysfunctional telomeres activate a DNA response pathway leading to different outcomes: DNA repair, cell senescence or apoptosis. During the last 10 years, studies on the telomere/telomerase system in autoimmune and/or systemic immune-mediated diseases have revealed its involvement in relevant physiopathological processes. Here, we present a literature review of telomere and telomerase homeostasis in systemic inflammatory diseases including systemic lupus erythematosus, rheumatoid arthritis and granulomatous diseases. The available data indicate that both telomerase activity and telomere length are modified in various systemic immune-mediated diseases and appear to be connected with premature immunosenescence. Studies on the telomere/telomerase system open new research avenues for the basic understanding and for therapeutic approaches of these pathologies.

Study 8.32 — The Telomere/Telomerase System in Chronic Inflammatory Diseases. Cause or Effect?

CONCLUSIONS AND FUTURE PROSPECTS:

Many chronic conditions in humans are associated with chronic inflammation, immune system impairment and accelerated aging. In addition, abnormalities in telomere/ telomerase system of these patients have been reported in many of these disorders. Since telomerase, an enzyme directly associated with aging, is inactive in most cell types in a mature organism and active in immune system cells, one can easily hypothesize that the immune system dysfunction/accelerated aging observed in chronic conditions is connected with telomeres and telomerase biology. Indeed, a connection of this nature seems to exist since shortened telomeres, observed in aged cells, cause an inflammatory cascade whereas, at the same time, NFκB, a master regulator of inflammation, seems to directly induce telomerase transcription as stated above. Moreover, many researchers documented correlations between lower telomerase activity and/or shorter telomeres in immune system cells and elevated cytokines in blood serum from patients with chronic disorders. One should also bear in mind that, although aging is a multifactorial and complex procedure, healthy aging and longevity are believed to be associated with longer telomeres and lower inflammation profiles among older individuals. Despite all of the above, and despite the accumulating data of a strong interconnection between telomerase regulation/ activity and inflammation, the mechanistical details and the molecular pathways of this connection have not been uncovered yet.

Due to the emergence of chronic inflammation as a prominent risk factor of many human disorders, researchers hypothesize that harnessing inflammation can have many beneficiary and longevity effects. Interestingly, many of the interventions used so far to regulate and diminish inflammation also seem to positively affect telomere biology as well. For example, inhibition of one of the major cytokines produced by senescent cells, TNF-a, increases telomerase activity and proliferative potential. Another finding worth noting is the pleiotropic effects of statins and angiotensin converting enzyme inhibitors (ACEIs). Statins are lipid lowering drugs and ACEIs are anti-hypertension drugs; both have been used effectively in many patient categories for decades. Both drugs are also considered anti-inflammatory agents as it has been observed to lower circulating cytokines in patients' blood serum. Additionally, both agents have also been found to promote telomerase activity and/or *hTERT* gene transcription. It is also worth noting that in certain disorders such as CKD, the possibility of targeted anti-inflammatory therapy is studied extensively with interleukin receptor antagonists and other agents like pentoxifylline already showing promising results in systematically lowering the inflammatory profile of these patients. Lifestyle habits and interventions are also another important factor that needs to be taken into account. A healthy diet, frequent exercise and a low everyday stress profile has been associated with a healthier inflammatory status as many studies have shown. As stated above, the same lifestyle factors are also connected with longer telomeres and/ or higher telomeraseactivity while psychiatric disorders, obesity, etc. are associated with deregulated telomere/telomerase physiology. It should also be noted that meditation has been reported to reduce stress, downregulate inflammatory genes and increase telomerase activity by up to 43% , while older married adults with high income are associated with longer telomeres.

Study 8.33   Inflammation and premature aging in advanced chronic kidney disease.

ABSTRACT:

Systemic inflammation in end-stage renal disease is an established risk factor for mortality and a catalyst for other complications, which are related to a premature aging phenotype, including muscle wasting, vascular calcification, and other forms of premature vascular disease, depression, osteoporosis, and frailty. Uremic inflammation is also mechanistically related to mechanisms involved in the aging process, such as telomere shortening, mitochondrial dysfunction, and altered nutrient sensing, which can have a direct effect on cellular and tissue function. In addition to uremia-specific causes, such as abnormalities in the phosphate-Klotho axis, there are remarkable similarities between the pathophysiology of uremic inflammation and so-called "inflammaging" in the general population. Potentially relevant, but still somewhat unexplored in this respect, are abnormal or misplaced protein structures, as well as abnormalities in tissue homeostasis, which evoke danger signals through damage-associated molecular patterns, as well as the senescence-associated secretory phenotype. Systemic inflammation, in combination with the loss of kidney function, can impair the resilience of the body to external and internal stressors by reduced functional and structural tissue reserves, and by impairing normal organ crosstalk, thus providing an explanation for the greatly increased risk of homeostatic breakdown in this population. In this review, the relationship between uremic inflammation and a premature aging phenotype, as well as potential causes and consequences, are discussed.

Study 8.34   **Chronic Inflammation: Accelerator of Biological Aging.**

ABSTRACT:

Biological aging is characterized by a chronic low-grade inflammation level. This chronic phenomenon has been named "inflamm-aging" and is a highly significant risk factor for morbidity and mortality in the older persons. The most common theories of inflamm-aging include redox stress, mitochondrial dysfunction, glycation, deregulation of the immune system, hormonal changes, epigenetic modifications, and dysfunction telomere attrition. Inflamm-aging plays a role in the initiation and progression of age-related diseases such as type II diabetes, Alzheimer's disease, cardiovascular disease, frailty, sarcopenia, osteoporosis, and cancer. This review will cover the identification of pathways that control age-related inflammation across multiple systems and its potential causal role in contributing to adverse health outcomes.

Inflamm-aging is a new term. We can error-check ourselves one more time on telomeres and inflammation. We can check to see if the same things that increase the telomere length can also decrease inflammation. If the two have nothing in common, we can assume inflammation and telomere length are not related.

Here are the steps taken in the Dean Ornish study on prostate cancer patients to lengthen telomeres:

1. Diet: Low-fat, plant-based diet emphasizing whole foods (aka real foods, in their original forms).

2. Exercise: thirty minutes of aerobic exercises, six days a week.

3. Stress reduction: meditation or yoga for up to sixty minutes a day.

4. Increased social support: weekly support groups.

Let us compare this list to what we know can reduce inflammation:

1. A healthy diet high in antioxidants and foods considered to be whole or real foods.

2. Exercise.

3. Stress reduction.

4. Positive outlook and/or social support.

5. Weight kept under control.

We can see that these lists are almost identical, with the exception of weight. The message here is that we may be able to change our outcomes. We can make changes.

One might ask "What is the best way to lengthen our telomeres?" A study compared exercise, weight loss, a combination of weight loss and exercise, and a plant-based diet. No change in the telomere length with weight loss, exercise, or the combination group was found. However, the group on the plant-based diet experienced a 28% increase in the telomere length. Exercise and weight loss are important, but did not slow down aging at the same rate as the plant-based diet. Could it be that the plant-based diet has the ability to turn on or off the right cells?

Think about this for a second. Losing weight and exercising while eating the same foods did not work. What worked was a diet that turned the right cells on and off. This is, perhaps, why the low-protein diets don't have a great track record. If you are still eating bad foods, but less of them, we don't change our odds.

This was my experience on the Walser diet at Johns Hopkins. Almost any food was allowed, no matter how bad it was for you, if it had a low protein content. If we switch from one inflammatory food to another, we aren't treating the problem.

We can lengthen or shorten our telomeres based on diet and lifestyle. Dr. Dean Ornish proved that diet, exercise, stress management, and social support worked to increase the telomere length. The study was on men with prostate cancer.

The is important because we started this chapter with a discussion on inflammation and stress. Lowering or managing stress increased the telomere length. This confirms the data we discussed earlier in this chapter, that stress may be a big factor in our disease progression. The Ornish diet is a healthy diet that has fruits, vegetables, and grains, but is low in fats and refined or processed foods. Exercise also increased the telomere length in some studies.

The Good Stuff

We have a lot of data including microRNA and telomeres confirming that diet changes the most basic parts of our body—our DNA, or chromosomes. We can look at the other side of the argument and see if we can find evidence that different foods change the cells from inflammatory to anti-inflammatory.

An example is retinoic acid, a component of vitamin A. Retinoic acid increases the anti-inflammatory activity in macrophages and pushes more cells toward the anti-inflammatory side. However, depletion of vitamin A pushed the same anti-inflammatory M2 macrophages into the inflammatory range. That's the opposite of what they are supposed to do. We saw this in an earlier chart. The anti-inflammatory cells were so low, they were not detected.

Lack of vitamin A can turn anti-inflammatory cells into inflammatory cells.[39]

Could this explain why the inflammatory response is missing in some diseases as previously mentioned? Is a needed nutrient missing from our diet or in short supply? We eat a lot of calories that have very little nutrition.

Think about fast foods, restaurant foods, and packaged foods. Most of these are calorie- and fat-dense, but have little in the way of vitamins, minerals, and antioxidants.

Plant-based diets may have stopped, slowed, or reversed heart disease and prostate cancer in research studies by giving our bodies different instructions based on the diet choices. Exercise and weight loss won't work by themselves. We have to change the instructions we give to our body. Computer code gives instructions for a program to execute. Similarly, our food choices give instructions to our bodies to execute functions.

Summary

Let's review the following concepts about inflammation:

1. High-fat diets tell our body to produce more inflammation.

2. High-fructose (or sugar) diets tell our body to produce more inflammation.

3. High-animal-protein diets produce inflammation.

4. Diets rich in fat, artificial sugars, and animal protein contribute to diseases like heart and kidney disease.

5. Nutrient-poor and calorie-dense diets may not give our bodies enough of the necessary vitamins, antioxidants, and minerals, which may tell our bodies to produce more inflammation.

6. Inflammation is the symptom. We have to treat the cause, not the symptoms.

7. The cause, or at least some of the causes, of our diseases is the food we eat.

VS

1. Plant-based diets may help our bodies to produce anti-inflammatory cells, or do not contribute to inflammation.

2. Plant-based diets have been proven to reduce, stop, or reverse heart diseases and some cancers.

3. Nutrient-dense diets that are high in fibers, vitamins, and antioxidants may lengthen our telomeres and slow the aging process.

4. Plant-based diets have been proven to be safe.

5. Plant-based diets have had the highest success rates when it comes to slowing the progression of kidney diseases.

Which Diet Do We Want to Bet Our Lives On

That is really the question for us. I am not trying to be dramatic.

We have to try to cut off inflammation at the source and stop treating symptoms. The emphasis has to be on treating the cause, not the symptoms.

Post-prandial inflammation is another subject I will deal with in this book. This chapter was just too big to include this subject.

If you don't have a virus, bacterial infection, or injury, your body should have inflammation under control. The source of chronic inflammation might be your diet until inflammation becomes a runaway inflammation. I did not start getting better until I took the approach of reducing inflammation while increasing albumin at the same time. Albumin and inflammation are tied together in many ways.

The diet and treatment plan discussed later in this book are heavily focused on reducing, and hopefully stopping, inflammation.

Kidney disease is an inflammatory disease. Don't let anyone tell you anything different. Yes, kidney disease is multifactorial and complicated in many ways. However, all evidence points to inflammation as the single biggest factor responsible.

References

1. Libby P. Inflammatory mechanisms: the molecular basis of inflammation and disease. *Nutrition Reviews*. 2007;65(suppl_3):S140-S146.

2. Krishnamoorthy S, Honn KV. Inflammation and disease progression. *Cancer and Metastasis Reviews*. 2006;25(3):481-491.

3. Segerstrom SC, Miller GE. Psychological stress and the human immune system: a meta-analytic study of 30 years of inquiry. *Psychological Bulletin*. 2004;130(4):601-630.

4. Yamamoto Y, Gaynor RB. Therapeutic potential of inhibition of the NF-κB pathway in the treatment of inflammation and cancer. *Journal of Clinical Investigation*. 2001;107(2):135-142.

5. Abou-Raya A, Abou-Raya S. Inflammation: a pivotal link between autoimmune diseases and atherosclerosis. *Autoimmunity Reviews*. 2006;5(5):331-337. 6. Calle M, Fernandez M. Inflammation and type 2 diabetes. *Diabetes & Metabolism*. 2012;38(3):183-191.

6. Landray MJ, Wheeler DC, Lip GY, et al. Inflammation, endothelial dysfunction, and platelet activation in patients with chronic kidney disease: the chronic renal impairment in Birmingham (CRIB) study. *American Journal of Kidney Diseases*. 2004;43(2):244-253.

7. Stojanovich L, Marisavljevich D. Stress as a trigger of autoimmune disease. *Autoimmunity Reviews*. 2008;7(3):209-213.

8. Rampton DS. The influence of stress on the development and severity of immune-mediated diseases. *The Journal of Rheumatology Supplement*. 2011;88:43-47.

9. Powell ND, Sloan EK, Bailey MT, et al. Social stress up-regulates inflammatory gene expression in the leukocyte transcriptome via β-adrenergic induction of myelopoiesis. *Proceedings of the National Academy of Sciences*. 2013;110(41):16574-16579.

10. Cohen S, Janicki-Deverts D, Doyle WJ, et al. Chronic stress, glucocorticoid receptor resistance, inflammation, and disease risk. *Proceedings of the National Academy of Sciences*. 2012;109(16):5995-5999.

11. Hackett RA, Steptoe A. type 2 diabetes mellitus and psychological stress—a modifiable risk factor. *Nature Reviews Endocrinology*. 2017;13(9):547-560.

12. Kelly SJ, Ismail M. Stress and type 2 diabetes: a review of how stress contributes to the development of type 2 diabetes. *Annual Review of Public Health*. 2015;36:441-462.

13. Ackerman KD, Heyman R, Rabin BS, et al. Stressful life events precede exacerbations of multiple sclerosis. *Psychosomatic Medicine*. 2002;64(6):916-920.

14. Steptoe A, Kivimäki M. Stress and cardiovascular disease. *Nature Reviews Cardiology*. 2012;9(6):360-370.

15. Dinarello CA, Novick D, Kim S, Kaplanski G. Interleukin-18 and IL-18 binding protein. *Frontiers in Immunology*. 2013;4(Article 289):1-10.

16. Johnston C. Functional foods as modifiers of cardiovascular disease. *American Journal of Lifestyle Medicine.* 2009;3(1_ Suppl):39S-43S.

17. Kugler E, Cohen E, Goldberg E, et al. C reactive protein and long-term risk for chronic kidney disease: a historical prospective study. *Journal of Nephrology.* 2015;28(3):321-327.

18. Silverstein DM. Inflammation in chronic kidney disease: role in the progression of renal and cardiovascular disease. *Pediatric Nephrology.* 2009;24(8):1445-1452.

19. Tonelli M, Sacks F, Pfeffer M, Jhangri GS, Curhan G. Biomarkers of inflammation and progression of chronic kidney disease. *Kidney International.* 2005;68(1):237-245.

20. Sharain K, Hoppensteadt D, Bansal V, Singh A, Fareed J. Progressive increase of inflammatory biomarkers in chronic kidney disease and end-stage renal disease. *Clinical and Applied Thrombosis/Hemostasis.* 2013;19(3):303-308.

21. Shi B, Ni Z, Cao L, et al. Serum IL-18 is closely associated with renal tubulointerstitial injury and predicts renal prognosis in IgA nephropathy. *Mediators of Inflammation.* 2012;2012.

22. Kraydaschenko O, Berezin A, Dolinnaya M, Swintozelsky A. Serum Interleukin-18 as a Biomarker of Tubular Kidney Damage in Patients with Chronic Glomerulonephritis. *Biological Markers and Guided Therapy.* 2016;3(1):185-191.

23. Formanowicz D, Wanic-Kossowska M, Pawliczak E, Radom M, Formanowicz P. Usefulness of serum interleukin-18 in predicting cardiovascular mortality in patients with chronic kidney disease–systems and clinical approach. *Scientific Reports.* 2015;5(18332):1-13.

24. Marsik C, Kazemi-Shirazi L, Schickbauer T, et al. C-reactive protein and all-cause mortality in a large hospital-based cohort. *Clinical Chemistry.* 2008;54(2):343-349.

25. Don BR, Kaysen G. Poor nutritional status and inflammation:

26. serum albumin: relationship to inflammation and nutrition. *Seminars in Dialysis.* 2004;17(6):432-437.

27. Hanafusa N, Nitta K, Okazaki M, et al. Serum albumin level adjusted with C-reactive protein predicts hemodialysis patient survival. *Renal Replacement Therapy.* 2017;3(1):1-9.

28. Hingorani S, Gooley T, Pao E, Sandmaier B, McDonald G. Urinary cytokines after HCT: evidence for renal inflammation in the pathogenesis of proteinuria and kidney disease. *Bone Marrow Transplantation.* 2014;49(3):403-409.

29. Martínez-Moreno JM, Herencia C, de Oca AM, et al. High phosphate induces a pro-inflammatory response by vascular smooth muscle cells. Modulation by vitamin D derivatives. *Clinical Science.* 2017:CS20160807.

30. Benz K, Varga I, Neureiter D, et al. Vascular inflammation and media calcification are already present in early stages of chronic kidney disease. *Cardiovascular Pathology.* 2017;27:57-67.

31. Roubicek T, Bartlova M, Krajickova J, et al. Increased production of proinflammatory cytokines in adipose tissue of patients with end-stage renal disease. *Nutrition.* 2009;25(7):762-768.

32. Devaraj S, Jialal I. C-reactive protein polarizes human macrophages to an M1 phenotype and inhibits transformation to the M2 phenotype. *Arteriosclerosis, Thrombosis, and Vascular Biology.* 2011;31(6):1397-1402. 33. Tian S, Chen S-Y. Macrophage polarization in kidney diseases. *Macrophage.* 2015;2(1):1-10.

33. Li C, Ding XY, Xiang DM, et al. Enhanced M1 and impaired M2 macrophage polarization and reduced mitochondrial biogenesis via inhibition of AMP kinase in chronic kidney disease. *Cellular Physiology and Biochemistry.* 2015;36(1):358-372.

34. Kraakman MJ, Murphy AJ, Jandeleit-Dahm K, Kammoun HL. Macrophage polarization in obesity and type 2 diabetes: weighing down our understanding of macrophage function? *Frontiers in Immunology.* 2014;5(Article 470).

35. Tarallo S, Pardini B, Mancuso G, et al. MicroRNA expression in relation to different dietary habits: a comparison in stool and plasma samples. *Mutagenesis.* 2014;29(5):385-391.

36. Sud N, Zhang H, Pan K, Cheng X, Cui J, Su Q. Aberrant expression of microRNA induced by high-fructose diet:

37. implications in the pathogenesis of hyperlipidemia and hepatic insulin resistance. *The Journal of Nutritional Biochemistry.* 2017;43:125-131.

38. Wolfson B, Zhang Y, Gernapudi R, et al. A high-fat diet promotes mammary gland myofibroblast differentiation through microRNA 140 downregulation. *Molecular and Cellular Biology.* 2017;37(4):e00461-00416.

39. Okabe Y, Medzhitov R. Tissue-specific signals control reversible program of localization and functional polarization of macrophages. *Cell.* 2014;157(4):832-844.

CHAPTER 9

Uremia

Uremia is a condition that arises due to the build-up of waste products from amino acid and protein metabolism. We talked about uremic toxins in Chapter 8. If left untreated, these toxic waste products can prove detrimental to your health.

The chapter on uremic toxins provided good information about this subject, but here I present some additional information.

In the simplest terms, uremia develops when you eat more protein than your body and kidneys can process. The protein can be of any kind, not just animal protein. The waste products build up faster than your kidneys can filter them, and they eventually excrete in your urine. Dialysis is the current treatment for uremia. Uremia is sometimes referred as "protein overload."[1]

The average American male consumes 102 grams of protein per day. Now let's calculate the actual amount of protein required. A 75 kg (165 lb) person needs 60 grams of protein a day according to the USDA, which implies 0.8 grams per kilogram of body weight.[2] The European Food Safety Authority recommends 0.83 grams of protein per kilogram.[3]

For most of the dialysis patients, these recommendations vary from 1 to 1.2 grams of protein per kg a day, or 75 grams or more in total per day. The increase in protein intake values is an attempt to increase protein nutrition. 75 to 90 grams would be the current recommendation for dialysis patients.[4]

Right off the bat, you can see the average consumption is 42 grams higher than necessary. The average American is found to eat 70% more protein than necessary to maintain good health. These statistics imply that the protein or uremic workload on your kidneys is 70% higher than necessary. To overcome this health hazard, eating 60 grams of protein per day will dramatically lessen the load on your kidneys and should reduce uremia or uremic symptoms.

However, contradictory notions persist in the community with regard to the benefits of low protein consumption. On the one hand, Dr. Walser reported that any protein consumption over 50 grams a day does not appear to slow down kidney disease progression. Consuming 60 grams of protein a day instead of 102 grams may reduce uremia and uremic symptoms slightly, but will likely not reduce the progression of kidney disease. According to Dr. Walser: "50 grams might as well be 100" concerning kidney disease progression. Remember the 'moderation kills' mantra. The reason low-protein diets have such a mixed track record is likely because protein restriction was not strict enough.[5]

Another problem is that available research suggests that consuming a higher amount of protein accelerates kidney disease progression. In fact, eating a large amount of protein does not work, for several reasons. First, it increases the chances and severity of uremia. Second, protein or albumin loss may occur due to other factors besides dietary consumption. Inflammation and oxidative stress are the two reasons why, despite adequate dietary protein intake, albumin still counts low. Eating more protein may increase protein synthesis in the liver, but this process may be obstructed due to oxidative stress, inflammation, and proteinuria, and subsequently result in increased uremia, which eventually favors kidney disease progression.[6]

What if you reduced your protein intake to 25 grams a day? The load on your kidneys would be a quarter of the load from 102 grams of protein. On paper, this represents a 75% reduction in protein workload. Doing the math, it appears that increasing your protein intake from 25 grams a day to 102 grams a day leads to a drastic 300% increase in kidney workload.

Let's say that again, eating 25 grams of protein versus 102 grams reduces kidney workload by over 300%. This example is not 100% correct because your body also produces waste products every day regardless of diet. Creatinine clearance usually measures this smaller but constant workload.

Let's look at this example in another way. You are putting 25 miles on your kidney engine a day as opposed to 102 miles per day. Kidney disease disproportionally affects older adults, so let's assume you are 65 years old and have been eating this way since you were 25 years old. 40 years of 102 kidney miles per day equals 1,124,200 kidney miles. At 25 miles per day, your total miles are 365,000. Which kidney do you think would be in better shape? Is it the one with more than a million miles, or the one with less than 400,000 miles?

This is a metaphor, but I want you to start thinking about kidney workload when it comes to protein and uremia. You want to live a healthy and long life, and you certainly want your kidneys to last as long as possible. This can be achieved only by putting as few miles on your kidneys as you can.

Presently, there are only two basic options for the treatment of uremia. The first and most proven option is dialysis.[7] The second and less proven option is a low-protein diet.[8] In some ways, this makes uremia treatment easier, as we do not have many choices. However, we have to watch out for uremic malnutrition. Uremic malnutrition puts us in a catch-22 situation.

It's black and white and not up for argument or debate. If your blood urea nitrogen levels and/or creatintine levels are higher than the normal range, you are eating more protein than your kidneys can handle. It should be kidney 101 to understand this and start lowering dietary protein intake immediately.

Uremic malnutrition is a term used to describe uremia combined with low serum albumin. Uremia reflects that we are eating more protein than our kidneys can handle. Low albumin tells us we are excreting too much protein in our urine, or that inflammation and oxidative stress are reducing albumin levels. Hence, the underlying truth behind this scenario is that eating more protein to increase albumin levels increases uremia, inflammation, and oxidative stress, which in turn works to further lower albumin levels. Unfortunately, we end up accelerating kidney disease progression while trying to treat low albumin levels.[9] You might say uremic malnutrition is nephrotic syndrome combined with uremia.

If we go on a low-protein diet without the right supplement, we risk not getting enough protein nutrition or adequate calories. Inadequate protein nutrition or calories can also lead to lower albumin levels. Fetuin-A, which protects your arteries from calcification, is also lowered. Uremia thereby lessens at the cost of overall nutrition and health.

The only viable solution other than dialysis is a low-protein diet supplemented with keto or amino acids. Let's look at the 25 gram protein example combined with the appropriate amount of keto acids. Keto acids are "broken down amino acids." The nitrogen has already been taken out, so kidneys do not produce nitrogen waste products. Keto acids go right into our bloodstream and do not require further breaking down. Keto acids contribute little to uremia or acid load and have been used successfully for over thirty years.

Uremic malnutrition is rarely treated, and this is the reason I have shed light on this topic in this chapter. Dialysis can treat uremia, but there is no treatment available for the nutrition abnormality. Some kidney diets recommend low protein, but the protein level is still too high. We know from Walser's work that anything over 50 grams is too much. Patients also need to be on an anti-inflammatory and high-antioxidant diet to reduce inflammation and oxidative stress. This allows albumin levels to rise if the patient is on a low-protein diet supplemented with keto acids.

The combination of a low-protein, healthy diet with keto acids for protein nutrition is currently the only treatment other than dialysis that has had any measurable success. The following chart[10] shows survival rates for patients with uremia and quartiles based on serum albumin levels.

FIGURE 9.1: **Kaplan-Meier Survival Curves for Quartiles of Mean Serum Albumin During the Study Period**

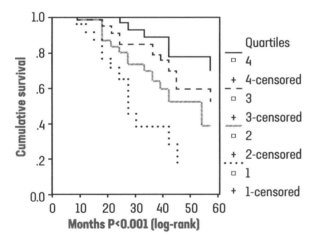

A study from the chapter on albumin estimated that 10,000 lives could be saved a year if we could successfully treat low albumin, and this chart explicitly shows why this is so important.

Incremental Dialysis

Incremental dialysis is a relatively new treatment idea. Uremic toxins are removed as in normal dialysis, but dialysis is done much earlier. The goal is to preserve renal function longer by reducing the effect of uremia or uremic toxins. This experiment hence puts forth a fundamental question:

Does removing uremic toxins earlier delay the progress of kidney disease?

The answer is yes, it may slow disease progression, based on the following pieces of evidence.

Study 9.1   Incremental dialysis: review of recent literature.[11]

RECENT FINDINGS:

Small studies suggested, then a larger study corroborated, that incremental hemodialysis was associated with preservation of residual kidney function whenever compared with conventional hemodialysis. The well tolerated nutritional status of incremental hemodialysis was questioned in a small study but a larger study was more reassuring. The mortality rate of patients undergoing incremental hemodialysis is similar to that in conventional hemodialysis, but only if the comorbidity burden is low.

SUMMARY:

<u>Incremental hemodialysis in incident patients can be performed safely, and probably is associated with preserved residual kidney function and a similar mortality rate to convention initiation of hemodialysis.</u> Patients must be prudently selected and managed for this approach to the initiation of dialysis.

Study 9.2   Incremental Hemodialysis, Residual Kidney Function, and Mortality Risk in Incident Dialysis Patients: A Cohort Study.[12]

CONCLUSIONS:

<u>Among incident hemodialysis patients with substantial RKF (residual kidney function), incremental hemodialysis may be a safe treatment regimen and is associated with greater preservation of RKF,</u> whereas higher mortality is observed after the first year of dialysis in those with the lowest RKF. Clinical trials are needed to examine the safety and effectiveness of twice-weekly hemodialysis.

The exact reason for the delay in progression is not known yet, but it is assumed the reason is an early reduction in uremia and or uremic toxins.

Current State of Kidney Diets and Nutrition

Let's take a look at diet and uremia. I was recently forwarded an email from a dialysis company with a recipe for chicken marsala served with rice.

Let's take a look at the ingredients and the effects on our kidneys:

> Olive oil

> White enriched flour

> Butter

> Mushrooms

> White Rice

> Seasonings/spices like garlic, parsley, etc.

> Marsala wine

Olive oil, wine, and butter contain no protein, and we will not worry about the spices. The combination of 1 cup of chicken, 1 cup of rice, ½ cup of mushrooms, and 2 tablespoons of flour gives us a total of 52 grams of protein. You could lower the protein level by manipulating the serving size. However, one cup is still a small portion for many of us.

52 grams of protein is consumed in one meal. Let's assume you consume half this amount, 25 grams of protein, for each breakfast and lunch. We are back to the 102 gram number again.

Besides the protein load do you see any of the following:

> Antioxidants?

> Anti-inflammatory substances?

> Low acid load?

> Low methionine?

> Low saturated fat?

> Fiber?

The 52 gram protein estimate assumes no other food was consumed with the meal: just the chicken, mushrooms, sauce, and rice.

This recipe was recommended for the following reasons:

> Low salt

> Low potassium

Does anyone think this kind of diet will help anyone with kidney disease? Have we all lost our minds? A high acid meal with almost zero antioxidants, low fiber, low nutritional value, and no anti-inflammatory ingredients will help us get better? Your odds of winning the lottery may be better. We know with 99.9% certainty that this kind of diet accelerates kidney disease progression. Yes, the recipe was low salt and potassium, but at what cost? I will say it over and over, we have to stop managing symptoms and start trying to slow or stop our disease.

The inflammatory response from a combination of rice and chicken was actually studied, believe it or not.

Study 9.3 **Effect of chicken, fat and vegetable on glycaemia and insulinaemia to a white rice-based meal in healthy adults[13]**

CONCLUSIONS:

Co-ingesting chicken, oil or vegetables with white rice considerably influences its glycemic and insulinemic responses. <u>Co-ingesting white rice with all three components attenuates the GR to a greater degree than when it is eaten with any single one of them</u>, and that this is not at the cost of an increased demand for insulin.

Why is this important? Blood glucose levels spike with this kind of meal, which in turns increases oxidative stress and inflammation. Here is what it looks like on a chart.

FIGURE 9.2: Insulin Response to Chicken and Rice

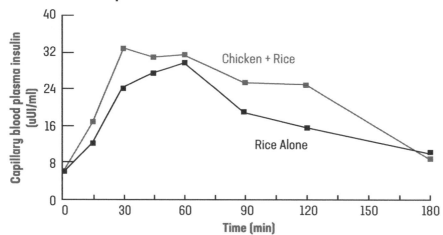

As you can see, chicken combined with rice caused an insulin response that lasted about three hours. You will likely eat your next meal four to five hours later. Our body will get back to normal for an hour or two before the following meal's response.

This is why treating uremia with diet is so important, whether you are on dialysis or not. Each meal gives us a choice whether we increase or decrease inflammation response, oxidative stress, and uremic toxins. Uremia is only a part of the story. No one ever talks about the related issues to kidney diets. Just reducing salt and phosphorus is like kindergarten concerning kidney diets. Trying for remission or to stop or dramatically slow disease progression is a Ph.D. in kidney diets. We all need degrees in kidney disease diet and management to improve our odds.

I am not picking on this company, but it shows what is considered acceptable today. Companies with almost unlimited resources still recommend these diets in 2018 using diet advice from the 1950's. In defense of this kind of advice, these companies cannot recommend keto acids and a low protein diet because keto acids are not available to patients in the U.S. These recipes are trying to include what they think is a high-quality protein to provide nutrition. No viable alternatives have existed in the U.S.

Another issue is dietary compliance. Chicken marsala tastes pretty great, and I would like to be able to eat foods like this. No one wants to be a party pooper or downer and tell you you can't eat foods you love. Many companies and doctors have concluded that appropriate diets for kidney health are just too difficult. While writing this book, I released chapters as they were available. The chapter on sodium was met with two angry emails. I personally feel managing salt is pretty easy; I just don't eat it. I was told, "it was not easy by any standard." Once this reader accurately started measuring salt in their diet, they found it was more than 2.5 times what they had expected. Another reader put it this way: "I cooked one full day with no salt, and food is not worth eating without salt."

I mention this because changing your diet to stop or reduce uremia will require some real changes on your part. I can't eat salty or greasy foods anymore. My taste buds have changed over time. Yours will too. It is insanity to choose salt over years of life. While it's not that simple, that is how I think of it. The question worth asking is: Is any food worth days or years of your life?

I hope this kind of diet logic will change with the arrival of keto acids. I have been working on bringing keto acids to the U.S. for two years. We now have access to keto acids for the first time in 2018. Check www. stoppingkidneydisease.com or www.albutrix.com for updates on availability and additional information.

Keto acids and a low-protein, high-antioxidant, anti-inflammatory, and nutrient-rich diet are the best remedy to reduce or cure uremic malnutrition other than dialysis. We need to shrink inflammation, reduce oxidative stress, and reduce the number of uremic toxins in our bloodstreams.

How else can we reduce uremic symptoms or uremic toxins?

| Study 9.4 | Nutritional intervention in uremia—myth or reality?[14] |

ABSTRACT:

Nutritional intervention in uremia, specifically the restricted protein diet, has been under debate for decades. The results of various clinical trials have not been concordant, as some studies have reported positive effects of the low-protein diets, whereas others have shown no benefit. Recently published data show that the restricted protein diets seem to be effective and safe in ameliorating nitrogen waste products retention and the disturbances in acid-base and calcium-phosphorus metabolism, and in delaying the initiation of renal replacement therapy (RRT), without any deleterious effect on the nutritional status of patients with chronic kidney disease. The nutritional support and particularly the supplemented very low protein diet could be a new link to the RRT-integrated care model. A possible delay in RRT initiation through nutrition could have a major economic effect, particularly in developing countries, where the dialysis facilities still do not meet the requirements. However, a careful selection of motivated patients who could benefit from such a diet, closer nutri-tional monitoring, and dietary counseling are required.

Study 9.5   Effects of a supplemented hypoproteic diet in chronic kidney disease.[15]

CONCLUSION:

SVLPD (Supplemented very low protein diet) seems to ameliorate the nitrogen waste products retention and acid-base and calcium-phosphorus metabolism disturbances and to postpone the renal replacement therapy initiation, preserving the nutritional status in patients with CKD.

Study 9.6   How to manage elderly patients with chronic renal failure: conservative management versus dialysis.[16]

ABSTRACT:

Over the past decade the number of elderly patients reaching end-stage renal disease has more than doubled. A fundamental medical decision that nephrologists commonly have to make is when to start dialytic treatment in elderly patients. Evidence is needed to inform about decision-making for or against dialysis, in particular in those patients frequently affected by multiple comorbidities for which dialysis may not increase survival. In fact, this decision affects quality of life, incurs significant financial costs, and finally mandates use of precious dialysis resources. The negative consequence of initiating dialysis in this group of patients can be deleterious as elderly people are sensitive to lifestyle changes. Furthermore, among dialysis patients, the elderly suffer the highest overall hospitalization and complication rates and most truncated life expectancy on dialysis of any age group. Studies of the factors that affect outcomes in elderly patients on dialysis or the possibility in postponing in a safe way the start of a dialytic treatment, were lacking until recent years. Recently in the literature, papers have been published that address these questions: the effects of dialysis on morbidity and mortality in elderly patients and the use of a supple-mented very low protein diet (sVLPD) in postponing the start of dialysis in elderly. The first study demonstrated that, although dialysis is generally associated with longer survival in patients aged >75 years, those with multiple comorbidities, ischemic heart disease in particular, do not survive longer than those treated conservatively. The second one is a randomized controlled study that compared a sVLPD with dialysis in 112 non-diabetic patients aged >70 years. Survival was not different between the two groups and the number of hospitalizations and days spent in hospital were significantly lower in those on a sVLPD. These studies add to the limited evidence that is currently available to inform elderly patients, their carers and their physicians about the risk and the benefit of dialysis.

Note: This article is relevant because it suggests that a supplemented very low-protein diet (SVLPD) was as effective as dialysis, and the number of hospitalizations was lower using diet compared to dialysis. Quality of life might be higher as well, with no visits to the dialysis clinic.

Think in Terms of Protein Workload

We need to go easy on high-mileage kidneys. Uremia and uremic toxins contribute to kidneys disease progression. The first step for all of us should be limiting protein so we prevent "protein overload." Put the brakes on uremia, and you automatically reduce related oxidative stress and inflammation. In kidney disease, everything is connected.

Many, if not most, of us are over-eating protein and increasing the speed at which our kidneys will fail. Once you start eating below your kidneys' ability to process, your kidneys will clean up your blood a little more every day.

If your kidneys can efficiently process 40 grams of protein a day and you eat 41 grams of protein, your kidneys cannot catch up. Each day, you will get a little farther behind, and this will show in your blood and urine tests. Your numbers will progressively worsen over time. Yes, the pace will be slow, but you may still be on a downward trajectory.

In the same example, if you consume 30 grams of protein a day, which is below the level of protein your kidneys can process (40 grams), then consequently over time your blood and urine tests should get better. The results will not be measurable for the first week or month, but you will find the difference gradually over time.

Sticking with your diet routine all week by eating 30 grams of protein a day and then falling off the wagon with a visit to your favorite steakhouse or barbeque joint erases the gains you made that week. One steak could have 62 grams of protein. By adding two sides with 5 of grams protein each and an appetizer, you could easily be at 77 grams of protein in one meal.

Assume you eat 20 grams of protein for the rest of the day. In total, 97 grams of protein will take days and weeks for your ailing kidneys to process. Let's assume you go back on a diet with 30 grams of protein a day. Your kidneys still have to catch up on the 77 gram workload. It could take seven to nine days for your kidneys to catch back up to where you were, even if you stayed with 30 grams of protein a day.

During this seven-day period, your blood tests will get worse. You will be back in a uremic state (if you have uremia). Oxidative stress and inflammation will also increase. You can see that one bad meal per week wrecks your progress.

This concept is misunderstood by almost everyone giving us advice. Eating more protein than your kidneys can process every day adds to uremia. Again, this is an example, not an exact science, but it is pretty close. Uremia is a result of too much protein workload. Eating below your kidneys' workload capacity allows your kidneys to catch up and lets your body try to get back to normal.

How do you know if you are eating too much protein? It's pretty simple. Your numbers will be the same or worse at the next checkup. The blood urea nitrogen, or BUN, test determines the amount of urea in your bloodstream, which will continue to stay the same or rise. If you eat below your capacity, then your BUN levels should drop slowly over time.

The diagnosis of uremia involves more than BUN testing, but BUN is the simplest way to reflect kidney workload. BUN levels usually are 7 to 20 mg/dl. You should see a drop in BUN levels after a few months if you are eating correctly for your current kidney function.

Again, BUN is not the only tool used to diagnose uremia, but we will use it later due to its simplicity.

Summary

One last note: Kidney workload is cumulative. Again, this is a metaphor, but as you eat more protein than you can handle, waste products build up over time. As you eat less, your blood gets cleaner over time. Think about it this way: Assume you have one pump filling a pond at a rate of 10 gallons per hour and another pump draining the same pond at 5 gallons per hour. The pond will fill up and overflow because you are not taking the water out quickly enough compared to the input. The net gain is 5 gallons per hour.

It's not so different with your kidneys and protein. If you fill your kidneys the waste from 100 grams of protein and your kidneys can only filter the waste from 40 grams of protein a day, your BUN and creatinine tests will keep getting worse over time, along with other related symptoms.

This is why 50 grams or more of protein per day does not slow progression of kidney disease. 50 grams is still more than we can process when we have low GFR. We have to get in the range of 25 to 35 grams per day to witness changes over several months.

This idea is confirmed by people with GFR below 60 who have trouble processing the load from a high-acid and high-protein meal.

Think of uremia as protein workload in excess of your kidneys' capacity. It is that simple. A low-protein diet may be considered as effective as dialysis in some cases. That is a compelling statement.

If your blood urea nitrogen (BUN) and/or creatinine blood tests are getting worse, the treatment is very simple: eat less protein. Uremia is simply a product of eating more protein than your kidneys can handle.

References

1. Eddy AA, Geary DF, Balfe JW, Clark W, Baumal R. Prolongation of acute renal failure in two patients with hemolytic-uremic syndrome due to excessive plasma infusion therapy. *Pediatric Nephrology*. 1989;3(4):420-423.

2. Irwin MI, Hegsted DM. A conspectus of research on protein requirements of man. *The Journal of Nutrition*. 1971;101(3):385429.

3. van der Zanden LD, van Kleef E, de Wijk RA, van Trijp HC. Knowledge, perceptions and preferences of elderly regarding protein-enriched functional food. *Appetite*. 2014;80:16-22.

4. Piccoli GB, Vigotti FN, Leone F, et al. Low-protein diets in CKD: how can we achieve them? A narrative, pragmatic review. *Clinical Kidney Journal*. 2015;8(1):61-70.

5. Walser M, Thorpe B. *Coping with kidney disease: A 12-step treatment program to help you avoid dialysis*. John Wiley & Sons; 2010.

6. Mitch WE, Remuzzi G. Diets for patients with chronic kidney disease, should we reconsider? *BMC Nephrology*. 2016;17(1):80.

7. Kusiak A, Dixon B, Shah S. Predicting survival time for kidney dialysis patients: a data mining approach. *Computers in Biology and Medicine*. 2005;35(4):311-327.

8. Wingen A-M, Fabian-Bach C, Schaefer F, Mehls O. Randomised multicentre study of a low-protein diet on the progression of chronic renal failure in children. *The Lancet*. 1997;349(9059):11171123.

9. Bamgbola FO, Kaskel FJ. Uremic malnutrition-inflammation syndrome in chronic renal disease: a pathobiologic entity. *Journal of Renal Nutrition*. 2003;13(4):250-258.

10. Pupim LB, Caglar K, Hakim RM, Shyr Y, Ikizler TA. Uremic malnutrition is a predictor of death independent of inflammatory status. *Kidney International*. 2004;66(5):2054-2060.

11. Golper TA. Incremental dialysis: review of recent literature. *Current Opinion in Nephrology and Hypertension*. 2017;26(6):543-547.

12. Obi Y, Streja E, Rhee CM, et al. Incremental hemodialysis, residual kidney function, and mortality risk in incident dialysis patients: a cohort study. *American Journal of Kidney Diseases*. 2016;68(2):256-265.

13. Sun L, Ranawana DV, Leow MK-S, Henry CJ. Effect of chicken, fat and vegetable on glycaemia and insulinaemia to a white rice-based meal in healthy adults. *European Journal of Nutrition*. 2014;53(8):1719-1726.

14. Garneata L, Mircescu G. Nutritional intervention in uremia—myth or reality? *Journal of Renal Nutrition*. 2010;20(5):S31-S34.

15. Mircescu G, Gârneaţă L, Stancu SH, Căpuşă C. Effects of a supplemented hypoproteic diet in chronic kidney disease. *Journal of Renal Nutrition*. 2007;17(3):179-188.

16. Brunori G, Viola BF, Maiorca P, Cancarini G. How to manage elderly patients with chronic renal failure: conservative management versus dialysis. *Blood Purification*. 2008;26(1):36-40.

CHAPTER 10

Oxidative Stress and Free Radicals

Most of us have probably heard of antioxidants and free radicals, so the following definition, published in a resource from Rice University,[1] may be familiar:

> Free radicals are atoms or groups of atoms with an odd (unpaired) number of electrons and can be formed when oxygen interacts with certain molecules. Once formed these highly reactive radicals can start a chain reaction, like dominoes. Their chief danger comes from the damage they can do when they react with important cellular components such as DNA, or the cell membrane. Cells may function poorly or die if this occurs. To prevent free radical damage the body has a defense system of *antioxidants.*

> Antioxidants are molecules which can safely interact with free radicals and terminate the chain reaction before vital molecules are damaged. Although there are several enzyme systems within the body that scavenge free radicals, the principle micronutrient (vitamin) antioxidants are vitamin E, beta-carotene, and vitamin C. Additionally, selenium, a trace metal that is required for proper function of one of the body's antioxidant enzyme systems, is sometimes included in this category. The body cannot manufacture these micronutrients so they must be supplied in the diet.

When we look at studies[2-4] for healthy people, we can see that antioxidant intake is correlated with heart disease and diabetes risk. The higher the antioxidant intake, the lower the risk. Lester Packer, Ph.D., at the University of California at Berkeley, wrote in his book *The Antioxidant Miracle:*

> Scientists now believe that free radicals are causal factors in nearly every known disease, from heart disease to arthritis to cancer and cataracts to the aging process itself. Free radicals can interfere with the biological components of our healthy cells and literally dismantle the body's essential cellular proteins, fatty cell membranes, and DNA.[5]

This may be one of the reasons kidney disease can cause accelerated aging. Oxidative stress, which is an imbalance between the production of damaging free radicals and the ability of the body to neutralize their ill effects with antioxidants, is much higher in people with kidney disease than the average person, and it accelerates a decline in kidney function. Increased oxidative stress may also be the reason for accelerated heart disease in people with kidney disease. Kidney disease reduces antioxidant capacity and increases oxidant activity. This dysfunction increases as kidney disease progresses. Inflammation, which is also present in CKD, further amplifies the oxidant generation process. This dysfunction also impairs amino acid metabolism.

The bottom line is when our bodies are not functioning properly, oxidative damage increases.

One of the major causes of free radicals is the digestion process. As we digest foods, free radicals are produced as a by-product of breaking down and digesting foods. When we eat foods that contribute only to creating free radicals and not to our antioxidant capacity, we end up in oxidative debt or oxidative stress. When free radicals outnumber antioxidants in our bodies, oxidative damage ensues and continues until antioxidants outnumber free radicals. Oxidative damage accumulates over time and has been implicated in aging, and age-dependent diseases such as cardiovascular disease, cancer, neurodegenerative disorders, and kidney disease.

I wanted to see this proof of the relationship between oxidative stress and kidney disease progression for myself:

Study 10.1 **Chronic Kidney Disease Influences Multiple Systems: Describing the Relationship between Oxidative Stress, Inflammation, Kidney Damage, and Concomitant Disease.[6]**

CKD is characterized by differing levels of oxidative stress[7] and inflammation,[7,8] as well as varying levels of risk in regard to the development of comorbidities such as type 2 diabetes[9] and CVD.[10]

Oxidative stress[7] and inflammation[8] influence the development and subsequent progression of CKD. Moreover, oxidative stress and inflammation are the primary reasons why CKD is often accompanied by comorbidities such as type 2 diabetes[11] and CVD.[12] Due to the potentially self exacerbating and cyclical nature of oxidative stress and inflammation, diseases characterized by these two risk factors (diseases such as CKD, type 2 diabetes, and CVD) are necessarily intertwined in that the progression of one disease may lead to the development or progression of another.

Study 10.2 **Oxidative stress in chronic kidney disease.[13]**

Structural characteristics in CKD, loss of renal energy, and uremia result in an imbalance between free radical production and antioxidant defenses. Also, CKD patients usually have multiple cardiovascular risk factors like diabetes mellitus, dyslipidemia, and hypertension. These conditions are associated with oxidative stress, which can trigger the inflammatory process and accelerate renal injury progression.

Study 10.3 **Oxidative stress and autophagy: crucial modulators of kidney injury.[14]**

Both acute kidney injury (AKI) and chronic kidney disease (CKD) that lead to diminished kidney function are interdependent risk factors for increased mortality. If untreated over time, end stage renal disease (ESRD) is an inevitable outcome. Acute and chronic kidney diseases occur partly due to an imbalance between the molecular mechanisms that govern oxidative stress, inflammation, autophagy and cell death. Oxidative stress refers to the cumulative effects of highly reactive oxidizing molecules that cause cellular damage.

Study 10.4 **What we know about oxidative stress in patients with chronic kidney disease on dialysis—clinical effects, potential treatment, and prevention.[15]**

Patients with chronic kidney disease (CKD) experience accelerated atherosclerosis leading to excessive cardiovascular death. This cannot be fully explained by traditional cardiovascular risk factors. Oxidative stress is currently receiving attention as an important pathogenetic mediator of tissue damage. Oxidative stress is highly prevalent in patients with CKD. Increased pro-oxidant activity (age, diabetes, hypertension, inflammation, incompatibility of dialysis membranes, and solutions) goes together with reduced antioxidant defense (reduced activity of the glutathione system, low levels of vitamin E, C). Oxidative stress has been linked to several surrogate markers of atherosclerosis in patients with CKD, such as endothelial dysfunction and intima-media thickness.

Study 10.5 **Oxidative stress in end-stage renal disease: an emerging threat to patient outcome.**[16]

ESRD patients are subjected to enhanced oxidative stress, as a result of reduced antioxidant systems (vitamin C and selenium deficiency, reduced intracellular levels of vitamin E, reduced activity of the glutathione system) and increased pro-oxidant activity (advanced age, high frequency of diabetes, chronic inflammatory state, uraemic syndrome, bio-incompatibility of dialysis membranes and solutions). Oxidative stress and inflammation are deeply interrelated, as different oxidant free radicals are generated by phagocytic cells in response to inflammatory stimuli: both are related to endothelial dysfunction, as the endothelium is a source and a target of oxidants and participates in the inflammatory response. There is growing evidence, from experimental and clinical studies, that oxidative stress may be implicated in the pathogenesis of atherosclerosis and other complications of ESRD, namely dialysis-related amyloidosis, malnutrition, and anemia.

Study 10.6 **Oxidative stress and inflammation, a link between chronic kidney disease and cardiovascular disease.**[17]

Renal disease is associated with a graded increase in oxidative stress markers even in early CKD. This could be the consequence of an increase in reactive oxygen species as well as a decrease in antioxidant defense. This oxidative stress can accelerate renal injury progression. Inflammatory markers such as C reactive protein and cytokines increase with renal function deterioration suggesting that CKD is a low-grade inflammatory process. In fact, inflammation facilitates renal function deterioration. Several factors can be involved in triggering the inflammatory process, including oxidative stress.

For further proof, we can check to see if antioxidant consumption is renoprotective or slows any decline in kidney function:

Study 10.7 **Associations of proanthocyanidin intake with renal function and clinical outcomes in elderly women**[18]

Note: Proanthocyanidins are a class of polyphenols found in a variety of fruits and veggies.

RESULTS:

Compared to participants with low consumption, participants in the highest tertile of proanthocyanidin intake had a 9% lower cystatin C concentration (P<0.001). High proanthocyanidin consumers were at 50% lower risk of moderate chronic kidney insufficiency, and 65% lower risk of experiencing a 5-year renal disease event (P<0.05). These relationships remained significant following adjustment for renal disease risk factors and diet-related potential confounders.

CONCLUSION:

Increased consumption of proanthocyanidins was associated with better renal function and substantially reduced renal associated events, which has been supported by mechanistic and animal model data. Proanthocyanidin intake should be further examined as a dietary contributor to better renal health.

Study 10.8 Anthocyanin/polyphenolic-rich fruit juice reduces oxidative cell damage in an intervention study with patients on hemodialysis.[19]

Hemodialysis patients face an elevated risk of cancer, arteriosclerosis, and other diseases, ascribed in part to increased oxidative stress. Red fruit juice with high anthocyanin/polyphenol content had been shown to reduce oxidative damage in healthy probands. To test its preventive potential in hemodialysis patients, 21 subjects in a pilot intervention study consumed 200 mL/day of red fruit juice (3-week run-in; 4-week juice uptake; 3-week wash-out). Weekly blood sampling was done to monitor DNA damage (comet assay +/- formamidopyrimidine-DNA glycosylase enzyme), glutathione, malondialdehyde, protein carbonyls, trolox equivalent antioxidant capacity, triglycerides, and DNA binding capacity of the transcription factor nuclear factor-kappaB. Results show a significant decrease of DNA oxidation damage (P < 0.0001), protein and lipid peroxidation (P < 0.0001 and P < 0.001, respectively), and nuclear factor-kappaB binding activity (P < 0.01), and an increase of glutathione level and status (both P < 0.0001) during juice uptake. We attribute this reduction in oxidative (cell) damage in hemodialysis patients to the especially high anthocyanin/polyphenol content of the juice. This provides promising perspectives into the prevention of chronic diseases such as cancer and cardiovascular disease in population subgroups exposed to enhanced oxidative stress in hemodialysis patients.

From these studies, we can see that certain antioxidants may be more protective of our kidneys than others. A 50% lower risk of renal insufficiency, as was demonstrated in the first of the two studies above, is a staggering number, especially when you consider that modern drugs do not come close to this kind of protection.

While we can say with certainty that we need high levels of antioxidants in our bodies, how much is enough? Can we get too much? Dietary Oxygen Radical Absorbency Capacity (ORAC) is a measurement of the antioxidant level or capacity of a food. ORAC has its critics and is likely not a perfect measurement of antioxidant capacity. However, ORAC information is freely available and has not been replaced by anything better at this writing, so we will use ORAC for antioxidant capacity when it comes to diets.[20]

The following two graphs give us some clues about what the ideal ORAC intake levels might be.

FIGURE 10.1: **Influence of Dietary ORAC Intake for Diastolic and Systolic Blood Pressure**

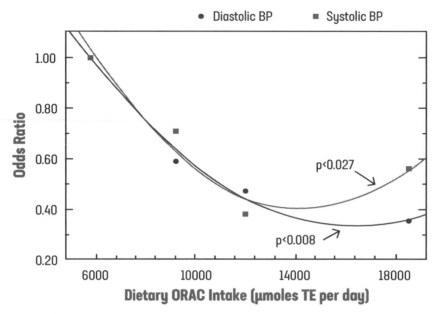

Influence of dietary ORAC (peroxyl radical) intake (μmol TE per day) on multivariate odds ratios across quartiles for diastolic (>140 mm Hg) and systolic (>90 mm Hg) blood pressure. Further adjustment for energy, protein and sodium intakes did not change the results materially. *Adapted from Farvid et al. (2013)*

FIGURE 10.2: **ORAC Intake and Risk of Stroke or Myocardial Infarction**

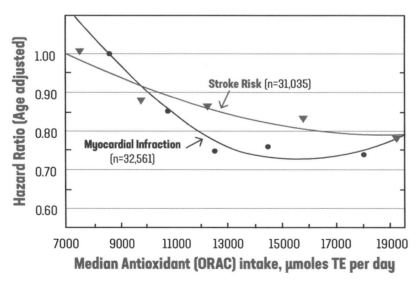

Median antioxidant (ORAC) intake (μmol Trolox Equivalent per day) and risk for stroke or myocardial infarction in Swedish mammography cohort (*n*=31,035-31,561 subjects. *Adapted from Rautianinen et al. (2021a; 2012b)*

We can see in both studies that a sweet spot of ORAC intake for healthy adults is between 15,000 and 17,000 (much higher than the traditional recommendation of 5,000 to 10,000 ORAC) a day. The benefits start to decline beyond this point. Again, these results are for healthy adults whose kidneys are working properly. For us, the number may need to be higher.

Ideal ORAC to Avoid Oxidative Stress

The aftereffect of eating a meal is called postprandial oxidative stress. Every time you eat, free radicals are created from digesting food. Based on a 2,000-calorie diet, a healthy person needs 9,000 to 10,000 ORAC just to offset the oxidative stress from eating three meals a day. As calorie intake increases, so do the ORAC required to offset the calories. The more calories you eat, the higher the potential for oxidative stress. We can think of 10,000 ORAC units or just ORAC as the breakeven point, so to speak. This matches with the recommended daily intake. We can see from the other studies that 10,000 ORAC is the starting point for real drops in heart attack and stroke risk. Once again, moderation kills. On top of that 10,000, my experience is we need more, likely another 5,000 to 7,000, to get ahead and have a surplus of antioxidants on call ready to take on bad guys.

Again, this is for healthy people. Just like our kidney function would ideally have excess capacity, the same is true for antioxidants. What we don't know is how much higher oxidative stress is in people with kidney disease. We just know it starts higher and very likely increases as your kidney function declines. Since no studies have quantified this number, we have to guess what our minimum antioxidant intake needs to be.

I was eating 40,000 to 50,000 ORAC units a day on one diet I tried. Based on the studies above, this may be a little too much. It is also very hard to do using real food. We don't know what the upper limit is or should be. Some studies indicate you can consume too many antioxidants, but these studies are related to supplements and pills, not real food. I don't think you can eat too many apples or blueberries in a day. You can, however, take too many pills. (More on this in Chapter 26.)

If the average healthy adult needs 15,000 to 17,000 ORAC units, then we can safely assume we need more. I personally feel that a good number for us is 30,000 plus per day as cooking reduces ORAC by some amount. This gives us an extra 10,000+ units a day to help deal with increased free radicals. You don't have to buy supplements or exotic foods to hit these numbers. You can get 30,000 from your local grocery store, which is a big plus. However, we can't eat just any foods to hit this level. It does take some planning. I want to be clear, this is an educated guess on my part. I could find no studies stating the correct antioxidant intake for people with kidney disease.

Next, I wanted to find an ideal daily amount of antioxidants and to understand how they affect us. Smokers, like people with kidney disease, have increased oxidative stress. Researchers studied what happens when smokers change to a higher antioxidant diet.[21] They found that a high-antioxidant diet changed the gene expression, or the signals that cells send to each other. Remember, in autoimmune diseases, our bodies send signals to attack our kidneys. Maybe changing the signals that we send cell-to-cell makes a difference. In the study, subjects ate either a diet heavy in various antioxidant-rich foods, a kiwifruit diet (three kiwifruits per day added to the regular diet), or a standard diet (the control group).

Here are the genes that were significantly regulated in the kiwifruit group when compared to controls:

Probe ID	Z-Score	Gene Symbol	Gene Title
204810_s_at	-3.3	CKM	Creatine kinase muscle
217034_at	-4.2	NTN3	Immunoglobulin-κ light chain variable region (IGKV gene), clone 25
221299_at	-3.9	GPR173	G protein-coupled receptor 173
1553633_s_at	4.3	NHEDC1	Na+/H+ exchanger domain containing 1
1557944_s_at	3.8	CTNND1	Catenin (cadherin-associated protein) -δ1

Five genes were affected by adding three kiwifruit a day to a regular diet. However, when a wide variety of antioxidants and higher amounts were consumed, more genes were affected. Don't worry about what the genes do here, just look at the numbers.

Here are the genes that were significantly upregulated (positive z-score) and downregulated (negative z-score) in the antioxidant-rich diet group when compared to controls:

Probe ID	Z-Score	Gene Symbol	Gene Title
208526_at	-4.4	OR2F1	Olfactory receptor, family 2, subfamily F, member 1
221444_at	-4.1	TAS2R16	Taste receptor, type 2, member 16
1559244_at	-4.0	FMN2	Formin 2
1553706_at	-4.0	HTRA4	HtrA serine peptidase 4
1553652_a_at	-3.8	C18orf54	Chromosome 18 open reading frame 54
1559270_at	-3.6	ZFHX4	Zinc finger homeobox 4
227401_at	-3.5	IL17D	Interleukin 17D
206644_at	-3.4	NROB1	Nuclear receptor subfamily 0, group B, member 1
229731_at	-3.3	FOXS1	Forkhead box S1
233897_at	-3.3	FEZF2	FEZ family zinc finger 2
233305_at	-3.3	NECAB1	N-terminal EF-hand calcium binding protein 1
213855_s_at	-3.2	LIPE	Lipase, hormone-sensitive
207817_at	-3.1	IFNW1	Interferon, omega 1

Probe ID	Z- Score	Gene Symbol	Gene Title
203059_s_at	-3.1	PAPSS2	3'-phosphoadenosine 5'-phosphosulfate synthase 2
205893_at	-2.9	NLGN1	Neuroligin 1
222041_at	-2.8	DPH1	DPH1 homolog (Saccharomyces cerevisiae)/// candidate tumor suppressor in ovarian cancer 2
215430_at	-2.8	GK2	Glycerol kinase 2
202855_s_at	6.6	SLC16A3	Solute carrier family 16, member 3 (monocarboxylic acid transporter 4)
202856_s_at	4.0	SLC16A3	Solute carrier family 16, member 3 (monocarboxylic acid transporter 4)
218505_at	3.7	WDR59	WD repeat domain 59
34726_at	3.5	CACNB3	Calcium channel, voltage-dependent, beta 3 subunit
211079_s_at	3.4	DYRK1A	Dual-specificity tyrosine-(Y)phosphorylation regulated kinase 1A
57163_at	3.1	ELOVL1	Elongation of very long-chain fatty acids (FEN1/Elo2, SUR4/Elo3, yeast)-like 1
225466_at	3.1	PATL1	Protein associated with topoisomerase II homolog 1 (yeast)
1569701_at	3.0	PER3	CDNA FLJ58931 complete cds, highly similar to Period circadian protein 3

I want to make a few points here:

Again, you don't need to understand the terms, but I wanted to emphasize how big the difference is between small and large doses of antioxidants, and the difference one type of fruit can make. Just look at the long list of genes affected by the antioxidant-rich diet.

The kiwi fruit diet regulated different genes than the high antioxidant diet. Not one of the regulated genes is the same. We need to eat a broad variety of antioxidants. Evidence also exists to suggest that a more diverse diet leads to increased gut flora diversity and health.

This study demonstrates that diet changes how our cells talk to each other. We can turn up the good and turn down the bad through diet. Crosstalk starts here at the most basic level, our genes. A few of these genes in particular need to be mentioned. Interleukin 17 is pro-inflammatory and was downregulated (that's good). HtrA proteins have been implicated in arthritis, tumor suppression, apoptosis, aging, and Parkinson's disease. It was also downregulated by the high-antioxidant diet.

Incidentally, eating any kind of food, not just antioxidants, can regulate gene expression. In animal models comparing milk, meat, and soy, the proteins were found to up- or downregulate different genes. Soy upregulated a gene that helps you burn fat for energy. Amino acid metabolism was also different for each protein.

In many ways, eating may be similar to giving instructions to your body. We can tell our bodies to crank up cholesterol or ask to crank it down. I think this is a very important concept. Genes are made up of DNA. Foods can tell the most basic building blocks of life what to do. Don't forget this!

The science regarding how diet affects our DNA and gene expression is still in its infancy. However, we can already see that what we eat not only provides nutrition but also tells our cells how to act and communicate with other cells.

Timing is Everything

When we eat antioxidants, most pass through our systems quickly. We can see that the antioxidant effect is lost after a few hours. This is important because it tells us we must constantly eat antioxidants—ideally with each meal—to offset the oxidative stress and post-meal oxidative stress. Assume we eat a high-antioxidant breakfast, but a not-so-great lunch. The antioxidants from breakfast may not be around to fight the bad guys from lunch. This means our bodies will have to dip into the antioxidant stores. Over time, these can become depleted as we use up more antioxidants than we eat.

Eating antioxidants with a meal lowers oxidative stress for several hours after a meal. Eating a bowl of berries with a meal reduces or eliminates post-meal oxidative stress:

| Study 10.9 | Plasma antioxidant capacity changes following a meal as a measure of the ability of a food to alter in vivo antioxidant status.[22] |

We have demonstrated that consumption of certain berries and fruits such as blueberries, mixed grapes, and kiwifruit, was associated with increased plasma AOC in the postprandial state and consumption of an energy source of macronutrients containing no antioxidants was associated with a decline in plasma AOC. However, without further long term clinical studies, one cannot necessarily translate increased plasma AOC into a potential decreased risk of chronic degenerative disease. Preliminary estimates of antioxidant needs based on energy intake were developed. Consumption of high-antioxidant foods with each meal is recommended in order to prevent periods of postprandial oxidative stress.

A list of high-antioxidant foods that are appropriate for people with kidney disease may look different than a high-antioxidant food list for healthy patients because we have to worry about issues like potassium and protein. We need to take into account all of the restrictions we have to deal with. Below is a table to give you an idea of the different antioxidants available in different foods.

TABLE 10.1: **Statistical Descriptives of the Antioxidant Food Table and Individual Categories**[23]

Antioxidant content in mmol/100g			
Name	**Average**	**Min**	**Max**
Plant based foods (a)	1943	0	2897.11
Animal based foods (b)	211	0	1
Mixed foods (c)	854	0	18.52
Categories			
1. Berries and berry products	119	0.06	261.53
2. Beverages	283	0	1347.83
3. Breakfast cereals	90	0.16	4.84
4. Chocolates and sweets	80	0.05	14.98
5. Dairy products	86	0	0.78
6. Desserts and cakes	134	0	4.1
7. Egg	12	0	0.16
8. Fats and oils	38	0.19	1.66
9. Fish and seafood	32	0.03	0.65
10. Fruit and fruit juices	278	0.03	55.52
11. Grains and grain products	227	0	3.31
12. Herbal/traditional plant medicine	59	0.28	2897.11
13. Infant foods and beverages	52	0.02	18.52
14. Legumes	69	0	1.97
15. Meat and meat products	31	0	0.85
16. Miscellaneous ingredients, condiments	44	0	15.54
17. Mixed food entrees	189	0.03	0.73
18. Nuts and seeds	90	0.03	33.29
19. Poultry and poultry products	50	0.05	1
20. Snacks, biscuits	66	0	1.17
21. Soups, sauces, gravies, dressing	251	0	4.67
22. Spices and herbs	425	0.08	465.32
23. Vegetables and vegetable products	303	0	48.07
24. Vitamins and dietary supplements	131	0	1052.44

A Word About Supplements

Before leaving the topic of antioxidants, a little education is in order on why real foods are better than supplements 99% of the time. When we eat fruit, like an apple, we get all of the antioxidants, fiber, vitamins, minerals, and so on. When we take a supplement, we get just the one on the label. Science has shown that isolating individual antioxidants is not as effective as getting a full range of antioxidants. A synergistic effect occurs when eating a large variety of antioxidants vs. taking a few pills of isolated compounds.

In addition, superfoods, aka high antioxidant foods, are expensive and may not be so super. A good example is acai berries. Dried acai berries are hailed as a superfood with an ORAC rating of 102,700, which is off the charts. However, actual human studies show that apples with an ORAC of 4,275 have a same or similar increase in antioxidant values measured in the bloodstream.[24] Save your money and don't spend it on antioxidant supplements unless they are proven.

Another reason to be careful is the dosage. Many times the dosage of a so-called superfood will be much higher than the amount any real person could eat in a day. One study on acai berries would require you to drink 400 glasses of berry pulp a day to see positive effects. Again, save your money. All that glitters is not gold.

Summary

No data suggests eating a diet low in antioxidants is good for us. Eating meals of empty calories with no or little antioxidants accelerates our disease and is detrimental to overall health.

All available evidence suggests a low-antioxidant diet increases the speed of kidney and heart disease.

High antioxidant consumption is another black-and-white issue for us. The evidence is overwhelming for a high-antioxidant diet for people with kidney disease. We can say that a diverse and high-antioxidant diet most likely protects our kidneys as long as it is low-protein and low-acid.

I will say it again, kidney diets focused on salt, potassium, and phosphorus are just managing symptoms, not helping us slow disease progression. Any advice that does not focus on increasing antioxidant consumption is 1950s diet advice.

References

1. Honig C. Antioxidants and Free radicals. 1996; http://www.rice. edu/~jenky/sports/antiox. html. Accessed 2nd June, 2017.

2. Hajhashemi V, Vaseghi G, Pourfarzam M, Abdollahi A. Are antioxidants helpful for disease prevention? *Research in Pharmaceutical Sciences.* 2010;5(1):1.

3. Hertog MG, Feskens EJ, Kromhout D, Hollman P, Katan M. Dietary antioxidant flavonoids and risk of coronary heart disease: the Zutphen Elderly Study. *The Lancet.* 1993;342(8878):1007-1011.

4. Montonen J, Knekt P, Järvinen R, Reunanen A. Dietary antioxidant intake and risk of type 2 diabetes. *Diabetes Care.* 2004;27(7):1845-1846.

5. Packer L, Colman C. *The Antioxidant Miracle: Your Complete Plan for Total Health and Healing.* Wiley; 1999.

6. Tucker PS, Scanlan AT, Dalbo VJ. Chronic kidney disease influences multiple systems: describing the relationship between oxidative stress, inflammation, kidney damage, and concomitant disease. *Oxidative Medicine and Cellular Longevity.* 2015;2015:1-8.

7. Dounousi E, Papavasiliou E, Makedou A, et al. Oxidative stress is progressively enhanced with advancing stages of CKD. *American Journal of Kidney Diseases.* 2006;48(5):752-760.

8. Oberg BP, McMenamin E, Lucas F, et al. Increased prevalence of oxidant stress and inflammation in patients with moderate to severe chronic kidney disease. *Kidney International.* 2004;65(3):1009-1016.

9. Ha H, Lee HB. Reactive oxygen species as glucose signaling molecules in mesangial cells cultured under high glucose. *Kidney International.* 2000;58(Supplement 77):S19-S25.

10. Go AS, Chertow GM, Fan D, McCulloch CE, Hsu C-y. Chronic kidney disease and the risks of death, cardiovascular events, and hospitalization. *New England Journal of Medicine.* 2004;351(13):1296-1305.

11. Drews G, Krippeit-Drews P, Düfer M. Oxidative stress and beta-cell dysfunction. *Pflügers Archiv-European Journal of Physiology.* 2010;460(4):703-718.

12. Cottone S, Lorito MC, Riccobene R, et al. Oxidative stress, inflammation and cardiovascular disease in chronic renal failure. *Journal of Nephrology.* 2008;21(2):175-179.

13. Modaresi A, Nafar M, Sahraei Z. Oxidative stress in chronic kidney disease. *Iranian Journal of Kidney Diseases.* 2015;9(3):165-179.

14. Sureshbabu A, Ryter SW, Choi ME. Oxidative stress and autophagy: crucial modulators of kidney injury. *Redox Biology.* 2015;4:208-214.

15. Del Vecchio L, Locatelli F, Carini M. What we know about oxidative stress in patients with chronic kidney disease on dialysis—clinical effects, potential treatment, and prevention. *Seminars in Dialysis.* 2011;24(1):56-64.

16. Locatelli F, Canaud B, Eckardt KU, Stenvinkel P, Wanner C, Zoccali C. Oxidative stress in end-stage renal disease: an emerging threat to patient outcome. *Nephrology Dialysis Transplantation.* 2003;18(7):1272-1280.

17. Cachofeiro V, Goicochea M, De Vinuesa SG, Oubiña P, Lahera V, Luño J. Oxidative stress and inflammation, a link between chronic kidney disease and cardiovascular disease. *Kidney International.* 2008;74:S4-S9.

18. Ivey KL, Lewis JR, Lim WH, Lim EM, Hodgson JM, Prince RL. Associations of proanthocyanidin intake with renal function and clinical outcomes in elderly women. *PloS One.* 2013;8(8):e71166.

19. Spormann TM, Albert FW, Rath T, et al. Anthocyanin/ polyphenolic–rich fruit juice reduces oxidative cell damage in an intervention study with patients on hemodialysis. *Cancer Epidemiology and Prevention Biomarkers.* 2008;17(12):3372-3380.

20. Prior RL. Oxygen radical absorbance capacity (ORAC): New horizons in relating dietary antioxidants/bioactives and health benefits. *Journal of Functional Foods.* 2015;18:797-810.

21. Bøhn SK, Myhrstad MC, Thoresen M, et al. Blood cell gene expression associated with cellular stress defense is modulated by antioxidant-rich food in a randomized controlled clinical trial of male smokers. *BMC Medicine.* 2010;8(54):1-15.

22. Prior RL, Gu L, Wu X, et al. Plasma antioxidant capacity changes following a meal as a measure of the ability of a food to alter in vivo antioxidant status. *Journal of the American College of Nutrition.* 2007;26(2):170-181.

23. Carlsen MH, Halvorsen BL, Holte K, et al. The total antioxidant content of more than 3100 foods, beverages, spices, herbs and supplements used worldwide. *Nutrition Journal.* 2010;9(3):1-11.

24. Pastoriza S, Mesías M, Cabrera C, Rufian-Henares J. Healthy properties of Green and White teas: an update. *Food & Function.* 2017.

CHAPTER 11

Metabolic Acidosis

Since I have already covered this subject in Chapter 4 (the chapter on renal acid load), this will be a short chapter.

Among several types of acidosis that exist, we are most worried about renal tubular acidosis.[1] Our kidneys cannot excrete enough acid in our urine to keep up with acid production in our bodies. Therefore, our compromised kidneys cannot keep up with the demand. Just as uremia is protein overload, acidosis is acid overload.

Although acidosis affects most of us, it is treatable in most cases. The traditional treatment is sodium bicarbonate, also called baking soda.[2] The downside of sodium bicarbonate is the sodium content; one teaspoon has approximately 1,259 mg of salt. This is why many doctors are hesitant to recommend sodium bicarbonate. This is especially true in the presence of edema or high blood pressure. Potassium citrate and sodium citrate are also used sometimes. Sodium bicarbonate pills have a lower amount of sodium, but you have to take several pills. If you have to take sodium bicarbonate, take the pill form that is measured in grains, not the kind from the store. They are the same except for a lower salt content in the pills. Amazon has several brands.

A blood gas test is used to test for acidosis. This test will determine your blood's pH and the amount of bicarbonate in your blood.[3] Normal pH usually ranges from 7.38 to 7.42, and bicarbonate falls within the range of 22 to 28 mmol/L. Although pH 7 is considered a neutral pH, our bodies prefer a slightly alkaline environment of 7.4. If your pH is below 7.35 and bicarbonate levels are in the low range of 22-25 mmol/L, you may be diagnosed with acidosis. In such conditions, when your pH and bicarbonate levels fall in the lower range than normal, you must pay attention.

On the other hand, bicarbonate levels can also be too high. Metabolic alkalosis is the term for bicarbonate levels higher than normal. This is very rare in people with kidney disease. I mention it here because high bicarbonate levels also contribute to disease progression.

We know that untreated acidosis accelerates kidney disease progression. Plasma bicarbonate levels are correlated with mortality rates. The severity of acidosis is represented by the standards of plasma bicarbonate.

FIGURE 11.1: **Kaplan-Meier Survival Curve Based on Serum Bicarbonate Levels Among Chronic Kidney Disease Patients**

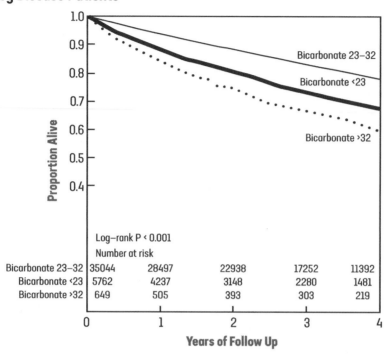

This chart is based on mortality rates of patients with stage 3 and 4 kidney disease. Bicarbonate levels above and below the normal range contribute to mortality rates for people with kidney disease.[4]

The following summary is a reasonable explanation of what happens to us:

Study 11.1   **Reducing the Dietary Acid Load: How a More Alkaline Diet Benefits Patients with Chronic Kidney Disease.[5]**

ABSTRACT:

It has been proposed that a low-protein diet will slow progression of chronic kidney disease although studies have not always supported this belief. The accepted practice is that 60% to 70% of protein comes from high biological value (HBV) protein, but this limits patient choice and patients struggle to follow the diet. When a diet with only 30% HBV protein was trialed, there was a significant increase in serum bicarbonate, and patients preferred the diet. The dietary advice given in predialysis clinics was changed. HBV protein was restricted to approximately 50% of total protein, bread and cereal foods were allowed freely, and fruits and vegetables (F&V) were encouraged. Patients who followed the diet have seen a slowing of progression and occasionally regression of their renal function. Both observations and scientific literature indicate that this is because of a reduction in the acid content of the diet. <u>When foods are metabolized, most proteins produce acid, and most F&V produce alkali.</u> A typical 21st-century diet produces 50 to 100 mEq H$^+$ per day which the kidney is challenged to excrete. Acid is excreted with phosphate and is lim-ited to about 45 mEq H$^+$ per day. With chronic kidney disease, this falls progressively to below 20 mEq H$^+$ per day. Historically, ammonium excretion was believed to be excretion of acid (NH$_3^+$ + H$^+$ → NH$_4^+$), but it is now understood to be a byproduct in the neutralization of acid by glutamine. The remaining acid is neutralized or stored within the body. Bone and muscle are lost in order to neutralize the acid. Acid also accumulates within cells, and serum bicarbonate falls. <u>The author postulates that reducing the acid load through a low-protein diet with greater use of vegetable proteins and increased F&V intake will slow progression or occasionally improve renal function while maintaining the nutritional status of the individual.</u>

Note: See how our ability to excrete acid dropped from 45 to 20 with kidney disease. This is a drop of over 50% in our ability to deal with acid and ammonia. If we don't decrease acid intake by 50%, then we get acidosis. This is another reminder that we have to do the workload for our kidneys.

Again, we correlate protein intake with renal acid load. As I keep saying, everything in kidney disease is related. Acidosis is related to the severity of albuminuria. The lower the bicarbonate levels, the greater the loss of protein in our urine.

Study 11.2 — Association between serum bicarbonate levels and albuminuria in stage 3 and stage 4 chronic kidney disease: a cross-sectional study.[6]

CONCLUSIONS:

<u>Low serum bicarbonate levels were associated with significant albuminuria, even at levels in the normal range, in CKD patients, especially with stage 3 disease.</u>

Note: Another reason we have to treat kidney disease early.

A summary of current bicarbonate studies.

Study 11.3 — Short- and long-term effects of alkali therapy in chronic kidney disease: a systematic review.[7]

CONCLUSIONS:

<u>Alkali therapy is associated with an improvement in kidney function, which may afford a long-term benefit in slowing the progression of CKD. However, differences in study protocols and small sample sizes preclude definitive conclusions.</u>

The last line in this study deserves some attention. The last three words, "precludes definitive conclusions," explicitly showcase that, like every issue in this book, it has not been researched perfectly. We have to look at the weight of the evidence. We also have to consider the risks and rewards of making a decision based on this incomplete, imperfect, and even inconclusive evidence.

This scenario applies to almost every subject in this book. I will use acidosis as an example. The weight of the evidence suggests that a high renal acid load or acidosis contributes to a decline in kidney function. We have checked both sides of the argument.

1. The weight of evidence suggests that low serum bicarbonate levels (aka acidosis) contributes to decline in kidney function.

2. The weight of evidence also suggests that bicarbonate therapy (treating acidosis) slows kidney disease progression.

3. No data can be found that states that treating acidosis leads us to take exceptional risks. Sodium bicarbonate is well tolerated and affordable. The pros and cons of additional salt intake must be considered.

4. It is better to consume natural bicarbonate foods like fruits and veggies than to take sodium bicarbonate, if you have a choice.

We have incomplete data based on dozens of studies, all pointing in the same direction. This is the nature of kidney disease research today. We must look into the gravity of the conclusions made in these studies and then evaluate pros and cons of treatment.

Diet

We don't need to worry about treatment methods if we adopt a diet high in alkaline foods (fruits and veggies) and low in renal acid load. Over time, we will build up our serum bicarbonate levels. We can see from a few studies that serum bicarbonate levels may continue to rise over two years with the right diet. Eating a kidney and heart-healthy diet will slowly allow your body to build up bicarbonate and lower the amount of acid your kidneys have to excrete.

The fact that your bicarbonate levels can rise consistently for over a year is also a reminder that we have to stay on these diets for a long time to get the full benefits.

One constant theme in this book is the importance of doing the work for your kidneys with the right diet choices. It's no different with acid load. Severe acidosis may require both appropriate diet and treatment with sodium bicarbonate. However, over time you should be able to reduce or stop the usage of sodium bicarbonate.

The bottom line is renal tubular acidosis is easily treatable through proper diet and/or an alkalizing agent like sodium bicarbonate. There is no reason for any of us to aid disease progression by not treating or managing acidosis. Putting our foot on the brake is not hard in this case.

For many of us, curing acidosis is as simple as eliminating high acid foods from our diet. It is that simple in many cases. It won't happen overnight, but eating alkaline foods will build your bicarbonate levels over time. Your bicarbonate levels can rise for years if you are eating the right diet.

Don't underestimate your power to cure acidosis.

Reread Predicted Renal Acid Load for more information.

References

1. Laing CM, Unwin RJ. Renal tubular acidosis. *Journal of Nephrology*. 2006;19:S46-52.

2. Szeto C-C, Wong TY-H, Chow K-M, Leung C-B, Li PK-T. Oral sodium bicarbonate for the treatment of metabolic acidosis in peritoneal dialysis patients: a randomized placebo-control trial. *Journal of the American Society of Nephrology*. 2003;14(8):21192126.

3. Burki NK. Arterial blood gas measurement. *Chest*. 1985;88(1):3-4.

4. Navaneethan SD, Schold JD, Arrigain S, et al. Serum bicarbonate and mortality in stage 3 and stage 4 chronic kidney disease. *Clinical Journal of the American Society of Nephrology*. 2011;6(10):2395-2402.

5. Passey C. Reducing the dietary acid load: How a more alkaline diet benefits patients with chronic kidney disease. *Journal of Renal Nutrition*. 2017;27(3):151-160.

6. Lee Y-J, Cho S, Kim SR. Association between serum bicarbonate levels and albuminuria in stage 3 and stage 4 chronic kidney disease: a cross-sectional study. *Clinical Nephrology*. 2014;81(6):405-410.

7. Susantitaphong P, Sewaralthahab K, Balk EM, Jaber BL, Madias NE. Short-and long-term effects of alkali therapy in chronic kidney disease: a systematic review. *American Journal of Nephrology*. 2012;35(6):540-547.

CHAPTER 12

High Blood Pressure

I am not going to spend a lot of time on this issue, as it is so well-known. Blood pressure is currently being treated in most people with kidney disease. The ways to reduce blood pressure are also well-known. However, less common issues like pulse pressure deserve some review.

We talked about ACE inhibitors and the benefits to people with kidney disease. ACE inhibitors have the effect of slowing kidney disease progression.

Blood pressure operates in a narrow range, like many things in our bodies.

Blood pressure is more likely to be too high, but it can be too low as well. A certain amount of pressure is needed to push the blood through the filters in our kidneys and avoid the normal side effects of low blood pressure like fainting and dizziness. Higher blood pressure equals more blood flow. Low blood pressure may result in your blood tests coming back a bit high because blood pressure is too low to force enough blood through the filters in your kidneys.[1]

When blood pressure is too high, we are forcing blood through the kidney filters at such high pressure that they are permanently damaged. Remember the colander/strainer example from Chapter 15. The kidney is a very vascular organ, and these tiny blood vessels are fragile.[2]

Understanding your blood pressure and keeping it under control is a part of life for everyone with kidney disease.

FIGURE 12.1: **A Graphic Explaining Blood Pressure Basics**

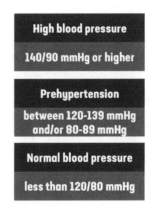

Normal Blood Pressure

The pressure of blood in the vessels when the heart beats: **systolic pressure**

The pressure between beats when the heart relaxes: **diastolic pressure**

less than
120/80 mmHg

millimeters of mercury

High blood pressure
140/90 mmHg or higher

Prehypertension
between 120-139 mmHg and/or 80-89 mmHg

Normal blood pressure
less than 120/80 mmHg

Another issue is pulse pressure (PP). Pulse pressure is the difference between systolic and diastolic numbers.

120/80 yields a pulse pressure of 40. 30 to 40 is the normal range for pulse pressure. If your pulse pressure is higher than 55 or 60, a doctor's visit is in order. Pulse pressure may be more accurate than traditional blood pressure for predicting kidney and heart disease progression.[3]

Study 12.1 — Pulse pressure and progression of chronic kidney disease.[4]

CONCLUSIONS:

Baseline PP was the only predictor of eGFR decline adjusted for age, baseline eGFR, diabetes, hemoglobin and use of angiotensin-converting enzyme inhibitors or angiotensin receptor blockers. PP >65 mm Hg was associated declining renal function (log rank chi-square; p<0.05). This study suggests that PP is a better predictor of adverse renal outcome, even in mild to moderate CKD, than DBP or even SBP.

Note: Pulse pressure greater than 65 was associated with declining kidney function.

Study 12.2 — Central Pulse Pressure in Chronic Kidney Disease—A Chronic Renal Insufficiency Cohort—Ancillary Study[5]

The low-resistance nature of the renal circulation predisposes the kidney to pressure-mediated damage. Brachial PP measures have been shown to predict both the development of CKD and the rate of loss of kidney function when CKD is already present. Knowledge of brachial PP is an imperfect predictor of CPPs, thus, measures of CPP may be useful in patients with CKD to quantify their risk of cardiovascular disease and CKD progression. The role of CPP in predicting progressive kidney function loss, as well as incident cardiovascular disease, in established mild-to-moderate CKD remains to be seen. Longitudinal data from CRIC and other studies pursuing the value of central blood pressure measures will clarify further this important issue.

Study 12.3 — Central Pulse Pressure and Aortic Stiffness Determine Renal Hemodynamics Pathophysiological Implication for Microalbuminuria in Hypertension[6]

Each 0.1 increase in renal RI (resistive index) was associated with a 5.4-fold increase in the adjusted relative risk of albuminuria. In conclusion, increased aortic pulse pressure causes renal microvascular damage through altered renal hemodynamics resulting from increased peripheral resistance and/or increased flow pulsation.

Note: The risk of albuminuria increased over 500% with each increase in resistance. Resistance requires our blood pressure to increase to compensate and may mean part of our kidneys are not able to get the required blood flow.

Pulse pressure is something we should all keep an eye on. The combination of blood pressure in excess of 130/80 and a high pulse pressure is a bad omen for us. The good news is that ACE inhibitors lower pulse pressure, and we can do several things to lower our blood pressure as well.

How important is keeping track of your blood pressure?

If you lower your blood pressure from 140/90 to 120/80, you will have:

> 38% lower relative risk of heart failure

> 43% lower relative risk of cardiovascular death

> 27% lower relative risk of mortality overall*
  *https://www.ncbi.nlm.nih.gov/pmc/articles/PMC4689591/

Lowering your blood pressure by 20 and 10 points, respectively, cuts your risk of heart attack by over 40%. Home blood pressure machines are available for reasonable prices. There's no excuse not to check your blood pressure frequently.

Study 12.4   Association Between More Intensive vs Less Intensive

Blood Pressure Lowering and Risk of Mortality in Chronic Kidney Disease Stages 3 to 5. A Systematic Review and Meta-analysis[7]

This study identified 30 RCTs that potentially met the inclusion criteria. The CKD subset mortality data were extracted in 18 trials, among which there were 1,293 deaths in 15,924 participants with CKD. The mean (SD) baseline systolic BP (SBP) was 148 (16) mm Hg in both the more intensive and less intensive arms. The mean SBP dropped by 16 mm Hg to 132 mm Hg in the more intensive arm and by 8 mm Hg to 140 mm Hg in the less intensive arm. More intensive vs less intensive BP control resulted in 14.0% lower risk of all-cause mortality (odds ratio, 0.86; 95% CI, 0.76-0.97; P = .01), a finding that was without significant heterogeneity and appeared consistent across multiple subgroups.

CONCLUSIONS AND RELEVANCE:

Randomization to more intensive BP control is associated with lower mortality risk among trial participants with hypertension and CKD. Further studies are required to define absolute BP targets for maximal benefit and minimal harm.

Note: Lowering blood pressure by eight points results in a 14% difference in mortality. This study suggests that staying on top of our blood pressure is mandatory.

Study 12.5   Effects of intensive blood pressure lowering on cardiovascular and renal outcomes: updated systematic review and meta-analysis.[8]

FINDINGS:

We identified 19 trials including 44,989 participants, in whom 2,496 major cardiovascular events were recorded during a mean 3.8 years of follow-up (range 1.0-8.4 years). Our meta-analysis showed that after randomization, patients in the more intensive blood pressure-lowering treatment group had mean blood pressure levels of 133/76 mm Hg, compared with 140/81 mm Hg in the less intensive treatment group. Intensive blood pressure-lowering treatment achieved RR reductions for major cardiovascular events (14% [95% CI 4-22]), myocardial infarction (13% [0-24]), stroke (22% [10-32]), albuminuria (10% [3-16]) and retinopathy progression (19% [0-34]). However, more intensive treatment had no clear effects on heart failure (15% [95% CI -11 to 34]), cardiovascular death (9% [-11 to 26]), total mortality (9% [-3 to 19]) or end-stage kidney disease (10% [-6 to 23]). The reduction in major cardiovascular events was consistent across patient groups, and additional blood pressure lowering had a clear benefit, even in patients with systolic blood pressure lower than 140 mm Hg. The absolute benefits were greatest in trials in which all enrolled patients had vascular disease, renal disease, or diabetes. Serious adverse events associated with blood pressure lowering were only reported by six trials and had an event rate of 1.2% per year in intensive blood pressure-lowering group participants, compared with 0·9% in the less intensive treatment group (RR 1/35 [95% CI 0.93-1.97]). Severe hypotension was more frequent in the more intensive treatment regimen (RR 2.68 [1.21-5.89], p=0.015), but the absolute excess was small (0.3% vs 0.1% per person-year for the duration of follow-up).

INTERPRETATION:

Intensive blood pressure lowering provided greater vascular protection than standard regimens. In high-risk patients, there are additional benefits from more intensive blood pressure lowering, including for those with systolic blood pressure below 140 mmHg. The net absolute benefits of intensive blood pressure lowering in high-risk individuals are large.

Study 12.6 **Blood pressure and chronic kidney disease progression in a multi-racial cohort: the Multi-Ethnic Study of Atherosclerosis.[9]**

ABSTRACT:

The relationship between blood pressure (BP) and kidney function among individuals with chronic kidney disease (CKD) remains controversial. This study evaluated the association between BP and estimated glomerular filtration rate (eGFR) decline among adults with nondiabetic stage 3 CKD. The Multi-Ethnic Study of Atherosclerosis participants with an eGFR 30-59 ml min (-1) per 1.73 m2 at baseline without diabetes were included. Participants were followed over a 5-year period. Kidney function change was determined by annualizing the change in eGFR using cystatin C, creatinine and a combined equation. Risk factors for progression of CKD (defined as a decrease in annualized eGFR>2.5 ml min (-1) per 1.73 m2) were identified using univariate analyses and sequential logistic regression models. There were 220 participants with stage 3 CKD at baseline using cystatin C, 483 participants using creatinine and 381 participants using the combined equation. The median (interquartile range) age of the sample was 74 (68-79) years. The incidence of progression of CKD was 16.8% using cystatin C and 8.9% using creatinine (P=0.002). Systolic BP>140 mm Hg or diastolic BP>90 mm Hg was significantly associated with progression using a cystatin C-based (odds ratio (OR), 2.49; 95% confidence interval (CI), 1.12-5.52) or the combined equation (OR, 2.07; 95% CI, 1.16-3.69), but not when using creatinine after adjustment for covariates. In conclusion, with the inclusion of cystatin C in the eGFR assessment hypertension was an important predictor of CKD progression in a multiethnic cohort with stage 3 CKD.

| Study 12.7 | Impact of visit-to-visit variability of blood pressure on deterioration of renal function in patients with non-diabetic chronic kidney disease.[10] |

ABSTRACT:

An association between visit-to-visit variability (VVV) of blood pressure (BP) and renal damage was recently reported in a cross-sectional study. We aimed to clarify the longitudinal effect of VVV of BP on deterioration of renal function in patients with non-diabetic chronic kidney disease (CKD). We retrospectively studied 56 patients with non-diabetic CKD (stage 3 or 4) who visited our nephrology clinic between September 1994 and May 2011. VVV of BP was defined as the standard deviation and coefficient of variation (CV) of office BP measured at 12 consecutive visits. Main outcomes were the annual decline in the estimated glomerular filtration rate (eGFR) and the composite renal end point defined as a doubling of serum creatinine or the need for dialysis. The median observation period was 83 months. Standard deviation and CV of office systolic BP (SBP) were significantly associated with the slope of the eGFR after adjustments for confounders. The adjusted risk for composite renal end points more than doubled for each increment of 1-standard deviation of the standard deviation of office SBP (hazard ratio (HR) 2.20, P=0.001), and for each increment of 1-standard deviation of the CV of office SBP (HR 2.12, P=0.002). The present study demonstrated that the visit-to-visit variability of BP is an independent determinant of deterioration of renal function in patients with non-diabetic CKD.

Note: This study shows that the stability of our blood pressure matters. If our blood pressure is going up and down all the time, our odds get worse.

The message for us is that a stable blood pressure of 120/80 or so, combined with a pulse pressure of less than 50, is where we want to be. As these numbers creep up, so does our risk of kidney and heart disease progression.

What Raises Our Blood Pressure

Most of the issues that raise blood pressure are well-known. Here are the most common:

1. Obesity

2. Smoking

3. Lack of exercise

4. Salt consumption

5. Alcohol consumption in excess of one drink a day

6. Aging

7. Family history

8. Kidney disease

Which Ones Can We Do Something About

> Obesity

> Smoking

> Exercise

> Salt intake

> Alcohol consumption: Limit alcohol to one drink per day

> Aging: Can't do much about this one, except try to age a little slower

> Family history: Can't do a thing, except be aware of it

> Kidney disease: If we have kidney disease, we have to manage it well

Five of the eight items can be managed with diet and exercise. One item (kidney disease) has to be managed aggressively, and two (aging and family history) are things we can't do anything about.

Kidneys are the major organs for fluid and electrolyte balance. If your kidneys are 100%, your body can handle excess salt. However, if your kidneys are functioning at 30%, that is a very different story. You have to help your kidneys maintain the right balance by diet. Most research doesn't apply to us. I have read new research that suggests that salt does not cause high blood pressure. Don't believe it for now. Stay with the salt restriction until we have more evidence. Salt also contributes to edema.

Study 12.8   **Altered dietary salt intake for people with chronic kidney disease.**[11]

AUTHORS' CONCLUSIONS:

We found a critical evidence gap in long-term effects of salt restriction in people with CKD that meant we were unable to determine the direct effects of sodium restriction on primary end-points such as mortality and progression to end-stage kidney disease (ESKD). We found that salt reduction in people with CKD reduced blood pressure considerably and consistently reduced proteinuria. If such reductions could be maintained long-term, this effect may translate to clinically significant reduc-tions in ESKD incidence and cardiovascular events. Research into the long-term effects of sodium-restricted diet for people with CKD is warranted, as is investigation into adherence to a low-salt diet.

The DASH diet is short for Dietary Approach to Stop Hypertension. The DASH diet has been very successful in reducing blood pressure. The diet is rich in fruits and vegetables, low or nonfat dairy, and lean meats, and is low in fat. The DASH diet is also low in sodium. A line of salt-free spices is available in most grocery stores under the "DASH" name.

Let's add up an example of what we can do to lower blood pressure in terms of points:

Activity	Points
Exercise (minimum of 35 minutes a day)	7.5
Salt restriction	5
Lose 9 pounds	4
Stop smoking	3.5
Reduce alcohol consumption	3.6
Total possible controllable reduction	23.6

A 23.6 reduction in systolic blood pressure is possible, depending on your current health and habits, without drugs. If you don't drink or smoke, and are not overweight, you can still reduce your blood pressure by 12.5 points.

ACE inhibitors reduce systolic blood pressure by an average of 11 points using a low dose. We can say that exercise and salt restriction are as effective as these drugs in managing high blood pressure.

People with kidney disease would do well to buy a home blood pressure monitor. Current models range from $15 to $100.

Checking your blood pressure once a week is a good habit. If you are struggling with high blood pressure, you should check it more often. Ideally, you should check your blood pressure first thing in the morning before eating or taking any medications. Pulse pressure is something else you should monitor.

Most of these machines have a memory feature that records your past tests. You can compare your current blood pressure with the past results very easily.

Aggressive blood pressure monitoring is associated with lower rates of heart attack and kidney disease progression. It takes less than five minutes. My current $30 blood pressure monitor is over six years old and still works well.

In summary, aggressive blood and pulse pressure monitoring and treatment yields big benefits for us over the long term. Blood pressure monitoring is relatively cheap, easy, and fast. The combination of diet, exercise, weight control, and drugs is usually enough to address even the worst cases of blood pressure.

References

1. Berglund G, Andersson O. Beta-blockers or diuretics in hypertension? A six-year follow-up of blood pressure and metabolic side effects. *The Lancet.* 1981;317(8223):744-747.

2. Zandi-Nejad K, Luyckx VA, Brenner BM. Adult hypertension and kidney disease. *Hypertension.* 2006;47(3):502-508.

3. Safar ME, Blacher J, Pannier B, et al. Central pulse pressure and mortality in end-stage renal disease. *Hypertension.* 2002;39(3):735-738.

4. Arulkumaran N, Diwakar R, Tahir Z, Mohamed M, Carlos Kaski J, Banerjee D. Pulse pressure and progression of chronic kidney disease. *JN Journal of Nephrology.* 2010;23(2):189-193.

5. Townsend RR, Chirinos JA, Parsa A, et al. Central Pulse Pressure in Chronic Kidney Disease. *Hypertension.* 2010;56(3):518-524.

6. Hashimoto J, Ito S. Central Pulse Pressure and Aortic Stiffness Determine Renal Hemodynamics. *Hypertension.* 2011(HYPERTENSIONAHA.111.177469).

7. Malhotra R, Nguyen HA, Benavente O, et al. Association between more intensive vs less intensive blood pressure lowering and risk of mortality in chronic kidney disease stages 3 to 5: a systematic review and meta-analysis. *JAMA Internal Medicine.* 2017;177(10):1498-1505.

8. Xie X, Atkins E, Lv J, et al. Effects of intensive blood pressure lowering on cardiovascular and renal outcomes: updated systematic review and meta-analysis. *The Lancet.* 2016;387(10017):435-443.

9. Bloomfield G, Yi S, Astor B, et al. Blood pressure and chronic kidney disease progression in a multi-racial cohort: the MultiEthnic Study of Atherosclerosis. *Journal of Human Hypertension.* 2013;27(7):421-426.

10. Yokota K, Fukuda M, Matsui Y, Hoshide S, Shimada K, Kario K. Impact of visit-to-visit variability of blood pressure on deterioration of renal function in patients with non-diabetic chronic kidney disease. *Hypertension Research.* 2013;36(2):151-157.

11. McMahon EJ, Campbell KL, Bauer JD, Mudge DW. Altered dietary salt intake for people with chronic kidney disease. *Cochrane Database of Systematic Reviews.* 2015;2015(2):Art. No.: CD010070.

CHAPTER 13

Advanced Glycation End Products (AGEs)

Before I began researching ways to improve my kidney function, I had never heard of something called AGE, despite hundreds of medical papers written about the topic. The burned, charred, blackened, and browned parts of foods like steak, hamburger, bread, or pizza crust are the source of most AGEs in our diet. AGE stands for advanced glycation end products, which are proteins or fats that become bonded or linked as a result of exposure to heat and sugars.[1] In most cases these proteins or fats become bonded as a result of direct heat.

AGE refers to a process more than a certain type of food. The Maillard reaction is the name of the chemical reaction between amino acids and sugars that give browned foods their taste and appearance.[2] The browning gives us better taste in many cases, but also much higher AGE levels. High levels of the compounds do exist in foods that are not grilled, fried, or charred. For instance, some fats also contain large amounts of AGEs even though they are not burned or heated during processing. Cigarette smoke is another source of AGEs.[3] But in general, AGE has a lot to do with how foods are cooked. I always thought the charred part of a brisket or steak was the best part. It seems I was wrong, very wrong.

AGE levels in your skin are strongly linked to aging. Patients with high AGE levels have older-looking skin. If you are looking for the fountain of youth, limiting AGEs in your diet might be a good start.[4]

Dietary advanced glycation end products (dAGEs) are known to contribute to increased oxidant stress and inflammation, which are linked to the recent epidemics of diabetes, cardiovascular disease, and now kidney disease. Research also shows that high consumption of well-done, fried, or barbecued meats is associated with increased risks of colorectal, pancreatic, and prostate cancer.[5]

Let's look at what the research says about people with kidney disease and foods high in AGEs:

Study 13.1   The low AGE diet: a neglected aspect of clinical nephrology practice?[6]

Over the past decade, several clinical trials have been performed in a variety of conditions demonstrating that the application of an AGE-restricted diet reduces not only the systemic levels of AGEs but also the levels of markers of oxidative stress and inflammation. This has been shown in CKD patients before and after the initiation of dialysis and either in the presence or absence of coexistent diabetes. Reduction of the AGE content in food is obtained by simple changes in culinary techniques and appears to be a feasible, easily applicable and safe intervention, even in advanced CKD patients.

Study 13.2 **Advanced glycation end product accumulation: a new enemy to target in chronic kidney disease?[7]**

Over the past three decades, <u>AGEs have been implicated in the progression of CKD, and specifically diabetic nephropathy.</u> Although numerous in vitro and in vivo studies highlight the detrimental role of AGEs accumulation in tissue injury, few prospective human studies or clinical trials show that inhibiting this process ameliorates disease. Nonetheless, <u>recent studies have focused on the novel mechanisms that contribute to end-organ injury because of AGEs accumulation, as well as novel targets of therapy in kidney disease.</u>

Study 13.3 **Dietary Advanced Glycation End Products and Risk Factors for Chronic Disease: A Systematic Review of Randomized Controlled Trials[8]**

<u>The findings of this review suggest that consumption of a high AGE diet increases circulating levels of TNFα(Tumor Necrosis Factor) and AGEs in healthy individuals and in individuals with chronic disease. Furthermore, there is evidence to suggest that dietary AGEs promote oxidative stress in healthy adults, and increase CVD markers in patients with diabetes. As such, dietary AGEs may play a role in the promotion of chronic conditions such as T2DM, CVD, and CKD through increased oxidative stress and inflammation.</u>

Given that the standard Western diet contains a high amount of AGEs, further research into the consequences of habitual high AGE diets is important. <u>The potential benefits of restricted AGE intake are promising and could offer a simple dietary therapy in the prevention and treatment of chronic conditions.</u>

Study 13.4 **Advanced glycation end products in renal failure.[9]**

In mild renal insufficiency, plasma glycation free adducts accumulated as renal clearance declined. In patients with end-stage renal disease, plasma glycation free adducts were increased up to 18-fold on peritoneal dialysis and up to 40-fold on hemodialysis.

Therefore, protein glycation free adducts normally excreted efficiently in urine show profound mishandling and accumulation in chronic renal failure. Their accumulation may impair vascular cell function and contribute to morbidity and mortality in renal disease.

Study 13.5 **Advanced Glycation End Products in Foods and a Practical Guide to Their Reduction in the Diet[1]**

AGEs in the diet represent pathogenic compounds that have been linked to the induction and progression of many chronic diseases. This report reinforces previous observations that high temperature and low moisture consistently and strongly drive AGE formation in foods, whereas comparatively brief heating time, low temperatures, high moisture, and/or pre-exposure to an acidified environment are effective strategies to limit new AGE formation in food (13). The potentially negative effects of traditional forms of cooking and food processing have typically remained outside the realm of health considerations. <u>However, accumulation of AGEs due to the systematic heating and processing of foods offers a new explanation for the adverse health effects associated with the Western diet, reaching beyond the question of over-nutrition.</u>

Our kidneys are the primary organs responsible for getting rid of AGEs. When our kidneys are not functioning in the normal range, AGEs accumulate more rapidly and lead to a faster decline in kidney function. You see the vicious circle? A decrease in kidney function reduces the excretion and increases the formulation of AGEs in our bodies. AGEs are also involved in the structural changes of progressive diseases such as glomerulosclerosis, interstitial fibrosis, and tubular atro-phy. This effect is seen in diabetic nephropathy, but also in other nondiabetic kidney diseases.

Here are the cons of eating AGEs:

1. Speeds kidney decline

2. Accelerates aging process

3. Is a cancer risk

4. Is a heart disease risk

5. Leads to more oxidative stress in our bodies

6. Turns on low-level inflammation

Pros of eating AGEs: None, except maybe taste.

I could not find any data suggesting AGEs had a positive effect on health. Like many issues in previous chapters, I could find no evidence or research that suggests AGEs are good for us in any way. AGEs must be limited for those of us with kidney disease. There's no way around it. Looking at the weight of the evidence, I could see no reason not to start limiting AGEs. The golden-brown surface of fried chicken and even the crusty edges of cornbread and lasagna are indications that cooking has increased the amount of these harmful chemicals. AGE levels in many foods have exponentially increased due to the industrial scale of food processing.[10]

I thought about my diet when I first started having symptoms. A sausage muffin on the way to work was high-acid, high-protein, high-AGE, and had few, if any, real antioxidants. A lunchtime meal of a burger, fries, and a soft drink was the same: high-acid, high-protein, high-AGE, and low antioxidants. Dinner might be out or at home, but in most cases, it was the same: high-acid, high-protein, high-AGE, and few real antioxidant combinations.

Maybe eating a diet high in acid, high in protein, high in AGEs, and low in antioxidants is the perfect storm for kidney disease. Could it be that a combination of factors caused my disease, not just one factor? Could it be that the convenience, availability, and low cost of these foods is driving the shocking increase in FSGS (focal segmental glomerulosclerosis) and other kidney diseases? These foods are contributors to high blood pressure, obesity, and type 2 diabetes, but that doesn't explain the ten-fold increase in FSGS over a twenty-year period.[11]

I still don't have all the answers, but I do know that a combination of high acid, high protein, high AGE, and low antioxidants in a diet is incredibly hard on your kidneys.

In fact, the idea of "kidney factors" that I discussed in Chapter 3 truly came to me when I was thinking about AGEs and how many factors were affecting my kidney function. How many issues were actually speeding the rate at which my kidneys' function declined?

Low-protein diets were a step in the right direction, but they addressed only a small portion of what was affecting my kidney disease decline, and we know now that we must treat every aspect of kidney workload, not just one part of it. By treating only protein, I was ignoring antioxidants, AGEs, renal acid load, and several other issues.

No standard exists for safe daily AGE consumption. I tried to find a well-researched level but had no success. AGE research appears to be too new to have resulted in a dietary standard. So, we should set our own dietary standard. This is just my opinion, but limiting AGEs should be easily achievable. Setting our daily limit for AGEs is a good start, but we also need to help our bodies and kidneys get rid of both new AGEs and any existing accumulation. We could set our limit to 1,000 or less, but that would make it hard to get enough calories in a day. Fats contain higher levels of AGEs than fruits and vegetables, but they're an essential part of daily caloric intake. To hit our target calorie amount for the day, we need to include some fats in our diet.

In addition to reducing the amount of AGEs in our diet, we can consume foods that help our bodies and (hopefully our kidneys) break down AGEs. Some antioxidants appear to help our bodies get rid of AGEs or protect against damage from AGEs:

Study 13.6 Cinnamon bark proanthocyanidins as reactive carbonyl scavengers to prevent the formation of advanced glycation endproducts.[12]

(Note: Proanthocyanidins are antioxidants present in berries and some spices like cinnamon)

Cinnamon bark has been reported to be effective in the alleviation of diabetes through its antioxidant and insulin-potentiating activities. In this study, the inhibitory effect of cinnamon bark on the formation of advanced glycation end products (AGEs) was investigated in a bovine serum albumin (BSA)-glucose model. Several phenolic compounds, such as catechin, epicatechin, and procyanidin B2, and phenol polymers were identified from the subfractions of aqueous cinnamon extract. These compounds showed significant inhibitory effects on the formation of AGEs. Their anti-glycation activities were not only brought about by their antioxidant activities but also related to their trapping abilities of reactive carbonyl species such as methylglyoxal (MGO), an intermediate reactive carbonyl of AGE formation. Preliminary study on the reaction between MGO and procyanidin B2 revealed that MGO-procyanidin B2 adducts are primary products which are supposed to be stereoisomers. This is the first report that proanthocyanidins can effectively scavenge reactive carbonyl species and thus inhibit the formation of AGEs. As proanthocyanidins behave in a similar fashion as aminoguanidine (AG), the first AGE inhibitor explored in clinical trials; they show great potential to be developed as agents to alleviate diabetic complications.

Study 13.7   **Inhibition of advanced glycation end products by red grape skin extract and its antioxidant activity.**[13]

RESULTS:

The results showed that the content of total phenolics, flavonoids and total anthocyanins in RGSE [red grape skin extract] was 246.3 ± 0.9 mg gallic acid equivalent/g dried extract, 215.9 ± 1.3 mg catechin equivalent/g dried extract, and 36.7 ± 0.8 mg cyanidin3-glucoside equivalent/g dried extract, respec-tively. In the DPPH radical scavenging activity, hydroxyl radical scavenging activity, and superoxide radical scavenging activity, RGSE had the IC50 values of 0.03 ± 0.01 mg/ml, 5.40 ± 0.01 mg/ml, and 0.58 ± 0.01 mg/ml, respectively. In addition, RGSE had Trolox equivalent antioxidant capacity assay (395.65 ± 1.61 mg Trolox equivalent/g dried extract), ferric reducing antioxidant power (114.24 ± 0.03 mM FeSO4/g dried extract), and ferrous ion chelating power (3,474.05 ± 5.55 mg EDTA/g dried extract), respectively. The results showed that RGSE at different concentrations (0.031-0.500 mg/ml) has significantly inhibited the formation of AGEs in terms of the fluorescence intensity of glycated BSA during 4 weeks of study. The RGSE markedly decreased the level of fructosamine, which is directly associated with the reduction of AGE formation and Nε-(carboxymethyl)lysine (CML). The results demonstrated the significant effect of RGSE on preventing protein oxidative damages, including effects on the thiol and protein carbonyl oxidation.

CONCLUSIONS:

The present study revealed that RGSE would exert beneficial effects by virtue of its antioxidants and anti-glycation. The findings could provide new insight into the naturally occurring anti-glycation properties of RGSE for preventing AGE-mediated diabetic complication.

Study 13.8   **Inhibitory effect of quercetin in the formation of advanced glycation end products of human serum albumin: An in vitro and molecular interaction study.**[14]

(Note: Blueberries, apples, cranberries, and hot peppers are high in quercetin.)

Non-enzymatic glycation entails the reaction between the carbonyl group of sugar with the amino group of a protein giving rise to Schiff base and Amadori products. The formation of advanced glycation end products (AGEs) leads to the generation of free radicals, which play an important role in the pathophysiology of aging and diabetes. Bioavailable dietary antioxidants like quercetin (QC) are thought to inhibit AGEs formation. This study was aimed to investigate the effect of quercetin on AGE formation and features the glycation of human serum albumin (HSA) and its characterization by various spectroscopic techniques. The effect of quercetin, against the formation of AGEs was stud-ied using a glycated human serum albumin product, hemoglobin-δ-gluconolactone, and aminoguanidine. The results were then corroborated with estimation of protein oxidation, lipid peroxidation, and comet assay. Based on the experimental data, computational docking studies were then per-formed to understand the location of the site of quercetin binding and its best-bound conformation with respect to human serum albumin. Through this study, we have demonstrated the mechanism of formation of AGE and its inhibition by quercetin. We have also suggested that the supplementation with dietary antioxidants like quercetin might protect against free radical toxicity.

We see that the type of foods we eat can limit or maybe even stop the damage done by AGEs. The foods in the previous studies are high in antioxidants and address AGE issues. They also happen to be low in protein and low in acid. We'll amend our guidelines to say that an ideal diet includes a daily limit of AGEs and a daily intake of proanthocyanins and antioxidants to help offset AGE intake.

Since AGE data is so hard to come by, I am including here a very large and long list of the AGE content of different foods. As we discuss the issues that can accelerate your disease, I think more information and education is always better.

Food item	AGE Content		
	AGE kU/100g	Serving size (g)	AGE kU/ serving
Fats			
Almonds, blanched slivered (Bazzini Nut Club)	5,473	30	1,642
Almonds, roasted	6,650	30	1,995
Avocado	1,577	30	473
Butter, whipped	26,480	5	1,324
Butter, sweet cream, unsalted, whipped (Land O'Lakes)	23,340	5	1,167
Cashews, raw (Bazzini Nut Club)	6,730	30	2,019
Cashews, roasted	9,807	30	2,942
Chestnut, raw	2,723	30	817
Chestnut, roasted, in toaster oven 350°F for 27 min	5,353	30	1,606
Cream cheese, Philadelphia whipped, (Kraft)	10,883	30	3,265
Cream cheese, Philadelphia original (Kraft)	8,720	30	2,616
Margarine, tub	17,520	5	876
Margarine, tub, I Can't Believe It's Not Butter (Unilever)	9,920	5	496
Margarine, tub, Smart Balance (CFA Brands, Heartbeat Foods)	6,220	5	311
Margarine, tub, Take Control (Unilever, Best Foods)	4,000	5	200
Mayonnaise	9,400	5	470
Mayonnaise, imitation (Diet Source)	200	5	10
Mayonnaise, low fat (Hellman's, Unilever Best Foods)	2,200	5	110
Olive, ripe, large (5 g)	1,670	30	501
Peanut butter, smooth, Skippy (Unilever)	7,517	30	2,255

Food item	AGE Content		
	AGE kU/100g	Serving size (g)	AGE kU/ serving
Peanuts, cocktail (Planters, Kraft)	8,333	30	2,500
Peanuts, dry roasted, unsalted (Planters, Kraft)	6,447	30	1,934
Peanuts, roasted in shell, salted (Frito-Lay)	3,440	30	1,032
Pine nuts (pignolias), raw (Bazzini Nut Club)	11,210	30	3,363
Pistachios, salted (Frito Lay)	380	30	114
Pumpkin seeds, raw, hulled (House of Bazzini)	1,853	30	556
Soybeans, roasted and salted (House of Bazzini)	1,670	30	501
Sunflower seeds, raw, hulled (House of Bazzini)	2,510	30	753
Sunflower seeds, roasted and salted (House of Bazzini)	4,693	30	1,408
Tartar Sauce, creamy (Kraft)	247	15	37
Walnuts, roasted	7,887	30	2,366
Fat, liquid			
Cream, heavy, ultrapasteurized (Farmland Dairies)	2,167	15	325
Oil, canola	9,020	5	451
Oil, corn	2,400	5	120
Oil, cottonseed (The B Manischewitz Company,)	8,520	5	426
Oil, diacylglycerol, Enova (ADM Kao LLC)	10,420	5	521
Oil, olive	11,900	5	595
Oil, olive, extra virgin, first cold pressed (Colavita)	10,040	5	502
Oil, peanut (Planters)	11,440	5	572
Oil, safflower (The Hain Celestial Group, Inc)	3,020	5	151
Oil, sesame (Asian Gourmet)	21,680	5	1084
Oil, sunflower (The Hain Celestial Group, Inc)	3,940	5	197
Salad dressing, blue cheese (Kraft)	273	15	41
Salad dressing, Caesar (Kraft)	740	15	111
Salad dressing, (H. J. Heinz Co)	113	15	17
Salad dressing, French, lite, (Diet Source)	0	15	0
Salad dressing, Italian (Heinz)	273	15	41
Salad dressing, Italian, lite (Diet Source)	0	15	0
Salad dressing, thousand islands (Kraft)	187	15	28

Food item	AGE Content		
	AGE kU/100g	Serving size (g)	AGE kU/ serving
Meats and meat substitutes			
Beef			
Beef, bologna	1,631	90	1,468
Beef, corned brisket, deli meat (Boars Head)	199	90	179
Beef, Frankfurter, boiled in water, 212° F, 7 min	7,484	90	6,736
Beef, Frankfurter, broiled 450°F, 5 min	11,270	90	10,143
Beef, ground, boiled, marinated 10 min w/lemon juice	1,538	90	1,384
Beef, ground, pan browned, marinated 10 min w/lemon juice	3,833	90	3,450
Beef, ground, 20% fat, pan browned	4,928	90	4,435
Beef, ground, 20% fat, pan/ cover	5,527	90	4,974
Beef, hamburger (McDonald's Corp)	5,418	90	4,876
Beef, hamburger patty, olive oil 180°F, 6 min	2,639	90	2,375
Beef, meatball, potted (cooked in liquid), 1 h	4,300	90	3,870
Beef, meatball, w/sauce	2,852	90	2,567
Beef, meatloaf, crust off, 45 min	1,862	90	1,676
Beef, raw	707	90	636
Beef, roast	6,071	90	5,464
Beef, steak, broiled	7,479	90	6,731
Beef, steak, grilled 4 min, George Foreman grill (Salton Inc)	7,416	90	6,674
Beef, steak, microwaved, 6 min	2,687	90	2,418
Beef, steak, pan fried w/ olive oil	10,058	90	9,052
Beef, steak, raw	800	90	720
Beef, steak, strips, 450°F, 15 min	6,851	90	6,166
Beef, steak, strips, stir fried with 1 T canola oil, 15 min	9,522	90	8,570
Beef, steak, strips, stir fried without oil, 7 min	6,973	90	6,276
Beef, stewed, shoulder cut	2,230	90	2,007
Beef, stewed	2,657	90	2,391
Beef, stewed, (mean)	2,443	90	2,199

Food item	AGE Content		
	AGE kU/100g	Serving size (g)	AGE kU/ serving
Poultry			
Chicken, back or thigh, roasted then BBQ	8,802	90	7,922
Chicken, boiled in water, 1 h	1,123	90	1,011
Chicken, boiled with lemon	957	90	861
Beef, salami, kosher (Hebrew National, ConAgra Foods)	628	90	565
Chicken, breast, skinless, roasted with BBQ sauce	4,768	90	4,291
Chicken, breast, skinless, breaded	4,558	90	4,102
Chicken, breast, skinless, breaded, reheated 1 min	5,730	90	5,157
Chicken, breast, boiled in water	1,210	90	1,089
Chicken, breast, breaded, deep fried, 20 min	9,722	90	8,750
Chicken, breast, breaded, oven fried, 25 min, with skin	9,961	90	8,965
Chicken, breast, breaded/ pan fried	7,430	90	6,687
Chicken, breast, grilled/George Foreman grill (Salton Inc)	4,849	90	4,364
Chicken, breast, pan fried, 13 min, high	4,938	90	4,444
Chicken, breast, pan fried, 13 min high/microwave 12.5 sec	5,417	90	4,875
Chicken, breast, poached, 7 min, medium heat	1,101	90	991
Chicken, breast, potted (cooked in liquid), 10 min medium heat	2,480	90	2,232
Chicken, breast, roasted, 45 min with skin	6,639	90	5,975
Chicken, breast, skinless, microwave, 5 min	1,524	90	1,372
Chicken, breast, skinless, poached, 15 min	1,076	90	968
Chicken, breast, skinless, raw	769	90	692
Chicken, breast, steamed in foil, 15 min, medium heat	1,058	90	952
Chicken, breast, strips, stir fried with canola oil, 7 min	4,140	90	3,726
Chicken, breast, strips, stir fried without oil, 7 min	3,554	90	3,199
Chicken, breast, with skin, 450°F, 45 min	8,244	90	7,420
Chicken, breast, skinless, broiled, 450°F, 15 min	5,828	90	5,245
Chicken, crispy (McDonald's)	7,722	90	6,950
Chicken, curry, cube skinless breast, pan fry 10 min, broiled 12 min	6,340	90	5,706

Food item	AGE Content		
	AGE kU/100g	Serving size (g)	AGE kU/ serving
Chicken, curry, cube skinless breast, steam 10 min, broiled 12 min	5,634	90	5,071
Chicken, dark meat, broiled, inside, 450°F, 15 min	8,299	90	7,469
Chicken, fried, in olive oil, 8 min	7,390	90	6,651
Chicken, ground, dark meat with skin, raw	1,223	90	1,101
Chicken, ground, dark w/ skin, pan fried, w/canola oil, 2.5 min, high heat	3,001	90	2,701
Chicken, ground, white meat, pan fried, no added fat, 5 min, high heat	1,808	90	1,627
Chicken, ground, white meat, pan fried, with oil	1,647	90	1,482
Chicken, ground, white meat, raw	877	90	789
Chicken, kebab, cubed skinless breast, pan fried, 15 min	6,122	90	5,510
Chicken, leg, roasted	4,650	90	4,185
Chicken, loaf, roasted	3,946	90	3,551
Chicken, loaf, roasted, crust off	1,420	90	1,278
Chicken, meatball, potted (cooked in liquid), 1 h	1,501	90	1,351
Chicken, nuggets, fast food (McDonald's)	8,627	90	7,764
Chicken, potted (cooked in liquid) with onion and water	3,329	90	2,996
Chicken, roasted	6,020	90	5,418
Chicken, selects (McDonald's)	9,257	90	8,331
Chicken, skin, back or thigh, roasted then BBQ	18,520	90	16,668
Chicken, skin, leg, roasted	10,997	90	9,897
Chicken, skin, thigh, roasted	11,149	90	10,034
Chicken, thigh, roasted	5,146	90	4,631
Turkey, burger, pan fried with cooking spray, 5 min, high heat	7,968	90	7,171
Turkey, burger, pan fried with cooking spray, 5 min, high heat, microwaved 13.5 sec, high heat	8,938	90	8,044
Turkey, burger, pan fried with 5 mL canola oil, 3.5 min, high heat	8,251	90	7,426
Turkey, ground, grilled, crust	6,351	90	5,716
Turkey, ground, grilled, interior	5,977	90	5,379
Turkey, ground, raw	4,957	90	4,461
Turkey, burger, broiled	5,366	90	4,829

Food item	AGE Content		
	AGE kU/100g	Serving size (g)	AGE kU/ serving
Turkey, breast, roasted	4,669	90	4,202
Turkey, breast, smoked, seared	6,013	90	5,412
Turkey, breast, steak, skinless, marinated w/ orange juice, broiled	4,388	90	3,949
Pork			
Bacon, fried 5 min no added oil	91,577	13	11,905
Bacon, microwaved, 2 slices, 3 min	9,023	13	1,173
Ham, deli, smoked	2,349	90	2,114
Liverwurst (Boar's Head)	633	90	570
Pork, chop, marinated w/ balsamic vinegar, BBQ	3,334	90	3,001
Pork, chop, raw, marinated w/balsamic vinegar	1,188	90	1,069
Pork, chop, pan fried, 7 min	4,752	90	4,277
Pork, ribs, roasted, Chinese take out	4,430	90	3,987
Pork, roast, Chinese take out	3,544	90	3,190
Sausage, beef and pork links, pan fried	5,426	90	4,883
Sausage, Italian, raw	1,861	90	1,675
Sausage, Italian, BBQ	4,839	90	4,355
Sausage, pork links, microwaved, 1 min	5,943	90	5,349
Lamb			
Lamb, leg, boiled, 30 min	1,218	90	1,096
Lamb, leg, broiled, 450°F, 30 min	2,431	90	2,188
Lamb, leg, microwave, 5 min	1,029	90	926
Lamb, leg, raw	826	90	743
Veal			
Veal, stewed	2,858	90	2,572
Fish/Seafood			
Crabmeat, fried, breaded (take out)	3,364	90	3,028
Fish, loaf (gefilte), boiled 90 min	761	90	685
Salmon, Atlantic, farmed, prev. frozen, microwaved, 1 min, high heat	954	90	859
Salmon, Atlantic, farmed, prev. frozen, poached, 7 min, medium heat	1,801	90	1,621

Food item	AGE Content		
	AGE kU/100g	Serving size (g)	AGE kU/ serving
Salmon, Atlantic, farmed, prev. frozen, steamed, 10 min, medium heat	1,212	90	1,091
Salmon, Atlantic, farmed, prev. frozen, steamed in foil, 8 min, medium heat	1,000	90	900
Salmon, breaded, broiled 10 min	1,498	90	1,348
Salmon, broiled with olive oil	4,334	90	3,901
Salmon, canned pink (Trident Seafoods)	917	90	825
Salmon, fillet, boiled, submerged, 18 min	1,082	90	974
Salmon, fillet, broiled	3,347	90	3,012
Salmon, fillet, microwaved	912	90	821
Salmon, fillet, poached	2,292	90	2,063
Salmon, pan fried in olive oil	3,083	90	2,775
Salmon, raw, previously frozen	517	90	465
Salmon, raw	528	90	475
Salmon, smoked	572	90	515
Scrod, broiled 450°F, 30 min	471	90	424
Shrimp frozen dinner, microwaved 4.5 min	4,399	90	3,959
Shrimp, fried, breaded (take out)	4,328	90	3,895
Shrimp, marinated raw	1,003	90	903
Shrimp, marinated, grilled on BBQ	2,089	90	1,880
Trout, baked, 25 min	2,138	90	1,924
Trout, raw	783	90	705
Tuna, patty, chunk light, broiled, 450°F, 30 min	747	90	672
Tuna, broiled, with soy, 10 min	5,113	90	4,602
Tuna, broiled, with vinegar dressing	5,150	90	4,635
Tuna, fresh, baked, 25 min	919	90	827
Tuna, loaf (chunk light in recipe), baked 40 min	590	90	531
Tuna, canned, chunk light, w/water	452	90	407
Tuna, canned, white, albacore, w/oil	1,740	90	1,566
Whiting, breaded, oven fried, 25 mins	8,774	90	7,897

Food item	AGE Content		
	AGE kU/100g	Serving size (g)	AGE kU/ serving
Cheese			
Cheese, American, low fat (Kraft)	4,040	30	1,212
Cheese, American, white, processed	8,677	30	2,603
Cheese, brie	5,597	30	1,679
Cheese, cheddar	5,523	30	1,657
Cheese, cheddar, extra sharp, made with 2% milk (Cracker Barrel, Kraft)	2,457	30	737
Cheese, cottage, 1% fat (Light & Lively, Kraft)	1,453	30	436
Cheese, feta, Greek, soft	8,423	30	2,527
Cheese, mozzarella, reduced fat	1,677	30	503
Cheese, parmesan, grated (Kraft)	16,900	15	2,535
Cheese, Swiss, processed	4,470	30	1,341
Cheese, Swiss, reduced fat (Alpine Lace, Alpine Lace Brands, Inc, Maplewood, NJ)	4,743	30	1,423
Soy			
Bacon bits, imitation, Bacos (Betty Crocker, General Mills)	1,247	15	187
Meatless jerky, Primal Strips (Primal Spirit Inc)	1,398	90	1,258
Soy burger, Boca Burger, 400°F, 8 min-4 each side (BOCA Foods Co)	130	30	39
Soy burger, Boca Burger, microwaved, 1.5 min (BOCA Foods Co)	67	30	20
Soy burger, Boca Burger, skillet, cook spray, 5 min (BOCA Foods Co)	100	30	30
Soy burger, Boca Burger, skillet, w/1 tsp olive oil, 5 min (BOCA Foods Co)	437	30	131
Soy burger, Boca Burger (BOCA Foods Co) (mean)	183	30	55
Tofu, broiled	4,107	90	3,696
Tofu, raw	788	90	709
Tofu, soft, raw	488	90	439
Tofu, sautéed, inside	3,569	90	3,212
Tofu, sautéed, outside	5,877	90	5,289
Tofu, sautéed (mean)	4,723	90	4,251
Tofu, soft, boiled 5 min, +2 min to return to boil	628	90	565
Tofu, soft, boiled 5 min, +2 min, + soy sauce, sesame oil	796	90	716

Food item	AGE Content		
	AGE kU/100g	Serving size (g)	AGE kU/ serving
Eggs			
Egg, fried, one large	2,749	45	1,237
Egg white powder (Deb-El Products, Elizabeth, NJ)	1,040	10	104
Egg white, large, boiled 10 min	43	30	13
Egg white, large, boiled 12 min	63	30	19
Egg yolk, large, boiled 10 min	1,193	15	179
Egg yolk, large, boiled 12 min	1,680	15	252
Egg, omelet, pan, low heat, cooking spray, 11 min	90	30	27
Egg, omelet, pan, low heat, corn oil, 12 min	223	30	67
Egg, omelet, pan, low heat, margarine, 8 min	163	30	49
Egg, omelet, pan, low, butter, 13 min	507	30	152
Egg, omelet, pan, low, olive oil, 12 min	337	30	101
Egg, poached, below simmer, 5 min	90	30	27
Egg, scrambled, pan, high, butter, 45 secs	337	30	101
Egg, scrambled, pan, high, cooking spray, 1 min	117	30	35
Egg, scrambled, pan, high, corn oil, 1 min	173	30	52
Egg, scrambled, pan, high, margarine, 1 min	123	30	37
Egg, scrambled, pan, high, olive oil, 1min	243	30	73
Egg, scrambled, pan, med-low, butter, 2 min	167	30	50
Egg, scrambled, pan, med-low, cooking spray, 2 min	67	30	20
Egg, scrambled, pan, med-low, corn oil, 1.5 min	123	30	37
Egg, scrambled pan, med-low, margarine, 2 min	63	30	19
Egg, scrambled, pan, med-low, olive oil, 2 min	97	30	29
Carbohydrates			
Bread			
Bagel, small, Lender's	133	30	40
Bagel, large	107	30	32
Bagel, toasted	167	30	50
Biscuit (McDonald's)	1,470	30	441
Biscuit, refrigerator, baked oven, 350°F, 17 min (Pillsbury Grands, General Mills)	1,343	30	403

Food item	AGE Content		
	AGE kU/100g	Serving size (g)	AGE kU/ serving
Biscuit, refrigerator, uncooked (Pillsbury Grands, General Mills)	823	30	247
Bread, 100% whole wheat, center, toasted (Wonder)	83	30	25
Bread, 100% whole wheat, center (Wonder)	53	30	16
Bread, 100% whole wheat, top crust (Wonder)	73	30	22
Bread, 100% whole wheat, top crust, toasted (Wonder)	120	30	36
Bread, Greek, hard	150	30	45
Bread, Greek, hard, toasted	607	30	182
Bread, Greek, soft	110	30	33
Bread, pita	53	30	16
Bread, white, Italian, center (Freihofer's)	23	30	7
Bread, white, Italian, center, toasted (Freihofer's)	83	30	25
Bread, white, Italian, crust (Freihofer's)	37	30	11
Bread, white, Italian, top crust, toasted (Freihofer's)	120	30	36
Bread, white, slice (Rockland Bakery)	83	30	25
Bread, white, slice, toasted (Rockland Bakery)	107	30	32
Bread, whole wheat, slice (Rockland Bakery)	103	30	31
Bread, whole wheat, slice, toasted, slice, (Rockland Bakery)	137	30	41
Croissant, butter (Starbucks)	1,113	30	334
Roll, dinner, inside	23	30	7
Roll, dinner, outside	77	30	23
Breakfast cereals			
Bran flakes, from Raisin Bran (Post, Kellogg Co)	33	30	10
Cinnamon Toast Crunch (General Mills)	1,100	30	330
Corn Flakes (Kellogg Co)	233	30	70
Corn Flakes, Honey Nut (Kellogg Co)	320	30	96
Corn Flakes, Sugar Frosted (Kellogg Co)	427	30	128
Corn Pops (Kellogg Co)	1,243	30	373
Cream of Wheat, instant, prepared (Nabisco)	108	175	189
Cream of Wheat, instant, prepared with honey (Nabisco)	189	175	331
Fiber One (General Mills)	1,403	30	421

Food item	AGE Content		
	AGE kU/100g	Serving size (g)	AGE kU/ serving
Froot Loops (Kellogg Co)	67	30	20
Frosted Mini Wheats (Kellogg Co)	210	30	63
Granola, Organic Oats & Honey (Cascadian Farms, Small Planet Foods)	427	30	128
Life, mean (Quaker Oats)	1,313	30	394
Puffed Corn Cereal (Arrowhead Mills)	100	30	30
Puffed Wheat	17	30	5
Rice Krispies (Kellogg Co)	2,000	30	600
Total, Wheat and Brown Rice (General Mills)	233	30	70
Oatmeal, instant, dry (Quaker Oats)	13	30	4
Oatmeal, instant, prepared (Quaker Oats)	14	175	25
Oatmeal, instant, prepared with honey (Quaker Oats)	18	175	31
Breakfast foods			
French toast, Aunt Jemima, frozen, microwaved 1 min (Pinnacle Foods)	603	30	181
French toast, Aunt Jemima, frozen, 10 min @ 400°F (Pinnacle Foods Corp)	850	30	255
French toast, Aunt Jemima, frozen, not heated (Pinnacle Foods Corp, Cherry Hill, NJ)	263	30	79
French toast, Aunt Jemima frozen, toaster medium-1 cycle (Pinnacle Foods)	613	30	184
Hot Cakes (McDonald's)	243	30	73
Pancake, from mix	823	30	247
Pancake, frozen, toasted (General Mills)	2,263	30	679
Pancake, homemade	973	30	292
Waffle, frozen, toasted (Kellogg Co)	2,870	30	861
Grains/legumes			
Beans, red kidney, raw	116	100	116
Beans, red kidney, canned	191	100	191
Beans, red kidney, cooked 1 h	298	100	298
Pasta, cooked 8 min	112	100	112
Pasta, cooked 12 min	242	100	242
Pasta, spiral	245	100	245

Food item	AGE Content		
	AGE kU/100g	Serving size (g)	AGE kU/ serving
Rice, white, quick cooking, 10 min	9	100	9
Rice, Uncle Ben's white, cooked, 35min (Mars, Inc, Houston, TX)	9	100	9
Rice, white, pan toasted 10 min, cooked 30 min	32	100	32
Starchy vegetables			
Corn, canned	20	100	20
Potato, sweet, roasted 1 h	72	100	72
Potato, white, boiled 25 min	17	100	17
Potato, white, roasted 45 min, with 5 mL oil/serving	218	100	218
Potato, white, French fries (McDonald's)	1,522	100	1,522
Potato, white, French fries, homemade	694	100	694
Potato, white, French fries, in corn oil, held under heat lamp	843	100	843
Potato, white, hash browns (McDonald's)	129	100	129
Crackers/snacks			
Breadsticks, Stella D'oro hard (Brynwood Partners)	127	30	38
Cheez Doodles, crunchy (Wise Foods Inc)	3,217	30	965
Chex mix, traditional (General Mills)	1,173	30	352
Chips, corn, Doritos (Frito Lay)	503	30	151
Chips, corn, Harvest Cheddar Sun Chips (Frito-Lay)	1,270	30	381
Chips, Platanitos, plantain (Plantain Products Co)	370	30	111
Chips, potato (Frito Lay)	2,883	30	865
Chips, potato, baked original potato crisps (Frito Lay)	450	30	135
Combos, nacho cheese pretzel (M&M Mars)	1,680	30	504
Cracker, chocolate Teddy Graham (Nabisco)	1,647	30	494
Cracker, Pepperidge Farms Goldfish, cheddar (Campbell Soup Co)	2,177	30	653
Cracker, Keebler honey graham (Kellogg Co)	1,220	30	366
Cracker, Old London Melba toast (Nonni's Food Co)	903	30	271
Cracker, oyster	1,710	30	513
Cracker, rice cake, corn (Taanug)	137	30	41
Cracker, saltine, hospital (Alliant)	937	30	281

Food item	AGE Content		
	AGE kU/100g	Serving size (g)	AGE kU/ serving
Cracker, Keebler sandwich, club+cheddar, (Kellogg Co)	1,830	30	549
Cracker, toasted wheat	917	30	275
Cracker, wheat, round	857	30	257
Cracker, KA-ME rice crunch, plain (Liberty Richter)	917	30	275
Popcorn, air popped, with butter	133	30	40
Popcorn, Pop Secret microwaved, fat-free, no added fat (General Mills)	33	30	10
Pretzel, minis (Snyder's of Hanover)	1,790	30	537
Pretzel, Q rolled	1,883	30	565
Pretzel, stick	1,600	30	480
Pretzel (mean)	1,757	30	527
Veggie Booty (Robert's American Gourmet)	983	30	295
Cookies, cakes, pies, pastries			
Bar, granola, chocolate chunk, soft (Quaker)	507	30	152
Bar, Nutrigrain, apple cinnamon (Kellogg Co)	2,143	30	643
Bar, Rice Krispies Treat (Kellogg Co)	1,920	30	576
Bar, Granola, peanut butter & choc chunk, hard (Quaker)	3,177	30	953
Cake, angel food, Danish Kitchen (Sam's Club)	27	30	8
Cookie, biscotti, vanilla almond (Starbucks)	3,220	30	966
Cookie, chocolate chip, Chips Ahoy (Nabisco)	1,683	30	505
Cookie, Golden Bowl fortune (Wonton Food, Inc)	90	30	27
Cookie, Greek wedding, nut cookie	960	30	288
Cookie, meringue, homemade	797	30	239
Cookie, Keebler oatmeal raisin (Kellogg Co)	1,370	30	411
Cookie, Oreo (Nabisco)	1,770	30	531
Cookie, Nilla vanilla wafer (Nabisco)	493	30	148
Croissant, chocolate (Au Bon Pain)	493	30	148
Danish, cheese (Au Bon Pain)	857	30	257
Donut, glazed devil's food cake (Krispy Kreme)	1,407	30	422
Donut, chocolate iced, crème filled (Krispy Kreme)	1,803	30	541
Fruit pop, frozen (Dole)	18	60	11

Food item	AGE Content		
	AGE kU/100g	Serving size (g)	AGE kU/ serving
Fruit roll up, sizzlin' red (General Mills)	980	30	294
Gelatin, Dole strawberry (Nestle)	2	125	2
Gelatin, Dole strawberry, sugar-free (Nestle)	1	125	1
Ice cream cone, cake (Häagen-Dazs, Oakland, CA)	147	30	44
Ice cream cone, sugar (Häagen-Dazs)	153	30	46
Muffin, bran (Au Bon Pain)	340	30	102
Pie, apple, individual, baked (McDonald's)	637	30	191
Pie, crust, frozen, baked per pkg, mean Mrs. Smith's Dutch Apple Crumb and Pumpkin Custard (Kellogg Co)	1,390	30	417
Pie, Mrs. Smith's Dutch apple crumb, deep dish, apple filling (Kellogg Co)	340	30	102
Pie, Mrs. Smith's Dutch apple crumb, deep dish, crumbs (Kellogg Co)	1,030	30	309
Pie, Mrs. Smith's Dutch apple crumb, deep dish, crust (Kellogg Co)	1,410	30	423
Pie, Mrs. Smith's Dutch apple crumb, deep dish, pie (Kellogg Co)	893	30	268
Pie, Mrs. Smith's pumpkin custard, bake it fresh, original recipe, crust (Kellogg Co)	1,373	30	412
Pie, Mrs. Smith's pumpkin custard, bake it fresh, original recipe, custard (Kellogg Co)	617	30	185
Pie, Mrs. Smith's pumpkin custard, bake it fresh, original recipe, pie (Kellogg Co)	880	30	264
Pop Tart, microwave-3 sec high power (Kellogg Co)	243	30	73
Pop Tart, microwave-6 sec medium high power (Kellogg's)	210	30	63
Pop Tart, not heated (Kellogg Co)	133	30	40
Pop Tart, toaster-low, 1 cycle (Kellogg Co)	260	30	78
Scone, cinnamon (Starbucks)	790	30	237
Sorbet, Edy's strawberry (Dryer's)	2	125	3
Sweet roll, cinnamon swirl roll (Starbucks)	907	30	272
Fruits			
Apple, baked	45	100	45
Apple, Macintosh	13	100	13
Banana	9	100	9

Food item	AGE Content		
	AGE kU/100g	Serving size (g)	AGE kU/ serving
Cantaloupe	20	100	20
Coconut cream, Coco Goya cream of coconut (Goya)	933	15	140
Coconut milk, leche de coco, (Goya)	307	15	46
Coconut, Baker's Angel Flake, sweetened (Kraft)	590	30	177
Dates, Sun-Maid California chopped (Sun-Maid, Kingsburg, CA)	60	30	18
Fig, dried	2,663	30	799
Plums, Sun-Maid dried pitted prunes (Sun-Maid)	167	30	50
Raisin, from Post Raisin Bran (Kellogg Co)	120	30	36
Vegetables (raw unless specified otherwise)			
Carrots, canned	10	100	10
Celery	43	100	43
Cucumber	31	100	31
Eggplant, grilled, marinated with balsamic vinegar	256	100	256
Eggplant, raw, marinated with balsamic vinegar	116	100	116
Green beans, canned	18	100	18
Portabella mushroom, raw, marinated with balsamic vinegar	129	100	129
Onion	36	100	36
Tomato	23	100	23
Tomato sauce (Del Monte Foods)	11	100	11
Vegetables, grilled (broccoli, carrots, celery)	226	100	226
Vegetables, grilled (pepper, mushrooms)	261	100	261
Other carbohydrates			
Sugar, white	0	5	0
Sugar substitute, aspartame as Canderel (Merisant,)	0	5	0
Liquids			
Milk and milk products			
Cocoa packet, Swiss Miss, prepared (ConAgra Foods)	262	250	656
Cocoa packet, Swiss Miss sugar-free, prepared (ConAgra Foods)	204	250	511

Food item	AGE Content		
	AGE kU/100g	Serving size (g)	AGE kU/ serving
Ice cream, America's Choice vanilla (The Great Atlantic and Pacific Tea Co)	34	250	84
Milk, fat-free (hospital)	1	250	2
Milk, Lactaid fat-free (McNeil Nutritionals)	10	250	26
Milk, fat-free (Tuscan Dairy Farms)	2	250	4
Milk, fat-free, with A and D	0	250	1
Milk, fat-free, with A and D (microwaved,1 min)	2	250	5
Milk, fat-free, with A and D (microwaved, 2 min)	8	250	19
Milk, fat-free, with A and D (microwaved, 3 min)	34	250	86
Milk, soy (Imagine Foods, The Hain Celestial Group)	31	250	77
Milk, whole (4% fat)	5	250	12
Pudding, instant chocolate, fat-free, sugar-free, prepared	1	120	1
Pudding, instant chocolate, skim milk	1	120	1
Pudding, Hunt Wesson snack pack, chocolate (ConAgra Foods)	17	120	20
Pudding, Hunt Wesson snack pack, vanilla (ConAgra Foods)	13	120	16
Yogurt, cherry, (Dannon, White Plains, NY)	4	250	10
Yogurt, vanilla, (Dannon)	3	250	8
Fruit juice			
Juice, apple	2	250	5
Juice, cranberry	3	250	8
Juice, orange	6	250	14
Juice, orange, from fresh fruit	0	250	1
Juice, orange, with calcium	3	250	8
Vegetable juice			
Vegetable juice, V8 (Campbell Soup Co)	2	250	5
Other carbohydrate liquids			
Fruit pop, frozen (Dole)	18	60	11
Honey	7	15	1
Sorbet, strawberry (Edy's)	2	125	3
Syrup, caramel, sugar-free	0	15	0

Food item	AGE Content		
	AGE kU/100g	Serving size (g)	AGE kU/ serving
Syrup, dark corn	0	15	0
Syrup, pancake, lite	0	15	0
Combination foods and solid condiments			
Combination foods			
Bacon Egg Cheese Biscuit (McDonald's)	2,289	100	2,289
Bacon, Egg and Cheese McGriddles (McDonald's)	858	100	858
Big Mac (McDonald's)	7,801	100	7,801
Casserole, tuna	233	100	233
Cheeseburger (McDonald's)	3,402	100	3,402
Chicken McGrill (McDonald's)	5,171	100	5,171
Corned beef hash, canned, microwaved 2 min, high power (Broadcast)	1,691	100	1,691
Corned beef hash, canned, stove top, medium heat, 12 min (Broadcast)	2,175	100	2,175
Corned beef hash, canned, unheated (Broadcast)	1,063	100	1,063
Double Quarter Pounder with Cheese (McDonald's)	6,283	100	6,283
Filet-O-Fish (McDonald's)	6,027	100	6,027
Gnocchi, potato/flour/ Parmesan cheese, 3 min	535	100	535
Gnocchi, potato/flour/Parmesan cheese, 4.5 min	2,074	100	2,074
Hot Pocket, bacon, egg, cheese, oven, 350°F, 20 min (Nestle)	1,695	100	1,695
Hot Pocket-bacon, egg, cheese, microwaved 1 min (Nestle)	846	100	846
Hot Pocket-bacon, egg, cheese, frozen-not heated (Nestle)	558	100	558
Hummus, commercial	733	100	733
Hummus, with garlic and scallions	884	100	884
Hummus, with vegetables	487	100	487
Hummus (mean)	701	100	701
Macaroni and cheese	2,728	100	2,728
Macaroni and cheese, baked	4,070	100	4,070
Pasta primavera	959	100	959
Pesto, with basil (Buitoni, Nestle)	150	100	150

Food item	AGE Content		
	AGE kU/100g	Serving size (g)	AGE kU/ serving
Pizza, thin crust	6,825	100	6,825
Salad, Italian pasta	935	100	935
Salad, lentil potato	123	100	123
Salad, tuna pasta	218	100	218
Sandwich, cheese melt, open faced	5,679	100	5,679
Sandwich, toasted cheese	4,333	100	4,333
Soufflé, spinach	598	100	598
Timbale, broccoli	122	100	122
Taramosalata (Greek style caviar spread)	678	100	678
Veggie burger, California burger, 400°F, 8 min-4 each side (Amy's Kitchen)	198	100	198
Veggie burger, California burger, skillet, with spray, 5 min (Amy's Kitchen)	149	100	149
Veggie burger, California burger, skillet, with 1 tsp olive oil, 5 min (Amy's Kitchen)	374	100	374
Veggie burger, California burger, microwave, 1 min (Amy's)	68	100	68
Won ton, pork, fried (take out)	2,109	100	2,109
Ziti, baked	2,795	100	2,795
Candies			
Ginger, crystallized	490	10	49
Candy, Hershey Special Dark Chocolate (The Hershey Co, Hershey, PA)	1,777	30	533
Candy, M & M's, milk chocolate (Mars)	1,500	30	450
Candy, Reese's Peanut Butter Cup (The Hershey Co)	3,440	30	1,032
Candy, Raisinets (Nestle)	197	30	59
Candy, Snickers (Nestle)	263	30	79
Pickle, bread, and butter	10	30	3
Soups, liquid condiments, and miscellaneous liquids			
Soups			
Soup, beef bouillon	0.4	250	1
Soup, chicken bouillon	1.2	250	3
Soup, College Inn chicken broth, (Del Monte)	0.8	250	2

Food item	AGE Content		
	AGE kU/100g	Serving size (g)	AGE kU/ serving
Soup, chicken noodle, (Campbell Soup Company)	1.6	250	4
Soup, couscous, and lentil (Fantastic World Foods)	3.6	250	9
Soup, Knorr vegetable broth, (Unilever)	1.6	250	4
Soup, summer vegetable	1.2	250	3
Condiments			
Ketchup	13.33	15	2
Mustard	0	15	0
Pectin	80	15	12
Soy sauce	60	15	9
Vinegar, balsamic	33.33	15	5
Vinegar, white	40	15	6
Miscellaneous			
SoBe Adrenaline Rush (South Beach Beverage Co)	0.4	250	1
Budweiser Beer (AnheuserBusch)	1.2	250	3
Breast milk, fresh	6.67	30	2
Breast milk, frozen	10	30	3
Coca Cola, classic (The Coca-Cola Co)	2.8	250	7
Coffee, with milk and sugar	2.4	250	6
Coffee, drip method	1.6	250	4
Coffee, heating plate >1 h	13.6	250	34
Coffee, Taster's Choice instant (Nestle)	4.8	250	12
Coffee, instant, decaf (mean, Sanka [Kraft] and Taster's Choice)	5.2	250	13
Coffee, Spanish	4.8	250	12
Coffee, with milk	6.8	250	17
Coffee, with sugar	7.6	250	19
Coke	6.4	250	16
Coke, Diet (The Coca-Cola Company)	1.2	250	3
Coke, Diet 2008 (The CocaCola Company)	4	250	10
Coke, Diet plus (The CocaCola Company)	1.6	250	4
Enfamil, old (Mead Johnson Nutritional)	486.67	30	146

Food item	AGE Content		
	AGE kU/100g	Serving size (g)	AGE kU/ serving
Ensure plus	12.8	250	32
Gelatin, Dole strawberry (Nestle)	1.6	125	2
Gelatin, Dole strawberry, sugar-free (Nestle)	0.8	125	1
Glucerna (Abbott Nutrition)	70	250	175
Malta (Goya)	1.2	250	3
NOFEAR Super Energy Supplement (Pepsico)	0.4	250	1
Pepsi, diet (Pepsico)	2.8	250	7
Pepsi, diet MAX (Pepsico)	3.2	250	8
Pepsi, diet, caffeine free (Pepsico)	2.4	250	6
Pepsi, regular (Pepsico)	2.4	250	6
Resource (Nestle)	72	250	180
Rum, Bacardi Superior, 80 proof	0	250	0
Sprite (The Coca-Cola Company)	1.6	250	4
Sprite, diet (The Coca-Cola Company)	0.4	250	1
Tea, apple (RC Bigelow, Inc)	0.4	250	1
Tea, Lipton Tea bag (Unilever)	2	250	5
Tea, Lipton Tea bag, decaf (Unilever)	1.2	250	3
Vodka, Smirnoff, 80 proof (Diageo)	0	250	0
Whiskey, Dewar's White Label (Dewar's)	0.4	250	1
Wine, pinot grigio (Cavit Collection, Port Washington, NY)	32.8	250	82
Wine, pinot noir (Cavit Collection)	11.2	250	28

As you can see, the worst offender on our list is skin-on BBQ chicken, which comes in at a whopping 16,668 AGEs per serving. A McDonald's Big Mac is 7,801, and if we add French fries with a value of 1,522, we get 9,323 in AGEs for a single meal.

A clear difference in AGE content can be seen when processed, precooked, or industrialized foods are compared with raw or uncooked foods. A boiled potato goes from 17 to 1,522 when it is turned into French fries.

Simpler is better when it comes to AGEs, as processing adds AGEs in almost every case. For example, traditional white rice has an AGE of 9, while Rice Krispies jump to an AGE value of 600, 66 times the level of plain rice.

In the past when I have heard that processed food is bad, I always doubted this idea. However, I find that it is true in almost every case. Processing rarely, if ever (maybe never), improves a food's nutritional value.

Limiting AGEs is not as easy as it seems due to the high concentration of AGEs in fats, so fats must be limited on an AGE-restricted diet. Virgin cold pressed olive oil is 502 AGEs per 5ml (1 teaspoon) serving. No doubt we will have to consume some AGEs in our diet, but we can limit the charred, burned, and fried foods.

Summary

AGEs mostly come from blackened and charred parts of food. The blackened part contains burned food products that are bad for us.

As our kidney function declines, so does our ability to get rid of AGEs in our bodies. People with kidney disease accumulate AGEs at a higher rate than the healthy public.

The good news is AGEs can easily be reduced by just changing the cooking method. Cooking with liquids vs dry heat is the solution.

As in previous chapters, no data could be found suggesting AGEs are good for us. Another open-and-shut case. AGEs increase the rate at which our bodies age and the rate of kidney disease progression. AGEs have no place in our diets.

References

1. Uribarri J, Woodruff S, Goodman S, et al. Advanced glycation end products in foods and a practical guide to their reduction in the diet. *Journal of the American Dietetic Association.* 2010;110(6):911-916. e912.

2. Ashoor S, Zent J. Maillard browning of common amino acids and sugars. *Journal of Food Science.* 1984;49(4):1206-1207.

3. Cerami C, Founds H, Nicholl I, et al. Tobacco smoke is a source of toxic reactive glycation products. *Proceedings of the National Academy of Sciences.* 1997;94(25):13915-13920.

4. Gkogkolou P, Böhm M. Advanced glycation end products: Key players in skin aging? *Dermato-endocrinology.* 2012;4(3):259-270.

5. Sinha R, Park Y, Graubard BI, et al. Meat and meat-related compounds and risk of prostate cancer in a large prospective cohort study in the United States. *American Journal of Epidemiology.* 2009;170(9):1165-1177.

6. Uribarri J, He JC. The low AGE diet: a neglected aspect of clinical nephrology practice? *Nephron.* 2015;130(1):48-53.

7. Mallipattu SK, Uribarri J. Advanced glycation end product accumulation: a new enemy to target in chronic kidney disease? *Current Opinion in Nephrology and Hypertension.* 2014;23(6):547-554.

8. Clarke RE, Dordevic AL, Tan SM, Ryan L, Coughlan MT. Dietary advanced glycation end products and risk factors for chronic disease: a systematic review of randomised controlled trials. *Nutrients.* 2016;8(3):125. 9. Thornalley PJ. Advanced glycation end products in renal failure. *Journal of Renal Nutrition.* 2006;16(3):178-184.

9. Poulsen MW, Hedegaard RV, Andersen JM, et al. Advanced glycation endproducts in food and their effects on health. *Food and Chemical Toxicology.* 2013;60:10-37.

10. Kiffel J, Rahimzada Y, Trachtman H. Focal segmental glomerulosclerosis and chronic kidney disease in pediatric patients. *Advances in chronic kidney disease.* 2011;18(5):332-338.

11. Peng X, Cheng K-W, Ma J, et al. Cinnamon bark proanthocyanidins as reactive carbonyl scavengers to prevent the formation of advanced glycation endproducts. *Journal of agricultural and food chemistry.* 2008;56(6):1907-1911.

12. Jariyapamornkoon N, Yibchok-anun S, Adisakwattana S. Inhibition of advanced glycation end products by red grape skin extract and its antioxidant activity. *BMC Complementary and Alternative Medicine.* 2013;13(1):171.

13. Alam MM, Ahmad I, Naseem I. Inhibitory effect of quercetin in the formation of advanced glycation end products of human serum albumin: An in vitro and molecular interaction study. *International Journal of Biological Macromolecules.* 2015;79:336-343.

CHAPTER 14

Phosphorus

Almost every diet for kidney disease will have a limit on phosphorus, as well as sodium, and usually potassium. We need to understand the role phosphorus plays so we can manage it better. Phosphorus is the second most abundant mineral in the body, after calcium. The two minerals work together to help build bone. Phosphorus also plays a role in growth and repair of cells and in energy production. At any time, blood phosphorus levels reflect the balance between movements of this mineral from and into the intestine, bone, intracellular space, and kidneys.

When phosphorus intake is low, the body compensates by enhancing phosphate absorption in the small intestine. Again, lowering dietary phosphate causes the body to act by increasing phosphate absorption. So, it is very, very hard to ingest too little phosphorus. Low phosphorus levels, or *hyperphosphatemia*, is rare in people with kidney disease.[1] On the other hand, high phosphorus levels, or *hyperphosphatemia*, is an independent mortality risk factor for healthy adults as well as people with kidney disease. As kidney disease progresses or when a diet is too high in phosphorus, the mineral begins to accumulate in our bloodstreams as our kidneys lose the ability to effectively manage it. Hyperphosphatemia is one of the most important non-traditional risk factors associated with vascular calcification in CKD patients.[2]

Vitamin D production is also impaired in CKD, which reduces calcium absorption.[3] As calcium is reduced, phosphorus levels increase. In turn, high phosphorus levels cause our bodies to pull calcium from our bones to offset it. The combination of high phosphorus and calcium levels is even worse, leading to calcium being deposited in our blood vessels, lungs, eyes, and heart.

Here's more on what the research says about the dangers of high phosphorus levels and the impact on people with kidney disease:

Study 14.1   **Serum phosphate levels and mortality risk among people with chronic kidney disease.[4]**

Elevated serum phosphate levels have been linked with vascular calcification and mortality in dialysis patients. The relationship between phosphate and mortality has not been explored among patients with chronic kidney disease (CKD). A retrospective cohort study was conducted from eight Veterans Affairs' Medical Centers located in the Pacific Northwest. CKD was defined by two continuously abnormal outpatient serum creatinine measurements at least 6 mo. apart between 1999 and 2002. Patients who received chronic dialysis, those with a present or previous renal transplant, and those without a recent phosphate measurement were excluded. The primary end point was all-cause mortality. Secondary end points were acute myocardial infarction and the combined end point of myocardial infarction plus death. A total of 95,619 veterans with at least one primary care or internal medicine clinic contact from a Northwest VA facility and two or more outpatient measurements of serum creatinine, at least 6 mo. apart, between January 1, 1999, and December 31, 2002, were identified. From this eligible population, 7021 patients met our definition of CKD. After exclusions, 6730 CKD patients were available for analysis, and 3490 had a serum phosphate measurement during the previous 18 mo. <u>After adjustment, serum phosphate levels >3.5 mg/dl were associated with a significantly increased risk of death. Mortality risk increased linearly with each subsequent 0.5mg/dl increase in serum phosphate levels. Elevated serum phosphate levels were independently associated with increased mortality risk among this population of patients with CKD.</u>

Study 14.2 **The Impact of Normal Range of Serum Phosphorus on the Incidence of End-Stage Renal Disease by A Propensity Score Analysis.[5]**

The propensity score analysis shows that even the normal range of serum phosphorus clearly accelerates CKD progression to ESRD. Our results encourage clinicians to target serum phosphorus to inhibit CKD progression in the manner of 'the lower, the better.'

Study 14.3 **Phosphate attenuates the anti-proteinuric effect of very low-protein diet in CKD patients.[6]**

Phosphate is an important modifier of the anti-proteinuric response to VLPD. Reducing phosphate burden may decrease proteinuria and slow the progression of renal disease in CKD patients, an issue that remains to be tested in specific clinical trials.

Study 14.4 **Phosphorus and the Kidney: What Is Known and What Is Needed[7]**

<u>Experimentally, high dietary phosphorus has been shown to initiate and/or worsen progression of kidney dysfunction, whereas dietary phosphate restriction reverses and/or restricts the dysfunction.</u> Although the most common explanation has been phosphorus-induced calcification, there are other potential proposed mechanisms including phosphorus-dependent podocyte injury due to overexpression of pituitary-specific positive transcription factor 1 (Pit-1) transporter in rats. <u>It is also possible that the deleterious effect of acute phosphorus loading on systemic endothelial function described above might also extend to the glomerular endothelium.</u>

The Role of Klotho[8]

Phosphorus also has an unexpected link to aging. Klotho, an age-suppressing gene, is involved in the metabolism of phosphorus and calcium and it naturally declines with age. People with kidney disease are deficient in klotho; kidney disease is basically a sustained state of klotho deficiency. The low klotho levels that contribute to the aging process are likely the cause for accelerated aging in people with kidney disease. Klotho deficiency also renders the kidneys more susceptible to acute injuries, delays kidney regeneration, and promotes renal fibrosis.

Study 14.5 **The emerging role of Klotho in clinical nephrology.[9]**

<u>There is real and systemic Klotho deficiency in both acute kidney injury (AKI) and chronic kidney disease (CKD). Klotho plummets very early and severely in AKI and represents a pathogenic factor that exacerbates acute kidney damage. In CKD, Klotho deficiency exerts a significant impact on the progression of renal disease and extra renal complications.</u>

Klotho levels may be an indicator of early disease and predict the rate of progression, and presence and severity of soft tissue calcification. The correction of Klotho deficiency may delay progression and forestall the development of extra renal complications in CKD. Rarely does one find a molecule with such broad potential applications in nephrology.

Fibroblast Growth Factor-23 and Klotho

Fibroblast growth factor-23 (FGF23) is related to Klotho levels. FGF23 is a bone-derived hormone known to suppress phosphate reabsorption and Vitamin D hormone production in the kidneys. FGF23 effectively increases the output and decreases the input of phosphorus because it directly increases phosphorus excretion and indirectly decreases intestinal phosphorus absorption. It does this by decreasing calcitriol values. Low FGF23 levels end up increasing our absorption of phosphorus.

FGF23 levels increase during early stages of kidney malfunction. Plasma FGF23 continues to increase as CKD progresses, increasing dramatically in ESRD. At the same time, our ability to respond to high levels of FGF23 declines as our kidney function declines, which is associated with reduced klotho.

As the graph below shows, the cumulative incidence of death of CKD stage 2–4 patients increases significantly with ascending quartiles of baseline FGF23 levels in unadjusted analyses. Patients with the highest FGF23 levels had much higher mortality rates than the quartile with the lowest FGF 23 levels.

FIGURE 14.1: **FGF23 is an Independent Risk Factor for Mortality in CKD Stages 2–4[10]**

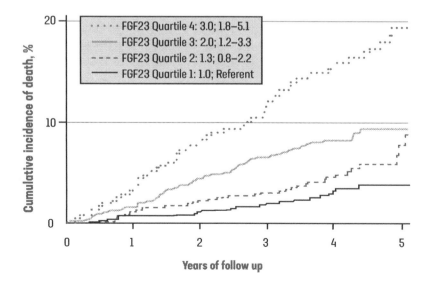

These studies show us that lowering phosphorus levels is a method for managing FGF23 and may also help increase klotho levels. Further, we need to think about lowering phosphorus levels as early as stage 2 kidney disease, and not wait until stage 4 or stage 5.

At this stage of my research, I recognized that an extra low phosphorus diet should be the goal, but I soon discovered that it might be harder to achieve than I had thought. The *type* of phosphorus we eat appears to matter more than I had realized. I didn't even know there were three different types of phosphorus. Three types of phosphorus exist from a dietary point of view, and they are absorbed at different rates by our bodies:

1. Plant-based phosphorus is not easily absorbed by our bodies. Absorption rate is 40% or less.

2. Animal-based phosphorus is more easily absorbed at rates of up to 80%.

3. Inorganic phosphorus used as a food additive is absorbed at a 80% to 100% rate. Study 14.2

Study 14.6   **Organic and inorganic dietary phosphorus and its management in chronic kidney disease.[11]**

Dietary phosphorus control is often the main strategy in the management of patients with chronic kidney disease. Dietary protein is a major source of phosphorus intake. Recent data indicate that imposed dietary phosphorus restriction may compromise the need for adequate protein intake, leading to protein-energy wasting and possibly to increased mortality. The two main sources of dietary phosphorus are organic, including animal and vegetarian proteins, and inorganic, mostly food preservatives. Animal based foods and plant are abundant in organic phosphorus. Usually, 40% to 60% of animal-based phosphorus is absorbed; this varies by degree of gastrointestinal vitamin D-receptor activation, whereas plant phosphorus, mostly associated with phytates, is less absorbable by human gastrointestinal tract. Up to 100% of inorganic phosphorus in processed foods may be absorbed; i.e., phosphorus in processed cheese and some soda (cola) drinks. A recent study suggests that a higher dietary phosphorus protein intake ratio is associated with incremental death risk in patients on long-term hemodialysis. Hence, for phosphorus management in chronic kidney disease, in addition to absolute dietary phosphorus content, the chemical structure (inorganic versus organic), type (animal versus plant), and the phosphorus-protein ratio should be considered. We recommend foods and supplements with no or lowest quantity of inorganic phosphorus additives, more plant-based proteins, and a dietary phosphorus protein ratio of less than 10 mg/g. Fresh (non-processed) egg white (phosphorus-protein ratio less than 2 mg/g) is a good example of desirable food, which contains a high proportion of essential amino acids with low amounts of fat, cholesterol, and phosphorus.

Study 14.7   **Management of natural and added dietary phosphorus burden in kidney disease.[12]**

Phosphorus retention occurs from higher dietary phosphorus intake relative to its renal excretion or dialysis removal. In the gastrointestinal tract, the naturally existing organic phosphorus is only partially (~60%) absorbable; however, this absorption varies widely and is lower for plant-based phosphorus including phytate (<40%) and higher for foods enhanced with inorganic phosphorus-containing preservatives (>80%). The latter phosphorus often remains unrecognized by patients and health care professionals, even though it is widely used in contemporary diets, in particular with low-cost foods.

This has big implications for us. Since phosphorus is not a required disclosure on food labels, the food we buy may contain large amounts of it without our knowing it. Further, from our perspective, not all phosphorus is created equal. We absorb inorganic phosphorus (the kind in pro-cessed foods) at twice the rate of plant-based phosphorus, so we must be very careful and adjust our diet accordingly. We could be meeting our daily phosphorus requirement based on our reading of food labels and still be going over our daily limit by a factor of two to five times.

If you think I am crying wolf when it comes to added inorganic phosphorus because no one has quantified how prevalent it is, read on:

Study 14.8 **The Prevalence of Phosphorus Containing Food Additives in Top Selling Foods in Grocery Stores[13]**

The labels of 2394 (80%) commonly purchased branded grocery products in northeast Ohio were reviewed for phosphorus additives.

FIGURE 14.2: **Percent of Foods with Phosphorus Additives**

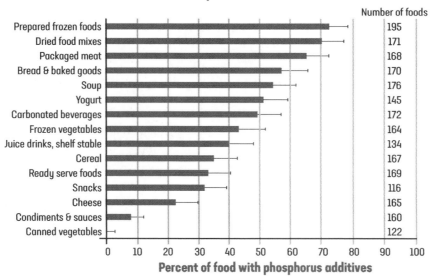

[As you can see in the chart above] <u>44% of the bestselling grocery items contained phosphorus additives.</u> The additives were particularly common in prepared frozen foods (72%), dry food mixes (70%), packaged meat (65%), bread & baked goods (57%), soup (54%), and yogurt (51%) categories. Foods containing phosphorus additives averaged 67 mg phosphorus/100 gm more than matched foods not containing phosphorus additives (p=.03). Sample meals comprised mostly of foods with phosphorus additives had 736 mg more phosphorus per day compared to meals consisting of only additive-free foods. Meals without phosphorus additives cost an average of $2.00 more per day.

Phosphorus additives are common in best-selling processed groceries and contribute significantly to their phosphorus content. Moreover, food with phosphorus additives are less costly than those without phosphorus additives. As a result, persons with chronic kidney disease may purchase these popular low-cost groceries and unknowingly increase their intake of highly bioavailable phosphorus.

In this study, almost 50% of the best-selling items in grocery stores had added phosphorus, and their sample meals resulted in an extra 736 mg of phosphorus per day. Remember that 800 mg to 1000 mg is the recommended daily allowance. You could be eating twice as much as the RDA if you are not careful, despite reading the labels carefully.

When reading labels (if phosphorus is disclosed), look for the word "phosphate" or even the root "phos-" in any word on the label. Here are some terms to look for:

> Calcium phosphate

> Disodium phosphate

> Phosphoric acid

> Monopotassium phosphate

> Sodium acid pyrophosphate

> Sodium tripolyphosphate

> Potassium phosphate

Every processed, frozen, or prepared food should be viewed with caution.

The Benefits of the Vegetarian or Vegan Diet

A vegetarian or vegan diet had a big effect on phosphorus levels in patients in this study. When a very low-protein vegan diet was used, calcium and phosphorus levels went back to the normal range. This did not happen with a low-protein diet including meats, dairy, eggs, or fish.

Study 14.9 **Vegetarian compared with meat dietary protein source and phosphorus homeostasis in chronic kidney disease.**[14]

Summary: Demonstrates that the source of protein has a significant effect on phosphorus homeostasis in patients with CKD. The results indicated that 1 week of a vegetarian diet led to lower serum phosphorus levels and decreased FGF23 levels.

Therefore, dietary counseling of patients with CKD must include information on not only the amount of phosphate but also the source of protein from which the phosphate derives.

Study 14.10 **Effects of a supplemented hypoproteic diet in chronic kidney disease.[15]**

In the SVLPD [severe hypoproteic diet, or vegan] group, serum urea significantly decreased (56 +/- 7.9 mmol/L vs. 43.2 +/- 10 mmol/L), and significant improvements in serum bicarbonate (23.4 +/- 2.1 mmol/L vs. 18.1 +/- 1.5 mmol/L), serum calcium (1.10 +/- 0.17 mmol/L vs. 1.00 +/- 0.15 mmol/L at baseline), serum phosphates (1.45 +/- 0.66 mmol/L vs. 1.91 +/- 0.68 mmol/L), and calcium-phosphorus product (1.59 +/- 0.11 mmol(2)/L(2) vs. 1.91 +/- 0.10 mmol(2)/L(2)) were noted after 48 weeks. No death was registered in any group. Significantly lower percentages of patients in group I required renal replacement therapy initiation (4% vs. 27%). After 48 weeks, estimated glomerular filtration rate did not significantly change in patients receiving SVLPD (0.26 +/- 0.08 mL/s vs. 0.31 +/- 0.08 mL/s at baseline), but significantly decreased in controls (0.22 +/- 0.09 mL/s vs. 0.30 +/- 0.07 mL/s). The compliance with the keto-diet was good in enrolled patients. No significant changes in any of the parameters of the nutritional status and no adverse reactions were noted.

SVLPD [a vegan diet] seems to ameliorate the nitrogen waste products retention and acid-base and calcium phosphorus metabolism disturbances and to postpone the renal replacement therapy initiation, preserving the nutritional status in patients with CKD.

My own results were like the second study above. When I was on a strict diet that eliminated processed foods, meat, eggs, and dairy, my phosphorus levels kept dropping each month until I was in the middle of the normal ranges.

But is phosphorus really the bad guy, or is it the protein consumption? We don't know, since most high-phosphorus foods are also high in protein.

It's worth noting that one theory for the reason kidney disease disproportionally affects people in lower income groups is that inorganic phosphorus is added to the cheapest foods, so those on tighter family budgets might consume more of these foods.[16] So could it be that the consumption of these cheaper foods with so much added inorganic phosphorus is a cause?

We don't have answers to many of these questions, but we do have *some* answers:

1. We should try to get phosphorus levels down below 3.0mg/dl if possible. We must reduce phosphorus intake to a level below our current kidney workload capacity. If we can do this, our balance of phosphorus and calcium may return to normal ranges.

2. If we stick to a vegetarian or vegan diet, we can eat more phosphorus because we absorb less. This allows our diet to expand compared to diets that contain meat products.

3. We need to find a way to increase klotho and reduce FGF 23. The main way we can do this is to reduce phosphorus levels to the low end of normal. Aerobic exercise may also increase klotho.[17]

4. If we cannot get our phosphorus levels low enough by diet alone, we should be using phosphate binders, which reduce the absorption of dietary phosphates. However, we should watch out for adding calcium supplements or binders to our diet. See Chapter 11.

5. Niacin may also help reduce phosphate absorption.[18]

6. New research shows that specific probiotics may also help reduce phosphorus levels.[19]

Summary

As mentioned earlier, reducing phosphorus should be done very early in your diagnosis – as early as stage 2. Remember, how we manage our disease in stage 2 is predictive of how fast we will progress to stage 3, and so on. If we don't manage stage 2 or 3 well, then stage 4 will come faster and likely with more health conditions to deal with. My conclusion is that a supplemented very low-protein vegan diet could reduce urea or nitrogen waste, help restore pH, and reduce phosphorus/calcium issues.

So, lowering your phosphorus load may slow the progression of kidney disease. As shown in this chapter, we need phosphorus to be on the low end of the normal range of 2.5 to 4.5 mg/dl for adults. We need to be below 3.0 mg/dl if possible. Normal phosphorus levels are bad for us and accelerate our disease. In this case, normal is bad.

One more reminder: We need to assume phosphorus is added to all prepackaged, prepared, frozen, and other commercial foods we buy. This also applies to food in restaurants. With no labeling requirements, there is no way to know how much or how little phosphorus has been added.

References

1. Uribarri J. PHOSPHORUS METABOLISM AND MANAGEMENT IN CHRONIC KIDNEY DISEASE: Phosphorus Homeostasis in Normal Health and in Chronic Kidney Disease Patients with Special Emphasis on Dietary Phosphorus Intake. *Seminars in Dialysis.* 2006;20(4):295-301.

2. Palit S, Kendrick J. Vascular calcification in chronic kidney disease: role of disordered mineral metabolism. Current pharmaceutical design. 2014;20(37):5829-5833. 3. Bosworth C, De Boer IH. Impaired vitamin D metabolism in CKD. *Seminars in Nephrology.* 2013;33(2):158-168.

3. Kestenbaum B, Sampson JN, Rudser KD, et al. Serum phosphate levels and mortality risk among people with chronic kidney disease. *Journal of the American Society of Nephrology.* 2005;16(2):520-528.

4. Chang WX, Xu N, Kumagai T, et al. The impact of normal range of serum phosphorus on the incidence of end-stage renal disease by a propensity score analysis. *PloS one.* 2016;11(4):e0154469.

5. Di Iorio BR, Bellizzi V, Bellasi A, et al. Phosphate attenuates the anti-proteinuric effect of very low-protein diet in CKD patients. *Nephrology Dialysis Transplantation.* 2012;28(3):632-640.

6. Ibels LS, Alfrey AC, Haut L, Huffer WE. Preservation of function in experimental renal disease by dietary restriction of phosphate. *New England Journal of Medicine.* 1978;298(3):122-126.

7. Kabat-Koperska J, Ciechanowski K. The Role of Klotho Protein in Chronic Kidney Disease: Studies in Animals and Humans. *Current Protein and Peptide Science.* 2016;17(8):821-826.

8. Hu MC, Kuro-o M, Moe OW. The emerging role of Klotho in clinical nephrology. *Nephrology Dialysis Transplantation.* 2012;27(7):2650-2657.

9. Wolf M. Update on fibroblast growth factor 23 in chronic kidney disease. *Kidney International.* 2012;82(7):737-747.

10. Noori N, Sims JJ, Kopple JD, et al. Organic and inorganic dietary phosphorus and its management in chronic kidney disease. *Iranian Journal of Kidney Diseases.* 2010;4(2):89.

11. Cupisti A, Kalantar-Zadeh K. Management of natural and added dietary phosphorus burden in kidney disease. *Seminars in Nephrology.* 2013;33(2):180-190.

12. León JB, Sullivan CM, Sehgal AR. The prevalence of phosphoruscontaining food additives in top-selling foods in grocery stores. *Journal of Renal Nutrition.* 2013;23(4):265-270. e262.

13. Moe SM, Zidehsarai MP, Chambers MA, et al. Vegetarian compared with meat dietary protein source and phosphorus homeostasis in chronic kidney disease. *Clinical Journal of the American Society of Nephrology.* 2011;6(2):257-264.

14. Mircescu G, Gârneaţă L, Stancu SH, Căpuşă C. Effects of a supplemented hypoproteic diet in chronic kidney disease. *Journal of Renal Nutrition.* 2007;17(3):179-188.

15. Gutiérrez OM. Sodium-and phosphorus-based food additives: persistent but surmountable hurdles in the management of nutrition in chronic kidney disease. *Advances in chronic kidney disease.* 2013;20(2):150-156.

16. Matsubara T, Miyaki A, Akazawa N, et al. Aerobic exercise training increases plasma Klotho levels and reduces arterial stiffness in postmenopausal women. *American Journal of Physiology-Heart and Circulatory Physiology.* 2014;306(3):H348-H355.

17. Maccubbin D, Tipping D, Kuznetsova O, Hanlon WA, Bostom AG. Hypophosphatemic effect of niacin in patients without renal failure: a randomized trial. *Clinical Journal of the American Society of Nephrology.* 2010;5(4):582-589.

18. George M, Joseph L, George D. Role of prebiotic and probiotic in the management of chronic kidney disease patients. *International Journal of Medical Research & Health Sciences.* 2016;5(2):50-53.

CHAPTER 15

Calcium

I will lead off with a headline to emphasize this chapter:

Vascular Calcification: The Killer of Patients with Chronic Kidney Disease[1]

Kidney disease causes heart disease to be greatly accelerated. In my eyes, the two cannot be separated. When I say greatly accelerated, I mean *really* accelerated. It is very likely that vascular calcification is the number one killer of people with kidney disease. We cannot talk about staying alive longer or things that accelerate kidney progression without talking about heart disease progression. Dietary calcium intake is not associated with kidney disease progression, but supplemental calcium appears to accelerate vascular calcification and heart disease.

If vascular calcification is the number one killer of people with kidney disease, why aren't we talking about this? Why aren't our recommended diets like the ones that have been proven to reduce heart disease? If kidney disease creates a perfect storm for heart disease via vascular calcification, why in the hell aren't we addressing this as early as possible? I feel like jumping up and down and screaming again.

Heart disease is a slow-moving progressive disease that starts very early in kidney disease patients. Heart disease progression can start as early as stage 2. Calcium and phosphorus combine to create something called phosphate-induced vascular calcification. The higher your phosphorus and calcium levels, the faster your heart disease progresses. While many other factors are at play, such as blood pressure, obesity, and exercise, calcium is something we can easily control with a little dietary planning.

Even in healthy patients, taking calcium supplements accelerates heart disease. Studies on healthy patients:

Study 15.1	Calcium Intake from Diet and Supplements and the Risk of Coronary Artery Calcification (CAC) and its Progression Among Older Adults: 10-Year Follow-up of the Multi-Ethnic Study of Atherosclerosis (MESA)[2]

CONCLUSIONS:

High total calcium intake was associated with a decreased risk of incident atherosclerosis over long-term follow-up, particularly if achieved without supplement use. However, calcium supplement use may increase the risk for incident CAC.

Study 15.2 **Dietary and supplemental calcium intake and cardiovascular disease mortality: The National Institutes of Health-AARP diet and health study.**[3]

Our findings suggest that high intake of supplemental calcium is associated with an excess risk of CVD death in men but not in women. Additional studies are needed to investigate the effect of supplemental calcium use beyond bone health.

Study 15.3 **Calcium intake and mortality from all causes, cancer, and cardiovascular disease: The Cancer Prevention Study II Nutrition Cohort.**[4]

In this cohort, associations of calcium intake and mortality varied by sex. For women, total and supplemental calcium intakes are associated with lower mortality, whereas for men, supplemental calcium intake ≥1000 mg/d may be associated with higher all-cause and CVD-specific mortality.

There are several other studies, but all lead to the same conclusion: In healthy men, high calcium intake from supplements more than 1,000 mg a day is associated with a higher mortality rate. High calcium intake from dietary foods seems to be okay in many cases. Women are less affected than men.

Remember, this data applies to healthy adults with normal phosphorus levels and normal kidney function.

Now let's look at data for people with kidney disease.

Study 15.4 **The relation of calcium-phosphorus metabolism related indexes with cardiac damages**[5]

CONCLUSIONS:

Calcium-phosphorus metabolism disorder in the context of kidney dysfunction may contribute to the damages of cardiac structure and functions.

Study 15.5 **Cardiac valves calcifications in dialysis patients**[6]

We found cardiac valve calcifications in 40 percent of patients on hemodialysis. We also found that CaxP (calcium and phosphorus) product is higher in patients with cardiac valve calcifications. We did not find a correlation between age, dialysis duration, BMI and cardiac valve calcifications. These findings support careful monitoring of calcium metabolism in end stage renal disease to reduce valvular calcifications and the risk of cardiovascular disease.

Study 15.6 **Valvular calcification and its relationship to atherosclerosis in chronic kidney disease.**[7]

CONCLUSION:

Valvular calcification is common in CKD and is closely associated with findings of intimal arterial disease. The presence of inflammation and the duration of dialysis treatment contribute to this complication. Diabetes is also a prominent risk factor for mitral annular calcification in CKD.

Study 15.7 Kidney Disease as a Risk Factor for Development of Cardiovascular Disease[8]

In 1998, the National Kidney Foundation (NKF) Task Force on Cardiovascular Disease in Chronic Renal Disease issued a report emphasizing the high risk of CVD in CKD.[5] <u>This report showed that there was a high prevalence of CVD in CKD and that mortality due to CVD was 10 to 30 times higher in dialysis patients than in the general population. The task force recommended that patients with CKD be considered in the "highest risk group" for subsequent CVD events and that treatment recommendations based on CVD risk stratification should take into account the highest-risk status of patients with CKD.</u>

Study 15.8 Pathophysiology of vascular calcification in chronic kidney disease.[9]

<u>Patients with chronic kidney disease (CKD) on dialysis have 2- to 5-fold more coronary artery calcification than age-matched individuals with angiographically proven coronary artery disease.</u> In addition to increased traditional risk factors, CKD patients also have many nontraditional cardiovascular risk factors that may play a prominent role in the pathogenesis of arterial calcification, including duration of dialysis and disorders of mineral metabolism.

Depending on which study you read, the increase in heart disease is 200% to 500%, or all the way to 3000% (30 times). The latter number comes from the American Heart Association statements from 1998 and 2003. Fifteen years ago, we knew these facts, but rarely do we get advice to manage heart disease as aggressively as kidney disease.

If we already have a 200% to 3,000% increase in heart disease on a normal diet, should we be taking calcium supplements? Hell no, we shouldn't. We should take calcium supplements only if we have no other choices. If we must take calcium, then we need to take the lowest amount possible. We should take calcium only if our doctors closely manage and supervise any supplemental calcium in our diet.

To be fair, several studies dispute the idea that calcium intake is associated with heart disease. The difference in these reports is the type of calcium. Dietary calcium naturally found in foods is fine, however supplemental calcium is the one we have to minimize.

Why is this such a big problem for us?

The first reason is calcium is added to many foods to increase nutrition for the public. We are usually getting more calcium every day than we think. Second, many phosphate or phosphorus binders used to lower phosphorus levels are calcium-based. Calcium carbonate is a very affordable and efficient phosphorus binder. It's a catch-22: we take calcium carbonate to reduce phosphorus, which is good, but are we doing it at the expense of accelerated heart disease? Lower phosphorus is good, but taking supplemental calcium is bad. There are better ways to lower phosphorus than calcium binders. The easiest way is to reduce your intake of phosphorus.

Does the lower phosphorus offset the higher calcium intake? No one knows at this point. It's a "damned if you do, damned if you don't" situation.

Another reason why we should be concerned is keto amino acid supplements. A supplement is used to provide protein nutrition with a lower nitrogen workload on the kidneys. However, the older keto acids are made from calcium. A normal daily dosage can be up to 1.20 mg from these keto acids alone. Again, a catch-22: we can extend kidney life and slow progression of kidney disease with keto acids, but we accelerate heart disease at the same time.

The double whammy is someone taking older keto acids with high calcium and a calcium phosphorus binder. 2,000 mg or more of calcium is possible and even likely in this situation. Now we are driving 100 mph toward heart disease instead of kidney disease.

Is there a solution? Can we stop calcification of our arteries? Maybe, but we can certainly slow it significantly in most cases. Stopping the progress of vascular calcification should be one of your treatment goals.

The solution is diet and magnesium. Magnesium reduces vascular calcification. Low magnesium is also associated with higher mortality rates, and high magnesium (slightly higher than the normal range) is associated with lower mortality rates. Magnesium also decreases inflammation. If we take a calcium supplement, we must take it with enough magnesium to offset the effect of calcium. The problem is when your GFR drops below 30; magnesium excretion may become impaired. We must manage magnesium well to do well.

Study 15.9   Magnesium prevents phosphate-induced calcification in human aortic vascular smooth muscle cells.[10]

CONCLUSIONS:

Increasing Mg (magnesium) concentrations significantly reduced VC (vascular calcification), improved cell viability and modulated secretion of VC markers during cell-mediated matrix mineralization clearly pointing to a cellular role for Mg (2+) and 2-APB further involved TRPM7 and a potential Mg (2+) entry to exert its effects. Further investigations are needed to shed light on the additional cellular mechanism(s) by which Mg (2+) can prevent VC.

Study 15.10   Magnesium and outcomes in patients with chronic kidney disease: focus on vascular calcification, atherosclerosis, and survival[11]

Magnesium and survival in hemodialysis patients: (partly based on data presented in abstract form only)

- Patients with slightly elevated serum magnesium concentrations may have a survival advantage.

- Low serum magnesium concentrations may be independent predictors of death.

CONCLUSIONS:

A growing body of evidence from in vitro investigations, animal models and both observational, as well as interventional clinical studies, point to the possibility that low magnesium levels are associated with vascular calcification. Moreover, several observational studies suggest a relationship between increased serum magnesium concentrations and better survival rates for patients receiving long-term dialysis treatment. Preliminary results from an uncontrolled interventional trial suggest that long-term intervention with magnesium in dialysis patients may retard arterial calcification.

FIGURE 15.1: **Effect of Diet on the Number of Calcifications for Different Diets**

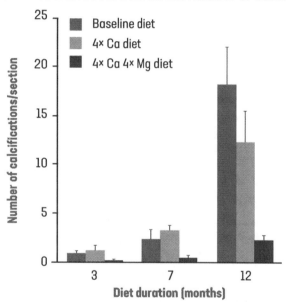

Effect of diet on the number of calcifications in blood vessels in the kidney cortex of *Abcc6-/-* mice. Histograms represent the average number of calcifications per kidney section as a function of diet and diet duration. Diets supplemented with calcium plus magnesium ('4 × Ca, 4 × Mg' diet) slowed down calcification significantly [compared with baseline unsupplemented diet or diet supplemented with calcium alone (4 × Ca diet)] after 3, 7 and 12 months [Kruskal–Wallis test, P<0.05 for all comparisons)] [53]. With kind permission from Springer Science+Business Media, Gorgels *et al.* [53] (Figure 2).

The chart above shows the number of calcifications for different diets. A normal diet, one with calcium supplements, and one with an equal amount of magnesium and calcium:

FIGURE 15.2: **Rate of Vascular Calcification**

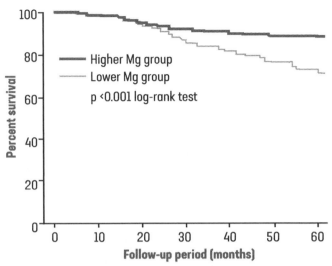

Kaplan-Meier analysis of all-cause mortality rates during a 51 month follow-up of 515 chronic haemodialysis patients. The relative risk of mortality was significantly greater in the group with lower baseline serum magnesium levels (<1.14 mmol/L, n = 261) than in that with the higher baseline serum magnesium levels (≥1.14 mmol/L; n = 254) [76]. All-cause mortality; P<0.001 (log-rank test); after adjustment by Cox multivariate analysis, P <0.05. Reprinted from Ishimura et al. [76], with permission

As you can see, after twelve months, the rate of vascular calcification was slowed dramatically using magnesium to offset the risks of calcium intake.

Mortality Rates

Patients with the highest magnesium levels had the best chances of survival over five years.

Let me caution you not to get carried away with magnesium or calcium. Hypomagnesemia and hypermagnesemia can be dangerous. We want magnesium to be at the very top of the normal range, maybe even slightly higher, but going higher than that can have serious health consequences. The same is true if magnesium gets too low.

Calcium is not the only culprit here. Diabetes, oxidative stress, uremia, high cholesterol, and high phosphorus levels also play a role. Kidney disease is a multifactorial disease. However, it is hard to deposit calcium in your arteries or heart valves when there isn't much calcium in your system. We will talk about magnesium more later, but it is so intertwined with calcium that I felt compelled to include in this chapter as well.

Kidney disease is a perfect storm for heart disease and vascular calcification. Heart disease is what kills us, but the accelerated heart disease was caused by our kidney disease. The heart health battle must be fought as hard as the kidney disease battle. They are inseparable.

Summary

What can we learn from this chapter? Dietary calcium is good and may be associated with a lower risk of heart disease, but supplemental calcium is bad unless it is reduced with magnesium. The highest sources of calcium are milk, kale, sardines, broccoli, watercress, cheese, bok choy, and okra. Many of these foods are very healthy, like kale, broccoli, watercress, bok choy, and okra. This may explain why dietary calcium intake is good and supplements are bad.

You should take calcium supplements only if you have no other choices and do so with you doctor's guidance. The lowest possible dose of calcium should be used if you must take supplemental calcium. Remember, the first step is always taking your foot off the gas. Stop taking calcium unless your doctor strongly recommends it and you have no other choices. This is a good conversation to have with your doctor.

Taking 1,000 mg of calcium a day and then trying to offset it with a large dose of magnesium is not recommended for several reasons. This could lead to a dangerous situation where you are trying to take 1,000 mg of magnesium (which you should never do) to offset 1,000 mg of calcium. This would be impossible to manage and could be dangerous. Stick with one of two options:

1. No supplemental calcium

2. Lower dose of supplemental calcium combined with low dose of magnesium

This will keep your risks low.

References

1. Mizobuchi M, Towler D, Slatopolsky E. Vascular calcification: the killer of patients with chronic kidney disease. *Journal of the American Society of Nephrology.* 2009;20(7):1453-1464.

2. Anderson JJ, Kruszka B, Delaney JA, et al. Calcium intake from diet and supplements and the risk of coronary artery calcification and its progression among older adults: 10-year follow-up of the Multi-Ethnic Study of Atherosclerosis (MESA). *Journal of the American Heart Association.* 2016;5(10):e003815.

3. Xiao Q, Murphy RA, Houston DK, Harris TB, Chow W-H, Park Y. Dietary and supplemental calcium intake and cardiovascular disease mortality: the National Institutes of Health–AARP diet and health study. *JAMA Internal Medicine.* 2013;173(8):639-646.

4. Yang B, Campbell PT, Gapstur SM, et al. Calcium intake and mortality from all causes, cancer, and cardiovascular disease: the Cancer Prevention Study II Nutrition Cohort. *The American Journal of Clinical Nutrition.* 2016;103(3):886-894.

5. Wu L, Bai Y, Chen T, et al. The relation of calcium-phosphorus metabolism-related indexes with cardiac damages. *Age (year).* 2016;56(2.79):51.06-53.02.

6. Klarić D, Klarić V, Kristić I. Cardiac valves calcifications in dialysis patients. *Acta Medica Croatica: Casopis Hravatske Akademije Medicinskih Znanosti.* 2011;65(Suppl 3):11-13.

7. Leskinen Y, Paana T, Saha H, et al. Valvular calcification and its relationship to atherosclerosis in chronic kidney disease. *The Journal of Heart Valve Disease.* 2009;18(4):429-438.

8. Sarnak MJ, Levey AS, Schoolwerth AC, et al. Kidney disease as a risk factor for development of cardiovascular disease. *Circulation.* 2003;108(17):2154-2169.

9. Moe SM, Chen NX. Pathophysiology of vascular calcification in chronic kidney disease. *Circulation research.* 2004;95(6):560-567.

10. Louvet L, Büchel J, Steppan S, Passlick-Deetjen J, Massy ZA. Magnesium prevents phosphate-induced calcification in human aortic vascular smooth muscle cells. *Nephrology Dialysis Transplantation.* 2012;28(4):869-878.

11. Massy ZA, Drüeke TB. Magnesium and outcomes in patients with chronic kidney disease: focus on vascular calcification, atherosclerosis, and survival. *Clinical Kidney Journal.* 2012;5(Suppl 1):i52-i61.

CHAPTER 16

Sodium

Salt restriction has been extensively researched. Limiting salt is very common for people with kidney disease. It is well-known that salt contributes to high blood pressure, which can lead to kidney disease.[1] What is less well-known is that salt can trigger inflammation and reduce the amount of oxygen our kidneys receive. Salt restriction is designed to address issues of high blood pressure and edema (swelling),[2] but there is more to it than blood pressure or swelling.

We want to treat the cause of kidney disease and not just the symptoms. Processed, prepackaged, and restaurant-prepared foods may have up to 100 times the salt content of home-cooked meals. Could salt be the cause of our woes?

The experience of the Yanomami, an isolated tribe in South America, may be informative. They have no access to salt in their normal diet, and it was found that their blood pressure did not increase as they aged.[3] For our part, it is simply assumed that, as we age, our blood pressure will rise. This may not need to be true, since it may be a result of constant salt consumption over many years. Issues such as autoimmune diseases may be linked to excess salt consumption as well.[4]

One of the most researched diets is the DASH diet, the "dietary approach to stopping hypertension." Salt restriction is the cornerstone of the DASH. The standard DASH diet has a sodium restriction of 2,300 mg but another version also exists with a 1,500 mg restriction. The DASH brand of spices is in most grocery stores and all of the DASH seasonings are salt-free.

Let's see what we can find on sodium, beginning with its role in inflammation:

Study 16.1   Variation in Dietary Salt Intake Induces Coordinated Dynamics of Monocyte Subsets and Monocyte-Platelet Aggregates in Humans: Implications in End Organ Inflammation[5]

In conclusion, for the first time, we demonstrated a rapid expansion of the CD14++CD16+ monocyte pool and platelet activation, as well as monocyte proinflammatory activation in response to increased dietary salt intake. In addition, monocyte recruitment and infiltration, presumably CD14++CD16+ monocytes, is associated with high-salt intake induced renal hypoxia. Our findings reveal novel pathophysiological links between dietary salt intake, innate immunity, and target organ inflammation. Future work is warranted to elucidate whether CD14++CD16+ monocytes may serve as a potential target for new therapeutic strategies in high-salt intake induced end organ injuries.

In other words, in the study above, high salt intake caused the kidneys to be starved for oxygen. This is something new for us to consider. And here's a second study showing the relationship between salt and inflammation. This is not something we hear about very often, as the research is new:

Study 16.2 — Induction of pathogenic Th17 cells by inducible salt sensing kinase SGK1[6]

Th17 cells are highly proinflammatory cells critical for clearing extracellular pathogens and for induction of multiple autoimmune diseases. IL-23 plays a critical role in stabilizing and reinforcing the Th17 phenotype by increasing expression of IL-23 receptor (IL-23R) and endowing Th17 cells with pathogenic effector functions. However, the precise molecular mechanism by which IL-23 sustains the Th17 response and induces pathogenic effector functions has not been elucidated. Here, we used transcriptional profiling of developing Th17 cells to construct a model of their signaling network and nominate major nodes that regulate Th17 development. We identified serum glucocorticoid kinase-1 (SGK1), a serine-threonine kinase, as an essential node downstream of IL-23 signaling. SGK1 is critical for regulating IL-23R expression and stabilizing the Th17 cell phenotype by deactivation of Foxo1, a direct repressor of IL-23R expression. SGK1 has been shown to govern Na+ transport and salt (NaCl) homeostasis in other cells. We here show that a modest increase in salt concentration induces SGK1 expression, promotes IL-23R expression and enhances Th17 cell differentiation in vitro and in vivo, accelerating the development of autoimmunity. Loss of SGK1 abrogated Na+-mediated Th17 differentiation in an IL23-dependent manner. These data demonstrate that SGK1 plays a critical role in the induction of pathogenic Th17 cells and provides a molecular insight into a mechanism by which an environmental factor such as a high salt diet triggers Th17 development and promotes tissue inflammation.

And then there's the risk of cardiovascular disease in CKD patients:

Study 16.3 — Sodium Excretion and the Risk of Cardiovascular Disease in Patients With Chronic Kidney Disease.[7]

Among 3757 participants (mean age, 58 years; 45% women), 804 composite CVD [cardiovascular disease] events (575 heart failures, 305 myocardial infarctions, and 148 strokes) occurred during a median 6.8 years of follow-up. From lowest (<2894 mg/24 hours) to highest (≥4548 mg/24 hours) quartile of calibrated sodium excretion, 174, 159, 198, and 273 composite CVD events occurred, and the cumulative incidence was 18.4%, 16.5%, 20.6%, and 29.8% at median follow-up. In addition, the cumulative incidence of CVD events in the highest quartile of calibrated sodium excretion compared with the lowest was 23.2% vs. 13.3% for heart failure, 10.9% vs. 7.8% for myocardial infarction, and 6.4% vs. 2.7% for stroke at median follow-up. Hazard ratios of the highest quartile compared with the lowest quartile were 1.36 (95% CI, 1.09-1.70; P = .007) for composite CVD events, 1.34 (95% CI, 1.03-1.74; P = .03) for heart failure, and 1.81 (95% CI, 1.08-3.02; P = .02) for stroke after multivariable adjustment. Restricted cubic spline analyses of the association between sodium excretion and composite CVD provided no evidence of a nonlinear association (P = .11) and indicated a significant linear association (P < .001).

Among patients with CKD, higher urinary sodium excretion was associated with increased risk of CVD.

And here's what the research says about what happens when salt intake is reduced:

| Study 16.4 | Salt intake in kidney disease—a missed therapeutic opportunity?[8] |

In renal patients, even a modest reduction of dietary sodium is associated with lower blood pressure, proteinuria and better outcome. Information on the impact of salt intake on the course of kidney disease is fragmentary but points to the direction that high salt aggravates long-term outcomes. All these data taken together support the call to avoid excessive high salt intake and underscore efforts to reduce dietary salt intake to recommended targets in CKD patients.

| Study 16.5 | Altered dietary salt intake for people with chronic kidney disease.[9] |

We found a critical evidence gap in long-term effects of salt restriction in people with CKD that meant we were unable to determine the direct effects of sodium restriction on primary endpoints such as mortality and progression to endstage kidney disease (ESKD). We found that salt reduction in people with CKD reduced blood pressure considerably and consistently reduced proteinuria. If such reductions could be maintained long-term, this effect may translate to clinically significant reductions in ESKD incidence and cardiovascular events. Research into the long-term effects of sodium-restricted diet for people with CKD is warranted, as is an investigation into adherence to a low salt diet.

| Study 16.6 | Role of Sodium Intake in the Progression of Chronic Kidney Disease[10] |

The relation of salt to hypertension and kidney disease had been well known at the turn of the last century, but the importance of salt has been grossly neglected more recently. There is a close link between salt intake and hypertension, as well as partially blood pressure–independent target organ damage including renal disease. In the general population, high salt intake is associated with hypertension and cardiovascular events. Salt loading also increases albuminuria in individuals without primary renal disease and raises excretion of albumin and protein in patients with renal disease. It aggravates proteinuria and glomerulosclerosis and accelerates progression in most animal models of renal damage. The effect of salt restriction cannot be reproduced by treatment with diuretics. Inappropriate increase of intrarenal angiotensin II and increased reactive oxygen species are the major culprits responsible for salt-related renal damage.

Summary

I am not going to spend much time on salt restriction, since it has been practiced for many decades and the benefits are so well-known. For us, sodium increases blood pressure, edema, inflammation, free radical damage, (maybe) renal hypoxia, and the risk for other illnesses like heart disease. Excessive or high salt consumption accelerates kidney disease progression. There is no question that we should be on a low-sodium diet. It's another black-and-white diet issue.

But how much sodium is too much? Your monthly blood test is the best guide to set your daily sodium limits. You should keep reducing sodium until your tests are in the middle or lower end of the normal range. Most of us start with a restriction of 2,000 to 2,200 mg a day. You can reduce your intake by 200 mg a month until you get into the normal range. Many people assume reducing salt in their diets will mean foods will taste bland. This is not the case, and you need not fear reducing salt as a part of your treatment plan. The DASH series of spices have no salt and have been popular for years.

Personally, my sodium levels went below the normal ranges when I prepared all meals at home with no added salt. My blood pressure went so low that I had to be taken off Vasotec, a blood pressure medication. This was after fifteen years on blood pressure medications.

It can be done!

References

1. Torres VE, Abebe KZ, Schrier RW, et al. Dietary salt restriction is beneficial to the management of autosomal dominant polycystic kidney disease. *Kidney International.* 2017;91(2):493-500.

2. Ohta Y, Kimura Y, Kitaoka C, Sakata T, Abe I, Kawano Y. Blood pressure control status and relationship between salt intake and lifestyle including diet in hypertensive outpatients treated at a general hospital. *Clinical and Experimental Hypertension.* 2017;39(1):29-33.

3. Mancilha-Carvalho JdJ. The Yanomami Indians in the INTERSALT study. *Arquivos brasileiros de cardiologia.* 2003;80(3):295-300.

4. Kleinewietfeld M, Manzel A, Titze J, et al. Sodium chloride drives autoimmune disease by the induction of pathogenic TH17 cells. *Nature.* 2013;496(7446):518-522.

5. Zhou X, Zhang L, Ji W-J, et al. Variation in dietary salt intake induces coordinated dynamics of monocyte subsets and monocyte-platelet aggregates in humans: implications in end organ inflammation. *PloS one.* 2013;8(4):e60332.

6. Wu C, Yosef N, Thalhamer T, et al. Induction of pathogenic Th17 cells by inducible salt sensing kinase SGK1. ***Nature.*** 2013;496(7446):513.

7. Mills KT, Chen J, Yang W, et al. Sodium excretion and the risk of cardiovascular disease in patients with chronic kidney disease. *Jama.* 2016;315(20):2200-2210.

8. Lambers Heerspink HJ, Navis G, Ritz E. Salt intake in kidney disease—a missed therapeutic opportunity? *Nephrology Dialysis Transplantation.* 2012;27(9):3435-3442.

9. McMahon EJ, Campbell KL, Bauer JD, Mudge DW. Altered dietary salt intake for people with chronic kidney disease. *Cochrane Database of Systematic Reviews.* 2015;2015(2):Art. No.: CD010070.

10. Ritz E, Koleganova N, Piecha G. Role of sodium intake in the progression of chronic kidney disease. *Journal of Renal Nutrition.* 2009;19(1):61-62.

CHAPTER 17

Hyperlipidemia/Dyslipidemia

High cholesterol and triglycerides (aka fats) in our blood are a very common issues for people with kidney disease.[1] When I was diagnosed with a kidney disorder, my total cholesterol was over 450. One of the confusing issues that arose over the past decade is conflicting data on the risks of high cholesterol for the public.

I assumed this would be a clear-cut issue. I was wrong (as usual). I thought treating high cholesterol is always beneficial. This might not be the case. It may still be the right thing to do, but whether we get the benefits from medication is not always clear. Intriguingly, certain patients may derive little to no benefit from cholesterol-lowering medications. This was very surprising to me.

We need to be very careful while looking at these studies and research papers. We need to focus on people with kidney disease and not the healthy public. When you read something about cholesterol, it may not apply to you.

Some basic definitions:

Lipids are a large group of fatty acids that occur naturally. For our purposes here, lipids are the fats in the bloodstream.[2]

LDL stands for the low-density lipoproteins. LDL is the type of cholesterol that we don't want in our body. Think of the L in LDL as low. We want lower levels of LDL.[3]

HDL stands for the high-density lipoproteins. HDL is what we want to be higher than LDL, as HDL carries LDL away from our arteries.[4] H is for High in HDL, and so, we want high HDL.

Triglycerides are the most common fats in our body. We want triglycerides to be low. We eat triglycerides, and our body makes them as well.[5]

Hyperlipidemia refers to the elevation of lipids or fats in our bloodstream above the normal range.[6]

Dyslipidemia is lipids above or below the average ranges. You can consider this to be a problem with lipids overall.[7]

Hypercholesterolemia refers to a high cholesterol level. This applies to total cholesterol. There is no absolute cutoff, but anything over 250 is considered high. The formula for calculating total cholesterol is LDL +HDL +(Triglycerides/5).[8]

Statins is the term used to describe the most popular cholesterol-lowering medications like Lipitor, with the generic name Atorvastatin.[9]

The first question we need to ask is, "Do high total cholesterol, HDL, LDL, or triglycerides contribute to kidney disease progression? Could it be that the lipids are related only to heart diseases?

I assumed that high cholesterol or high triglycerides levels contributed to the kidney disease progression.

Study 17.1   Dyslipidemia Associated with Chronic Kidney Disease[10]

CONCLUSIONS:

Dyslipidemia is a very common complication of CKD. Disturbances in lipoprotein metabolism are evident even at the early stages of CKD and usually follow a downhill course that parallels the deterioration in renal function. Recently published studies indicate that dyslipidemia in these patients may actively participate in the pathogenesis of CVD as well as in the deterioration of renal function. Thus, we believe that the current evidence dictates the use of statins in patients with mild to moderate CKD. On the other hand, in subjects with ESRD, the decision for the institution of lipid-lowering therapy should be individualized. Thus, in individuals with estab-lished CVD as well as in those who run a high risk for acute pancreatitis due to severe hypertriglyceridemia the administration of hypolipidemic drugs (statins and gemfibrozil, respectively) is a safe and reasonable approach. However, it should be kept in mind that further studies are needed to delineate the clinical efficacy of these interventions.

Study 17.2   Chronic kidney disease and dyslipidemia[11]

ABSTRACT:

Chronic kidney disease (CKD) must be considered as a high, or even very high-risk cardiovascular risk condition, since it leads to an increase in cardiovascular mortality that continues to increase as the disease progresses. An early diagnosis of CKD is required, together with an adequate identification of the risk factors, to slow down its progression to more severe states, prevent complications, and to delay, whenever possible, the need for renal replacement therapy. Dyslipidemia is a factor of the progression of CKD that increases the risk of developing atherosclerosis and its complications. Its proper control contributes to reducing the elevated cardiovascular morbidity and mortality presented by these patients. In this review, an assessment is made of the lipid-lowering therapeutic measures required to achieve to recommended objectives, by adjusting the treatment to the progression of the disease and the characteristics of the patient. In CKD, it seems that an early and intensive intervention of the dyslipidemia is a priority before there is a significant decrease in kidney function. Treatment with statins has been shown to be safe and effective in decreasing LDL-Cholesterol, and in the reduction of cardiovascular events in individuals with CKD, or after renal transplant, although there is less evidence in the case of dialyzed patients.

Study 17.3   Low levels of high-density lipoprotein cholesterol increase the risk of incident kidney disease and its progression.[12]

ABSTRACT:

Available experimental evidence suggests a role for high density lipoprotein cholesterol (HDL-C) in incident chronic kidney disease (CKD) and its progression. However, clinical studies are inconsistent. We, therefore, built a cohort of 1,943,682 male US veterans and used survival models to examine the association between HDL-C and risks of incident CKD or CKD progression (doubling of serum creatinine, eGFR decline of 30% or more), or a composite outcome of ESRD, dialysis, or renal transplantation. Models were adjusted for demographics, comorbid conditions, eGFR, body mass index, lipid parameters, and statin use over a median follow-up of 9 years. Compared to those with HDL-C of 40 mg/dl or more, low HDL-C (under 30 mg/dl) was associated with increased risk of incident eGFR under 60 ml/min/1.73 m (2) (hazard ratio: 1.18; confidence interval: 1.17-1.19) and risk of incident CKD (1.20; 1.18-1.22). Adjusted models demonstrate an association between low HDL-C and doubling of serum creatinine (1.14; 1.12-1.15), eGFR decline of 30% or more (1.13; 1.12-1.14), and the composite renal end (1.08; 1.061.11). Cubic spline analyses of the relationship between HDL-C levels and renal outcomes showed a U-shaped relationship, where the risk was increased in lowest and highest deciles of HDL-C. Thus, a significant association exists between low HDL-C levels and risks of incident CKD and CKD progression. Further studies are needed to explain the increased risk of adverse renal outcomes in patients with high HDL-C.

Note: A study of over one million patients indicated a link between low HDL and kidney disease progression.

Here's a study of the link between a high level of HDL and kidney disease progression to see if we can verify the idea that HDL is related to kidney disease progression.

Study 17.4   **High density lipoprotein cholesterol levels are an independent predictor of the progression of chronic kidney disease.[13]**

CONCLUSION:

CKD patients with low levels of plasma HDL-C have a poor prognosis. HDL functionality is also impaired in renal dysfunction. These data support the relevance of HDL in influencing CKD progression.

Study 17.5   **Impact of the Triglycerides to High-Density Lipoprotein Cholesterol Ratio on the Incidence and Progression of CKD: A Longitudinal Study in a Large Japanese Population.[14]**

CONCLUSION:

A higher TG: HDL-C ratio affects the decline in eGFR and incidence and progression of CKD in the Japanese population.

Note: TG:HDL-C refers to the ratio of triglycerides to HDL cholesterol.

Study 17.6   Non-HDL-cholesterol to HDL-cholesterol ratio as an independent risk factor for the development of chronic kidney disease.[15]

CONCLUSIONS:

Nonhle/HDLc ratio is an independent risk factor for the development of CKD. Assessment of NonHDLc/HDLc ratio may help identify high-risk groups with chronic kidney disease.

Note: This ratio is like the triglycerides ratio from the previous study.

These studies highlight the fact that HDL is protective of our bodies in some way. But, how can the way that HDL helps people with kidney disease still not be understood? We know raising HDL is a good strategy for slowing heart disease progression. HDL particles reduce the macrophage accumulation, prevent or delay the development of atherosclerosis, and transport the unhealthy fats out of our arteries.

How about LDL?

Study 17.7   Effects of Lowering LDL Cholesterol on Progression of Kidney Disease.[16]

ABSTRACT:

Lowering LDL cholesterol reduces the risk of developing atherosclerotic events in CKD, but the effects of such treatment on progression of kidney disease remain uncertain. Here, 6245 participants with CKD (not on dialysis) were randomly assigned to simvastatin (20 mg) plus ezetimibe (10 mg) daily or matching placebo. The main prespecified renal outcome was ESRD (defined as the initiation of maintenance dialysis or kidney transplantation). During 4.8 years of follow-up, allocation to simvastatin plus ezetimibe resulted in an average LDL cholesterol difference (SEM) of 0.96 (0.02) mmol/L com-pared with placebo. There was a nonsignificant 3% reduction in the incidence of ESRD (1057 [33.9%] cases with simvastatin plus ezetimibe versus 1084 [34.6%] cases with placebo; rate ratio, 0.97; 95% confidence interval [95% CI], 0.89 to 1.05; P=0.41). Similarly, allocation to simvastatin plus ezetimibe had no significant effect on the prespecified tertiary outcomes of ESRD or death (1477 [47.4%] events with treatment versus 1513 [48.3%] events with placebo; rate ratio, 0.97; 95% CI, 0.90 to 1.04; P=0.34) or ESRD or doubling of baseline creatinine (1189 [38.2%] events with treatment versus 1257 [40.2%] events with placebo; rate ratio, 0.93; 95% CI, 0.86 to 1.01; P=0.09). Exploratory analyses also showed no significant effect on the rate of change in eGFR. Lowering LDL cholesterol by 1 mmol/L did not slow kidney disease progression within 5 years in a wide range of patients with CKD.

Several studies on LDL have references to the same five-year study. Finding good data on LDL effects is hard. We have to say we don't know much about the effects of LDL on kidney disease progression.

What else can we find to help us know the facts about LDL?

Study 17.8   Relation of serum lipids and lipoproteins with progression of CKD: The CRIC study.[17]

CONCLUSION:

In this large cohort of patients with CKD, total cholesterol, triglycerides, VLDL-C, LDL-C, HDL-C, apoA-I, apoB, and Lp(a) were not independently associated with progression of kidney disease. There was an inverse relationship between LDL-C and total cholesterol levels and kidney disease outcomes in patients with low levels of proteinuria.

> **Note:** VLDL (very low-density lipoproteins) and apoA1 and apoB are the proteins involved in the lipid management and transport.

Study 17.9   Is Lipid Management Effective for All Stages of CKD?[18]

Note: This is a very well-done study, and everyone with kidney disease should read it: https://www.karger.com/Article/FullText/345932#ref28

I am going to summarize the findings here:

1. Overall, kidney patients benefit from statin therapy.

2. The benefits may not be seen if you are at ESRD, on dialysis, or are a transplant recipient.

3. Statins may help to slow the kidney disease progression.

4. Patients with high proteinuria appear to benefit more than those without this condition.

5. It is likely that atorvastatin (Lipitor) is the best statin for kidney patients at the time of this study.

What this study suggests that treating high cholesterol and triglycerides earlier is beneficial and the use of statins, especially atorvastatin, may be protective for the patients to a small extent. It also suggests that, once you have progressed to ESRD or dialysis, the benefits of using statins may not be effective.

The concept that the cholesterol-reducing medications work in only certain stages of kidney diseases is new to me. However, the research is pretty solid. Treating high cholesterol from stage 2 onward is beneficial and treating it over the long-term appears to be helpful. However, treating high cholesterol in stage 5 may not yield the same benefits. I wanted to know why.

Study 17.10   Low-dose atorvastatin in severe chronic kidney disease patients: a randomized, controlled endpoint study.[19]

CONCLUSIONS:

Although atorvastatin reduced total and LDL cholesterol efficiently it was not beneficial regarding the long-term outcomes of cardiovascular endpoints or survival. In contrast to other patient groups, <u>patients with severe chronic kidney disease, especially those on dialysis, seem to derive limited benefit from this lower dose of atorvastatin.</u>

The next study suggests the opposite.

Study 17.11 — Effect of statins on survival in patients undergoing dialysis access for end-stage renal disease.[20]

<u>Use of statins might halve the risk of all-cause mortality at 5 years in adult patients with vascular access for chronic dialysis.</u> Statins therapy should be considered in end stage renal disease populations requiring dialysis access placement.

How can this be? Lowering cholesterol should yield benefits for all of us, right? The issue seems to be calcium again. Calcification of our arteries takes place even with the statin treatment. In fact, the Cleveland Clinic reports that statins can increase calcification in our arteries. Hence, cholesterol is lowered, but calcification may be increased. This is bad news for most of us taking a statin (almost everyone) and those of us taking some form of supplemental calcium.

The following study is conducted on healthy patients.

Study 17.12 — Impact of statins on serial coronary calcification during atheroma progression and regression.[21]

CONCLUSIONS:

<u>Independent of their plaque-regressive effects, statins promote coronary atheroma calcification.</u> These findings provide an insight into how statins may stabilize plaque beyond their effects on plaque regression.

Note: Atheroma is the fatty material that forms plaques in the arteries.

In kidney transplant patients:

Study 17.13 — Effect of Statins on the Progression of Coronary Calcification (CAC) in Kidney Transplant Recipients.[22]

CONCLUSION:

<u>Although statins reduced the levels of cholesterol, triglycerides, inflammation and improve graft function, the dose adopted in the current study did not delay CAC progression within 12 months of follow up.</u>

Study 17.14 Does statins promote vascular calcification in chronic kidney disease?[23]

RESULTS:

Among 240 patients, 129 (53%) had a CAC score > 100 AUs. Multivariate analysis revealed that independent predictors of 1-SD higher CAC score were age, male gender, diabetes and use of statins. The association between CAC score and mortality remained significant after adjustment for age, gender, diabetes, CVD, use of statins, protein-energy wasting and inflammation. Repeated CAC imaging in 35 patients showed that statin therapy was associated with greater progression of CAC. In vitro synthesis of menaquinone-4 by hVSMCs was significantly impaired by statins.

CONCLUSION:

Elevated CAC score is a mortality risk factor in ESRD independent of inflammation. Future studies should resolve if statins promote vascular calcification and inhibition of vitamin K synthesis in the uremic milieu.

Study 17.15 Reasons for the lack of salutary effects of cholesterol lowering interventions in ESRD populations.[24]

ABSTRACT:

Cardiovascular disease (CVD) is the main cause of premature death in patients with chronic kidney disease (CKD). The underlying mechanisms of CVD in patients with mild to moderate CKD are different from those with end-stage renal disease (ESRD). While serum cholesterol is frequently elevated and contributes to atherosclerosis in many CKD patients particularly those with nephrotic proteinuria, it is usually normal, even subnormal in most ESRD patients receiving hemodialysis. CVD in the ESRD population is primarily driven by oxidative stress, inflammation, accumulation of the oxidation-prone intermediate density lipoproteins (IDL), chylomicron remnants and small dense LDL particles as well as HDL deficiency and dysfunction, hypertension, vascular calcification, and arrhythmias. Only a minority of hemodialysis patients have hypercholesterolemia which is most likely due to genetic or unrelated factors.

In addition, due to peritoneal losses of proteins which simulate nephrotic syndrome, peritoneal dialysis patients often exhibit hypercholesterolemia. Clearly when present, hypercholesterolemia contributes to CVD in CKD and ESRD population and justifies cholesterol lowering therapy. However, the majority of ESRD patients and a subpopulation of CKD patients with minimal proteinuria have normal or subnormal serum cholesterol levels and do not benefit from and can be potentially harmed by statin therapy. In fact, the lack of efficacy of statins in hemodialysis patients has been demonstrated in several randomized clinical trials. This review is intended to provide an overview of the mechanisms responsible for the failure of statins to reduce cardiovascular morbidity and mortality in most ESRD patients and to advocate the adoption of individualized care principal in the management of dyslipidemia in this population.

Study 17.16 — Effects of lipid-lowering therapy on reduction of cardiovascular events in patients with end-stage renal disease requiring hemodialysis.[25]

ABSTRACT:

In the general population, dyslipidemia is an established independent risk factor for cardiovascular disease. In patients with end-stage renal disease (ESRD), comorbid cardiovascular disease is present at alarming rates, and those who require hemodialysis and have cardiovascular disease continue to have a high mortality rate. Lipid abnormalities associated with chronic kidney disease (CKD) vary depending on the stage of disease (stages 1-5), but low-density lipoprotein cholesterol (LDL) has been established as the primary lipid treatment target. Guidelines support an LDL level of less than 100 mg/ dl in patients with all stages of CKD, except when the triglyceride level is above 500 mg/dl. As patients progress to stage 5 CKD (ESRD with hemodialysis), the high triglyceride, low high-density lipoprotein cholesterol, and increased lipoprotein(a) levels of the early stages become more pronounced, with increases in small dense LDL particles; however, total cholesterol and LDL values remain normal or decrease. In patients undergoing hemodialysis, lipid abnormalities are driven by an increase in hepatic secretion and delayed catabolism of very low-density lipoproteins, as well as a reduction in lipoprotein lipase and hepatic lipase. Epidemiologic data support the role of cholesterol lowering to lower cardiovascular events in the hemodialysis population. We conducted a literature search of various databases (1966-September 2009) to identify relevant clinical trials that evaluated the efficacy and safety of multiple lipid-lowering agents for the treatment of dyslipidemia in patients with ESRD requiring hemodialysis. Only those trials that used clinical primary end points of coronary heart disease (e.g., cardiovascular death, myocardial infarction, stroke) were included in this review. Evidence demonstrates that 3-hydroxy-3methylglutaryl coenzyme A reductase inhibitor (statin) therapy (i.e., atorvastatin and rosuvastatin) significantly reduces surrogate cardiovascular markers, particularly LDL, in patients with ESRD requiring hemodialysis; however, no statin has proved to reduce cardiovascular morbidity or mortality in this population. Trials evaluating omega-3 fatty acids did not show significant reductions in LDL or cardiovascular events in this population. Clinicians should appreciate these limitations when deciding whether to continue lipid-lowering pharmaco therapy in these patients, depending on their overall cardiovascular risk assessment.

The suggestion here is statins do not work at advanced stages of kidney diseases. By reading between the lines, we can see that vascular calcification is the killer at this stage and not high cholesterol. Statins may promote vascular calcification. Another viewpoint is statins can help repair the plaques or keep them in place. Back to a catch-22 situation! Using statins helps with cholesterol, but may increase the rate of vascular calcification, the number one killer of kidney patients.

Statins may produce an anti-inflammatory effect, which is why they may help patients with proteinuria. Proteinuria is related to inflammation. So, it makes sense that statins are anti-inflammatory agents and hence, can reduce proteinuria.

Study 17.17   Are statins anti-inflammatory?[26]

ABSTRACT:

Large scale clinical trials demonstrate significant reductions in cardiovascular event rates with sta-tin therapy. The observed benefit of statin therapy, however, may be larger in these trials than that expected on the basis of lipid lowering alone. Emerging evidence from both clinical trials and basic science studies suggest that statins have anti-inflammatory properties, which may additionally lead to clinical efficacy. Measurement of markers of inflammation such as high sensitivity C-reactive protein in addition to lipid parameters may help identify those patients who will benefit most from statin therapy.

Study 17.18   Role of preoperative atorvastatin administration in protection against postoperative atrial fibrillation following conventional coronary artery bypass grafting.[27]

Preoperative atorvastatin administration may inhibit inflammatory reactions to prevent atrial fibrillation following coronary artery bypass grafting with cardiopulmonary bypass.

Study 17.19   Postoperative statin therapy attenuates the intensity of systemic inflammation and increases fibrinolysis after coronary artery bypass grafting.[28]

Statin treatment caused a significant reduction in plasma IL-8 level (279.70 ± 3.42 ng/mL vs postop: 207.18 ± 3.63 ng/mL, $P < .05$), and TFPI (4.87 ± 2.05 ng/mL vs postop:

6.27 ± 1.25 ng/mL; $P < .05$). The results demonstrate that atorvastatin attenuates systemic inflammatory reaction after cardiac surgery.

In healthy adults, statins appear to be anti-inflammatory to some extent. If this is true, statins should reduce proteinuria or albumin in our urine.

Study 17.20   Potential benefit of statin therapy for dyslipidemia with chronic kidney disease: Fluvastatin Renal Evaluation Trial (FRET).[29]

CONCLUSION:

Fluvastatin reduces both UAE (Urinary albumin excretion) and the urinary L-FABP (urinary liver-type fatty acid binding protein) level, and thus, has renoprotective effects, independent of its lipid-lowering effects in dyslipidemic patients with CKD.

The weight of the evidence suggests the following:

1.   You must still treat vascular calcification, independent of statin use, by reducing supplemental calcium and lowering intake of cholesterol, phosphorus, and saturated fats. Statins may increase the rate of vascular calcification, which is already accelerated in people

with kidney disease. Treating high cholesterol but not treating vascular calcification may negate any benefits from statins when the kidney disease has progressed to the advanced stages. Inflammation and oxidative stress are also a few factors contributing to vascular calcification.

2. Statins may be anti-inflammatory and, hence, can help patients with proteinuria to a higher degree than the patients without proteinuria. This benefit is likely due to the anti-inflammatory properties that statins may have. (More proof reducing inflammation is key.)

3. It is unclear if high cholesterol contributes to the kidney disease progression, but high HDL appears to be beneficial.

4. Low LDL levels may contribute to the kidney disease progression, but supporting data is limited.

5. Higher HDL levels seem to improve our odds.

Diet Perspective on Cholesterol and Calcification

Dietary and serum recommendations from human studies of cardiovascular calcification are few. However, what we do know is the same diet that helps with other health issues may also reduce the vascular calcification.

Study 17.21   A Review of the Effect of Diet on Cardiovascular Calcification.[30]

ABSTRACT:

Cardiovascular (CV) calcification is known as sub-clinical atherosclerosis and is recognized as a predictor of CV events and mortality. As yet there is no treatment for CV calcification and conventional CV risk factors are not consistently correlated, leaving clinicians uncertain as to optimum management for these patients. For this reason, a review of studies investigating diet and serum levels of macro- and micronutrients was carried out. Although there were few human studies of macronutrients, nevertheless transfats and simple sugars should be avoided, while long chain ω-3 fats from oily fish may be protective. *__Among the micronutrients, an intake of 800 μg/day calcium was beneficial in those without renal disease or hyperparathyroidism, while inorganic phosphorus from food preservatives and colas may induce calcification. A high intake of magnesium (≥380 mg/ day) and phylloquinone (500 μg/day) proved protective, as did a serum 25(OH)D concentration of ≥75 nmol/L. Although oxidative damage appears to be a cause of CV calcification, the antioxidant vitamins proved to be largely ineffective, while supplementation of α-tocopherol may induce calcification. Nevertheless, other antioxidant compounds (epigallocatechin gallate from green tea and resveratrol from red wine) were protective. Finally, a homocysteine concentration >12 μmol/L was predictive of CV calcification, although a plasma folate concentration of >39.4 nmol/L could both lower homocysteine and protect against calcification.__*

In terms of a dietary program, these recommendations indicate avoiding sugar and the transfats and preservatives found in processed foods and drinks and adopting a diet high in oily fish and vegetables. The micronutrients magnesium and vitamin K may be worthy of further investigation as a treatment option for CV calcification.

Note: Back to the same issues we have talked about earlier: inorganic phosphorus, calcium, magnesium, and oxidative stress.

Study 17.22   Lowering LDL-cholesterol through diet: potential role in the statin era.[31]

SUMMARY:

Dietary recommendations may have an impressive impact on cardiovascular events because they can be implemented early in life and because the sum of the effect on LDL-cholesterol is far from being negligible: step 1 diet (-10%), dietary fibers (-5 to -10%), plant sterols/stanols (-10%), nut consumption (-8%), and soy protein (-3 to -10%).

Study 17.23   Dietary intervention to lower serum cholesterol.[32]

DISCUSSION:

Interventions that lower LDL-C lower the risk of cardiovascular disease. Comprehensive dietary intervention is indicated in all patients with an absolute 5-year risk for coronary disease of 10% or greater. Short-term trials indicate that these interventions have the potential to lower LDL-C by approximately 20%. A year-long trial has shown mean LDL-C lowering of 13%, with about one-third of subjects achieving a reduction greater than 20%, highlighting the importance of adherence to dietary advice. The most effective dietary strategies are replacing saturated and trans fatty acids with poly- and monounsaturated fats and increasing intake of plant sterols. Losing weight and increasing soluble fiber and soy protein intake can also lower serum choles-terol and may be considered when recommending a nutritionally balanced, cholesterol-lowering diet. Motivational interviewing by general practitioners can improve the effectiveness of brief, behavior orientated advice and dietary counseling to lower serum cholesterol.

In addition to a healthy diet, here are some known ways to increase the HDL levels.

1. Stop smoking

2. Start exercising, or exercise a little more

3. Lose weight

4. Have a drink a day (and I mean one)

5. Reduce or eliminate animal products such as meat and eggs

6. Be very careful with calcium intake (This seems to be a theme!)

7. Treat oxidative stress

8. Examine intake of niacin, which may increase HDL; data is mixed.

10. Manage your cholesterol. High cholesterol is not the smoking gun I once thought. However, if we don't manage cholesterol it "may" accelerate kidney and heart disease progression. I say "may" because the data is not one-sided like it has been for the other topics.

A healthy kidney and heart diet combined with exercise and possibly statin use is something we should all be doing. If you are not taking a statin now and have proteinuria, talk to your doctor.

References

1. Widiasta A, Pardede SO, Rachmadi D. Correlation between LDL, HDL, Total Cholesterol, and Triglyceride with the Degree of Chronic Kidney Disease in Children. *American Journal of Clinical Medicine Research*. 2017;5(1):1-5.

2. Am Fam Physician. Reducing the Lipid Levels in Your Blood. *American Academy of Family Physicians*. 1998;57(9):2207-2208.

3. Gotto AM, Grundy SM. Lowering LDL cholesterol. *Circulation*. 1999;99(8):e1-e7.

4. Barter P, Gotto AM, LaRosa JC, et al. HDL cholesterol, very low levels of LDL cholesterol, and cardiovascular events. *New England Journal of Medicine*. 2007;357(13):1301-1310.

5. Cox R, Garcia-Palmieri M. Cholesterol, Triglycerides, and Associated Lipoproteins. In: HK W, WD H, JW H, eds. *Clinical Methods: The History, Physical, and Laboratory Examinations*. 3rd ed. Boston: Butterworths; 1990.

6. Goldstein JL, Hazzard WR, Schrott HG, Bierman EL, Motulsky AG. Hyperlipidemia in coronary heart disease I. Lipid levels in 500 survivors of myocardial infarction. *Journal of Clinical Investigation*. 1973;52(7):1533.

7. Brown CD, Higgins M, Donato KA, et al. Body mass index and the prevalence of hypertension and dyslipidemia. *Obesity*. 2000;8(9):605-619.

8. Illingworth DR. Management of hypercholesterolemia. *Medical Clinics of North America*. 2000;84(1):23-42.

9. Unit ES. Efficacy and safety of cholesterol-lowering treatment: prospective meta-analysis of data from 90 056 participants in 14 randomised trials of statins. *Lancet*. 2005;366(9493):12671278.

10. Tsimihodimos V, Mitrogianni Z, Elisaf M. Dyslipidemia associated with chronic kidney disease. *The Open Cardiovascular Medicine Journal*. 2011;5:41-48.

11. Omran J, Al-Dadah A, Dellsperger KC. Dyslipidemia in patients with chronic and end-stage kidney disease. *Cardiorenal Medicine*. 2013;3(3):165-177.

12. Bowe B, Xie Y, Xian H, Balasubramanian S, Al-Aly Z. Low levels of high-density lipoprotein cholesterol increase the risk of incident kidney disease and its progression. *Kidney International*. 2016;89(4):886-896.

13. Baragetti A, Norata G, Sarcina C, et al. High density lipoprotein cholesterol levels are an independent predictor of the progression of chronic kidney disease. *Journal of Internal Medicine*. 2013;274(3):252-262.

14. Tsuruya K, Yoshida H, Nagata M, et al. Impact of the triglycerides to high-density lipoprotein cholesterol ratio on the incidence and progression of CKD: a longitudinal study in a large Japanese population. *American Journal of Kidney Diseases*. 2015;66(6):972-983.

15. Zuo P, Chen X, Liu Y, Zhang R, He X, Liu C. Non-HDL-cholesterol to HDL-cholesterol ratio as an independent risk factor for the development of chronic kidney disease. *Nutrition, Metabolism and Cardiovascular Diseases*. 2015;25(6):582-587.

16. Haynes R, Lewis D, Emberson J, et al. Effects of lowering LDL cholesterol on progression of kidney disease. *Journal of the American Society of Nephrology*. 2014;25(8):1825-1833.

17. Rahman M, Yang W, Akkina S, et al. Relation of serum lipids and lipoproteins with progression of CKD: The CRIC study. *Clinical Journal of the American Society of Nephrology*. 2014:CJN. 09320913.

18. Ku E, Campese V. Is lipid management effective for all stages of CKD. *Blood Purification*. 2013;35(1-3):26-30.

19. Stegmayr B, Brännström M, Bucht S, et al. Low-dose atorvastatin in severe chronic kidney disease patients: a randomized, controlled endpoint study. *Scandinavian Journal of Urology and Nephrology*. 2005;39(6):489-497.

20. De Rango P, Parente B, Farchioni L, et al. Effect of statins on survival in patients undergoing dialysis access for end stage renal disease. *Seminars in Vascular Surgery*. 2017;29(4):198-205.

21. Puri R, Nicholls SJ, Shao M, et al. Impact of statins on serial coronary calcification during atheroma progression and regression. *Journal of the American College of Cardiology*. 2015;65(13):1273-1282.

22. Yazbek DC, de Carvalho AB, Barros CS, Pestana JOM, Canziani MEF. Effect of statins on the progression of coronary calcification in kidney transplant recipients. *PloS One*. 2016;11(4):e0151797.

23. Chen Z, Qureshi AR, Parini P, et al. Does statins promote vascular calcification in chronic kidney disease? *European Journal of Clinical Investigation*. 2017;47(2):137-148.

24. Vaziri ND, Norris KC. Reasons for the lack of salutary effects of cholesterol-lowering interventions in end-stage renal disease populations. *Blood Purification*. 2013;35(1-3):31-36.

25. Marrs JC, Saseen JJ. Effects of Lipid-Lowering Therapy on Reduction of Cardiovascular Events in Patients with End-Stage Renal Disease Requiring Hemodialysis. Pharmacotherapy: *The Journal of Human Pharmacology and Drug Therapy*. 2010;30(8):823-829.

26. Blake GJ, Ridker PM. Are statins anti-inflammatory? *Trials*. 2000;1(3):161.

27. Sun Y, Ji Q, Mei Y, et al. Role of preoperative atorvastatin administration in protection against postoperative atrial fibrillation following conventional coronary artery bypass grafting. *International Heart Journal*. 2011;52(1):7-11.

28. Tetik S, Ak K, Sahin Y, et al. Postoperative statin therapy attenuates the intensity of systemic inflammation and increases fibrinolysis after coronary artery bypass grafting. *Clinical and Applied Thrombosis/Hemostasis*. 2011;17(5):526-531.

29. Inoue T, Ikeda H, Nakamura T, et al. Potential benefit of statin therapy for dyslipidemia with chronic kidney disease: Fluvastatin Renal Evaluation Trial (FRET). *Internal Medicine.* 2011;50(12):1273-1278.

30. Nicoll R, Howard JM, Henein MY. A review of the effect of diet on cardiovascular calcification. *International Journal of Molecular Sciences.* 2015;16(4):8861-8883.

31. Bruckert E, Rosenbaum D. Lowering LDL-cholesterol through diet: potential role in the statin era. *Current Opinion in Lipidology.* 2011;22(1):43-48.

32. Clifton P, Colquhoun D, Hewat C, et al. Dietary intervention to lower serum cholesterol. *Australian Family Physician.* 2009;38(6):424.

CHAPTER 18

Uremic Toxins

"Uremic toxins" was another term that was new to me before I began my research. Uremic toxins are related to uremia, the buildup of waste in the blood stream. However, these are somewhat different than normal waste produced from the breakdown of proteins. Uremic toxins are produced by bacteria in the bowels acting on proteins (amino acids) that escape digestion in the intestines. Hundreds of these toxins exist, yet we still don't know a lot about them.[1] These compounds are toxic to your kidneys and heart. Thanks to the crosstalk effect, they also influence other organs. Our kidneys normally process and excrete these toxic compounds, but damaged kidneys can't do this job as well, so the toxins build up in our systems over time. CKD patients have, on average, a concentration of toxins that's 5.2 times higher than levels in healthy subjects.[2] That's a 520% increase in uremic toxins compared to a healthy person.

Of the hundreds of uremic toxins, indoxyl sulfate (IS) and P-cresol sulfate (PCS) are the most studied to date. These result from the amino acids tryptophan and tyrosine, respectively. Indoxyl sulfate is toxic for the kidneys, heart, and bones. Some reports suggest that IS is directly associated with renal function loss and mortality in CKD patients. Indoxyl sulfate is also associated with heart disease. P-cresol sulfate is associated with renal disease progression and an increased risk of cardiovascular events.

Here's what the research says:

Study 18.1 — Serum Indoxyl Sulfate Is Associated with Vascular Disease and Mortality in Chronic Kidney Disease Patients.[3]

In the study presented here, we have demonstrated for the first time that there is a gradual rise in serum IS with the severity of CKD from the very earliest stages of the disease. Moreover, serum IS being directly associated with aortic calcification and vascular stiffness. Most importantly, higher serum IS was associated with an increased overall and cardiovascular mortality risk in the study cohort. This effect was independent of age, gender, diabetes mellitus, phosphate, albumin and hemoglobin levels, vascular stiffness, and aortic calcification.

Study 18.2 — p-Cresyl sulfate(PCS) and indoxyl sulfate predict progression of chronic kidney disease.[4]

Of 268 patients, 35 (13.1%) had renal progression, and 14 (5.2%) died after a mean follow-up of 21 ± 3 months. Univariate Cox regression analysis followed by multivariate analysis showed that high-serum PCS levels were associated with renal progression and all-cause mortality independent of age, gender, diabetes status, albumin levels, serum IS, serum creatinine, Ca × P product, intact parathyroid hormone, hemoglobin or high-sensitivity C-reactive protein level. Serum IS was only associated with renal progression; however, the predictive power of serum IS was weakened when serum PCS was also present in the analytical model.

In addition to traditional and uricemia-related risk factors such as renal function, serum IS, and PCS levels may help in predicting the risk of renal progression in patients having different stages of CKD.

Study 18.3 — The uremic toxin, indoxyl sulfate, signifies cardio-renal risk and intestinal-renal relationship.[5]

One of [the uremic toxins] is a member of the indol group, the indoxyl sulfate. This toxin is difficult to remove with dialysis and is an endogenous protein-bound uremic toxin. Today we know that indoxyl sulfate is a vascular-nephrotoxic agent, which can enhance the progression of cardiovascular and renal diseases. It is of particular importance that because of its redox potency, this toxin causes oxidative stress and antioxidant effects at the same time and, on top of that, it is formed in the intestinal system. Its serum concentration depends on the nutrition and the tubular function and, therefore, it can also signal the progression of chronic renal failure independently of glomerular filtration rate. Successful removal of indoxyl sulfate reduces the morbidity and mortality and improves survival.

Study 18.4 — Indoxyl sulfate and kidney disease: Causes, consequences, and interventions.[6]

At least 152 uremic retention solutes have been reported. This review focuses on indoxyl sulfate (IS), a protein-bound, tryptophan-derived metabolite that is generated by intestinal microorganisms (microbiota). Animal studies have demonstrated an association between IS accumulation and increased fibrosis, and oxidative stress. This has been mirrored by in vitro studies, many of which report cytotoxic effects in kidney proximal tubular cells following IS exposure. Clinical studies have associated IS accumulation with deleterious effects, such as kidney functional decline and adverse cardiovascular events, although causality has not been conclusively established.

Study 18.5 — Meta-Analysis of the Associations of p-Cresyl Sulfate (PCS) and Indoxyl Sulfate (IS) with Cardiovascular Events and All-Cause Mortality in Patients with Chronic Renal Failure.[7]

Elevated levels of PCS and IS are associated with increased mortality in patients with CKD, while PCS, but not IS, is associated with an increased risk of cardiovascular events.

Study 18.6 — p-Cresyl sulfate and indoxyl sulfate predict progression of chronic kidney disease.[4]

CONCLUSIONS:

In addition to traditional and uremia-related risk factors such as renal function, serum IS, and PCS levels may help in predicting the risk of renal progression in patients having different stages of CKD.

Uremic toxins may be another reason people with kidney disease have the highest rates of heart disease on the planet. Toxins like indoxyl sulfate cause plaque, or calcification of our arteries, which causes our arteries to become less flexible. These toxins do not cause the same amount of damage in healthy people because their kidneys get rid of them, but as people with kidney disease, these toxins build up in our bodies, causing accelerated cardiovascular disease. Uremic toxins also create more oxidative stress on our bodies, which causes more damage. It's yet another factor that can speed the decline of our kidney function.

Some research suggests that these toxins have effects very early in kidney disease—as early as stage 2. They may have negative effects on our brain function as well as our heart and kidneys:

Study 18.7 — Indoxyl sulfate, not p-cresol sulfate, is associated with cognitive impairment in early-stage chronic kidney disease.[8]

Our study showed that a higher serum IS level was associated with a poor executive function in the early stage of CKD. It would be worthwhile to investigate the effect of IS removal in early-stage CKD on the prevention of cognitive impairment in future studies.

Now that we know about the concept of uremic toxins, what can we do about them? We know they are bad for us in all kinds of ways, but can we stop or reduce the number of uremic toxins in our bodies?

Study 18.8 — The Production of p-Cresol Sulfate (PCS) and Indoxyl Sulfate(IS) in Vegetarians Versus Omnivores.[9]

Average PCS excretion was 62% lower (95% confidence interval [95% CI], 15–83) and average IS excretion was 58% lower (95% CI, 39–71) in vegetarians than in participants consuming an unrestricted diet. Food records revealed that lower excretion of PCS and IS in vegetarians was associated with a 69% higher (95% CI, 20–139) fiber intake and a 25% lower (95% CI, 3–42) protein intake. PCS and IS excretion rates varied widely among individual participants and were not closely correlated with each other but tended to remain stable in individual participants over 1 month.

PCS and IS production rates are markedly lower in vegetarians than in individuals consuming an unrestricted diet.

Study 18.9 — Effect of Increasing Dietary Fiber on Plasma Levels of Colon-Derived Solutes in Hemodialysis Patients.[10]

Increasing dietary fiber for 6 weeks significantly reduced the unbound, free plasma level of indoxyl sulfate (median –29% [25th percentile, 75th percentile, –56, –12] for fiber versus –0.4% [–20, 34] for control, P=0.02). The reduction in free plasma levels of indoxyl sulfate was accompanied by a reduction in free plasma levels of p-cresol sulfate (r=0.81, P<0.001). However, the reduction of p-cresol sulfate levels was of a lesser magnitude and did not achieve significance (median –28% [–46, 5] for fiber versus 4% [–28, 36] for control, P=0.05).

Increasing dietary fiber in hemodialysis patients may reduce the plasma levels of the colon-derived solutes indoxyl sulfate and possibly p-cresol sulfate without the need to intensify dialysis treatments. Further studies are required to determine whether such reduction provides clinical benefits.

Study 18.10 Very low protein diet reduces indoxyl sulfate levels in chronic kidney disease.[11]

IS serum concentration was significantly higher in the HD (43.4 ± 12.3 µM) and CKD (11.1 ± 6.6 µM) groups compared to the control group (2.9 ± 1.1 µM; $p < 0.001$). IS levels also correlated with creatinine values in CKD patients ($R(2) = 0.42$; $p < 0.0001$). <u>After only 1 week of a VLPD, even preceded by an LPD, CKD patients showed a significant reduction of IS serum levels (37%).</u>

VLPD supplemented with ketoanalogues reduced IS serum levels in CKD patients not yet on dialysis.

Here's what we can learn from these studies to help us manage or lower uremic toxin levels:

1. Eat less protein. If a smaller amount of protein reaches our bowels, then a lower number of uremic toxins may be produced. Very low-protein diets lowered indoxyl sulfate levels within a week.

2. Eat a high-fiber diet. Uremic toxins build up in the bowel while undigested protein is sitting around waiting to be excreted. High-fiber diets keep things moving and don't let these proteins sit around too long. This may also be one of the reasons high-fiber diets are known to reduce heart disease.

3. If you are using a protein supplement in addition to a low protein diet, use a supplement that contains only a small amount of tryptophan or tyrosine. A tryptophan-free formula may also be good, but malnutrition risks increase. Tyrosine is not needed in stage 3 patients, so stage 3 patients don't need to supplement tyrosine at all. Stage 4 patients may take a small amount. Stage 5 patients need more tyrosine. A small amount of each is likely the best answer so we don't increase our risks.

4. As with the previous topics, no data suggests that uremic toxins provide any benefit to us. Research proves the acceleration of cognitive decline in kidney and heart disease.

Summary

Above all, one fact stands out for me when considering uremic toxins: When it comes to kidney disease, everything is connected. The effects of our diet and our current kidney function, combined with our gut flora, determine the level of toxic substances produced by bacteria in our bowels. These, in turn, are toxic to our heart, kidneys, bones, and brain.

The bad news is uremic toxins affect us very early in kidney disease—as early as stage 2. The good news is a combination of a very low-protein and high-fiber diet, supplemented with the right probiotics, can dramatically reduce these toxins. This is yet another reason people with kidney disease should not wait to go on a kidney-friendly diet. Upon diagnosis, we all should take steps to reduce uremic toxins.

Our list is building: acid load, protein, AGEs, free radicals, and now uremic toxins. While this may seem a little overwhelming, many of these are related, and all of them can be handled by the same diet and treatment plan.

Uremia or uremic toxins should be treated by diet as early as possible. Stage 2 kidney disease is when we should start. Waiting until we are diagnosed with uremia is asking for trouble.

References

1. Vanholder R, De Smet R, Glorieux G, et al. Review on uremic toxins: classification, concentration, and interindividual variability. *Kidney International.* 2003;63(5):1934-1943.

2. de Loor H, Bammens B, Evenepoel P, De Preter V, Verbeke K. Gas chromatographic–mass spectrometric analysis for measurement of p-cresol and its conjugated metabolites in uremic and normal serum. *Clinical Chemistry.* 2005;51(8):1535-1538.

3. Barreto FC, Barreto DV, Liabeuf S, et al. Serum indoxyl sulfate is associated with vascular disease and mortality in chronic kidney disease patients. *Clinical Journal of the American Society of Nephrology.* 2009;4(10):1551-1558.

4. Wu I-W, Hsu K-H, Lee C-C, et al. p-Cresyl sulfate and indoxyl sulfate predict progression of chronic kidney disease. *Nephrology Dialysis Transplantation.* 2010;26(3):938-947.

5. Kiss I. The uremic toxin indoxyl sulfate reflects cardiorenal risk and intestinal-renal relationship. *Orvosi Hetilap.* 2011;152(43):1724-1730.

6. Ellis RJ, Small DM, Vesey DA, et al. Indoxyl sulfate and kidney disease: causes, consequences, and interventions. *Nephrology.* 2016;21(3):170-177.

7. Lin C-J, Wu V, Wu P-C, Wu C-J. Meta-analysis of the associations of p-cresyl sulfate (PCS) and indoxyl sulfate (IS) with cardiovascular events and all-cause mortality in patients with chronic renal failure. *PloS one.*2015;10(7):e0132589.

8. Yeh Y-C, Huang M-F, Liang S-S, et al. Indoxyl sulfate, not p-cresyl sulfate, is associated with cognitive impairment in early-stage chronic kidney disease. *Neurotoxicology.* 2016;53:148-152.

9. Patel KP, Luo FJ-G, Plummer NS, Hostetter TH, Meyer TW. The production of p-cresol sulfate and indoxyl sulfate in vegetarians versus omnivores. *Clinical Journal of the American Society of Nephrology.* 2012;7(6):982-988.

10. Sirich TL, Plummer NS, Gardner CD, Hostetter TH, Meyer TW. Effect of increasing dietary fiber on plasma levels of colon-derived solutes in hemodialysis patients. *Clinical Journal of the American Society of Nephrology.* 2014;9(9):1603-1610.

11. Marzocco S, Dal Piaz F, Di Micco L, et al. Very low protein diet reduces indoxyl sulfate levels in chronic kidney disease. *Blood Purification.* 2013;35(1-3):196-201.

CHAPTER 19

Depression and Anxiety

When it comes to healthcare, albumin and inflammation may grab most of the attention, but one certainly cannot skip the discussion on depression. Both albumin and depression go untreated in most patients. It is hard to take good care of yourself when you are depressed and feel as if you have been subjected to a death sentence. This book focuses on improving your health situation and your quality of life, hence, it becomes essential to shed some light on this topic.

It is terrible to be diagnosed with any form of disease. Being told the first treatment failed is even worse. However, after the second treatment fails, you get the "talk" about not being able to do anything else for you, which is downright devastating. A group of us numbering in the millions are left with the speech that goes something like this: "There is nothing else we can do for you right now. However, when you reach end-stage renal disease, you will be a candidate for dialysis or a kidney transplant." The time between this speech and dialysis or transplant might be ten years or more. What does this even imply? There's nothing that can be done for a decade to help me? Upon hearing this, how can you not be depressed?

Anxiety and depression are part of this disease, whether we like it or not. Not treating depression is a mistake. If you are depressed (and you will be some of the time), you stop taking care of yourself. Your decision-making may be impaired, which may adversely affect your general life as well. Not every blood test report is going to fit your expectation. There are going to be a lot of bumps and setbacks over the years.

I know depression or mental health is a taboo subject for some. Just because it can be uncomfortable to talk about doesn't mean we shouldn't talk about it. I grew up in that culture. We were all too tough to be depressed. It is considered as a sign of weakness, vulnerability, or may present you as less of a man if you need help. Conversations can be equally difficult for women. A lot of things have changed over the years, and the attitude toward mental health is better today. However, a lot of you (like me) will still be resistant to getting help. I hope I'm wrong about this.

I have talked about mortality rates and morbidity because that is how I approached my research. I wanted to know what was going to kill me first and start addressing each issue I could. I wanted to keep increasing my odds. In fact, if this book could be boiled down to one thought, we all want to improve our odds of survival.

Depression is known to occur commonly after a heart attack, heart surgery, or any life-threatening disease. Support groups and networks are common and are used extensively for some patient populations and especially for cancer patients. However, for us, the offerings are slim to non-existent.

Let's start with why you should treat depression and anxiety early in your disease or early in your diagnosis.

FIGURE 19.1: **Association of Depressive and Anxiety Symptoms with Adverse Events in Dutch Chronic Kidney Disease Patients: a Prospective Cohort Study**[1]

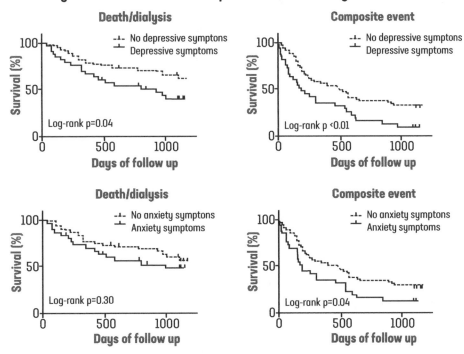

Kaplan-Meier survival curves for CKD patients with and without depressive or anxiety symptoms

The top two charts are based on depression, and the bottom two are based on anxiety symptoms. A composite event is a hospital stay or death.

As you can see, anxiety and depression lower your odds of survival over a period of three years. In the big picture, three years is a pretty short time. I assume that the difference would be even more significant over ten years.

Study 19.1 Association of symptoms of depression with progression of CKD.[2]

CONCLUSIONS:

Depressive symptoms in CKD are independent predictors of adverse clinical outcomes, including faster eGFR decrease, dialysis therapy initiation, death, or hospitalization. Depression should be evaluated early and treated in patients with CKD.

Study 19.2 Hopelessness, suicide ideation, and depression in chronic kidney disease patients on hemodialysis or transplant recipients.[3]

RESULTS:

BHS: 2% of each group scoring > 8 (p = 1.00). BSI: 4% in hemodialysis and 6% of the transplant patients scoring > 1 (p = 1.000). BDI: 20% in hemodialysis and 12% of transplant patients scoring > 14 (p = 0.275). Patients who did not have a labor activity presented more depressive symptoms (average BDI score: 10.5 vs. 7.3, p = 0.027). Transplant patients from deceased donor presented more depressive symptoms compared with those with the transplant from living donors (average BDI score: 11.0 vs. 6.7, p = 0.042).

CONCLUSION:

There was no difference in the intensity of hopelessness, suicide ideation and depression symptoms between stable hemodialysis and transplant patients. Not performing a labor activity and receiving the transplant from deceased donor lead to more depressive symptoms. The high prevalence of depressive symptoms and the finding of suicide ideation in both modalities of renal replacement therapy point to the need to monitor and care for those patients.

Patients who did not have a "labor activity," also known as a job, were more depressed than those who had a job. If we sit around and worry, our outcomes tend to be worse. Being active and engaged with family, friends, and your community will lead to a better quality of life and a better result.

In my former life as financial planner, I watched many newly-retired individuals and couples sink into a funk. In addition to their kids being on their own, couples suddenly find themselves without a job or much of anything to do each day. The lack of purpose is a bad thing. We all need to be needed in some ways. They turn inward and land in a bad place. These were healthy people without too much to worry about.

Imagine sitting at home all day, just thinking about being sick and not much else. You will land in a very bad place mentally. Taking care of yourself by doing something for others is great therapy.

Don't forget, this disease isn't just about you. How you feel will affect your spouse, kids, coworkers, friends, and so on. Getting help is good for everyone in your life. Don't forget about the other people your disease affects.

Study 19.3 Depression and chronic kidney disease: A review for clinicians.[4]

CONCLUSIONS:

Depression is common in CKD and is associated with a significant risk of adverse outcomes. Given the importance of this issue, there is now an urgent need for well-conducted randomized trials of interventions for depression in CKD to provide information on the safety and efficacy of treatments.

Study 19.4   **Association of depression and anxiety with reduced quality of life in patients with predialysis chronic kidney disease.**[5]

CONCLUSIONS:

<u>Patients with predialysis CKD have a high prevalence of depression and anxiety, which are associated with reduced quality of life (QOL).</u> Early detection of depression and anxiety and active interventions should be considered to improve the QOL of these patients.

Study 19.5   **Association between uremic toxins and depression in patients with chronic kidney disease undergoing maintenance hemodialysis.**[6]

RESULTS:

<u>Depressive patients had lower body mass index, lower serum creatinine, lower serum albumin and lower total IS. Univariate and multivariate logistic regression analyses that adjusted for age, gender, and other statistically significant variables indicated that depression was significantly and independently associated with lower serum albumin and lower total IS.</u> The levels of urea, $\beta2$ microglobulin and PCS were not significantly associated with depression.

CONCLUSION:

<u>Our results indicate that depression in patients with CKD was significantly and independently associated with lower serum albumin and lower total IS.</u> However, the pathological mechanisms underlying these associations are unknown.

I included the last study because it provides the link between depression and low serum albumin. Again, low serum albumin may reflect not taking care of ourselves.

We can debate how depression and anxiety are related to kidney disease progression and still never agree on the cause. Nevertheless, the reason doesn't matter. We already know with some certainty that depression and anxiety reduce our odds of survival.

The Struggle for Life

The Struggle for Life is a book about the psychology of living with kidney disease. I read this book because I wondered about something referred to as "medical noncompliance." Why don't we do the things necessary to live longer and live better? Why don't we follow the directions of healthcare providers? Why do I want a bacon cheeseburger when I know I should have the blueberry salad? I know on a logical basis what I should be eating, but emotionally the bacon cheeseburger is calling out my name. While my wife may think I am noncompliant all of the time, I shouldn't be when it comes to taking care of myself. A lot of people depend on me. It makes no sense to do things that are self-destructive or destructive to my kidneys.

Emotional eating is part of American culture. Somehow, eating things that are bad for us feels good. My diet goes down the drain when I am stressed. I am still not sure why this happens. I feel and look better when I am eating according to plan. I know what I should be doing, but I go through periods of falling off the wagon.

We make bad food choices when we are stressed, depressed, or overwhelmed by life; this makes following diets and treatment plans harder than ever.

From a dietary point of view, compliance is the holy grail. Following the plan is all you have. Every deviation from the plan reduces your odds. Noncompliance with chronic or life-threatening diseases is hard to understand from the outside looking in. From the patient's point of view, anger, rage, hopelessness, severe side effects from medications, cravings for a new diet, and so on, all work to reduce compliance with treatments plans. It could be summed up as a "What's the point?" attitude. Many of us reading this book have been in these shoes.

We must feel good or hopeful to make the right decisions daily for our health. I will be asking you to follow a diet and treatment plan with your doctors. It is going to take some discipline and a little willpower. Otherwise, depression and anxiety might derail your progress.

It took the loss of a sibling to wake me up. My younger sister was killed by a reckless driver speeding in a pouring rainstorm. A driver lost control and hydroplaned into her lane. I felt the pain of losing a sibling, but watching my parents bury a child was horrible. There are no deeper scars than burying a child. I promised myself they would never bury another child. My new goal was not to stop my disease, but to outlive my parents. It took this tragedy to get me moving. It gave me clarity, focus, discipline, and emotional power to do whatever it took to get better.

I don't want this for you. It shouldn't have taken the loss of a family member to wake me up. The fact that it did tells me I was in a funk for years and never knew it. We wait until it's too late to act because we don't feel any pain, and life isn't that bad. It took something horrible for me to make a change. Please, I am begging you, don't be like me. Take the bull by the horns today, not when you are on the transplant list or dialysis. Take control, and you will feel better and have a better outcome.

It is beyond the scope of this book to go into a detailed treatment plan for mental health. What I can tell you is your odds will improve if you get help. Your odds of sticking with a diet and treatment plan will also improve. In fact, it is likely that just about every aspect of your life will improve. I never thought to treat something like anxiety or depression. The first time I was asked about depression or mental health was at Johns Hopkins. I lied and said everything was fine. I was scared admitting that I was anxious and worried might keep me from being included in the dietary invention trial.

Prescription medicines have a success rate that is as high, or even higher, than traditional talk therapy. However, the combination of therapy and prescription medications appears to be the best. If a prescription drug can help you cope with the day-to-day stress and anxiety of a deadly disease, do it. A stoic idiot is still an idiot. If you have a personal objection, then just take the drug until you slow your disease and you are doing better.

Taking a pill is as easy as it gets. Don't be afraid to get help or else you are hurting yourself. Getting help for depression or anxiety should be part of any treatment plan. It doesn't make you weak, just human like the rest of us.

After giving it a long thought, I think a version of Alcoholics Anonymous (AA) is needed for people with kidney disease: "Kidneys Anonymous," if you will. It's a long fight, and we need support. I could call my sponsor when I have been sitting in the parking lot of a steakhouse for two hours, breaking into a cold sweat. The sponsor could talk me down from the dietary ledge. The sponsor could encourage me and help me not feel like I am fighting this battle alone. I could be part of a group of fellow patients standing up and fighting this disease.

The problem has no standard treatment plan, but support exists. One of my goals is to establish a treatment plan for kidney patients. Part of that treatment plan should be a support group. All of us should be working towards the same goal. We will be working on this in the future. It's a big project so it will take time. Sign up at **www.stoppingkidneydisease.com** for updates. Ideally, we would have online meetings several times a day so fellow patients can log in when they needed a little encouragement. Again, the AA model may not be ideal, but it may be the right place for us to start. Check the website and sign up to help us with this project.

In this online group, we can share tricks that helped us, like breaking everything into super small goals.

When you are depressed or anxious, everything seems overwhelming. Give yourself a break. You don't have to worry about the future or next year. Just make sure the next hour or this meal follows the diet and treatment plan. You win this war with thousands of tiny good decisions, not by one big decision. Commit this one to heart: Slowing or potentially stopping your disease will be the result of thousands of tiny decisions that add up over time. Every little good choice you make is a victory.

Don't worry about next year or the year after. Worry about the next hour, and take it hour by hour if you have to. I did. I was not treated for depression or anxiety because no one told me I needed to be. I probably should have been evaluated. I spent years going downhill, feeling like my future had been stolen. Looking back, I was probably depressed, and that is why it took a horrible event to wake me up.

Cognitive or group therapy may also help. Learn to recognize the good things and minimize or forget about the bad. The choice is yours, whether you view leading a better way of life as torture or as exciting.

Study 19.6 — Cognitive-behavioral group therapy is an effective treatment for major depression in hemodialysis patients.[7]

ABSTRACT:

Depression is an important target of psychological assessment in patients with the end-stage renal disease because it predicts their morbidity, mortality, and quality of life. We assessed the effectiveness of cognitive-behavioral therapy in chronic hemodialysis patients diagnosed with major depression by the Mini International Neuropsychiatric Interview (MINI). In a randomized trial conducted in Brazil, an intervention group of 41 patients was given 12 weekly sessions of cognitive-behavioral group therapy led by a trained psychologist over 3 months while a control group of 44 patients received the usual treatment offered in the dialysis unit. In both groups, the Beck Depression Inventory, the MINI, and the Kidney Disease and Quality of Life-Short Form questionnaires were administered at baseline, after 3 months of intervention or usual treatment, and after 9 months of follow-up. The intervention group had significant improvements, compared to the control group, in the average scores of the Beck Depression Inventory overall scale, MINI scores, and in quality-of-life dimensions that included the burden of renal disease, sleep, quality of social interaction, overall health, and the mental component summary. <u>We conclude that cognitive-behavioral group therapy is an effective treatment for depression in chronic hemodialysis patients.</u>

Perspective is everything. I have the chance to help thousands of people like me. I wouldn't have this opportunity if I didn't have a deadly disease. I am embarking on a new career in education and innvoation for people with kidney disease. This book is just the beginning. It seems very unfair to me that kidney patients in more than forty countries have access to one of the most proven supplements for kidney disease, but it is not available in the U.S. I met some wonderful people on this journey. It is an exciting new chapter in my life.

I could also look at this experience with a cynical or negative point of view and complain about long hours, crazy schedules, and the expense and risk of a new business at my age. But I choose to see the gains from this experience, which will potentially benefit everyone with kidney disease.

In the fight against kidney disease or any deadly disease, everything is on the table. The ends justify the means in our situation. Get help, even if you don't need it. The worst that can happen is you will end up with extra support. If you are old-school or stoic and refuse help, you are playing with your life.

If you think I was joking about the AA example and the steakhouse, let me clarify that those were indeed based on real-life experiences. I love Mexican food, especially a sauce called mole, pronounced mo-lay. Mole is a wonderful blend of nuts, spices, peppers, and chocolate. I know it sounds weird, but trust me it's crazy good. A local woman would make mole for a restaurant once a week. Every Friday was mole day. The restaurant would usually be sold out by 12:30. Chicken swimming in mole was always sold out, unless you got there early.

I was amazed at the number of ways I could rationalize making it to the restaurant every Friday to eat something I knew was very bad for my kidneys. I began to suspect someone was adding crack to the sauce. I felt a little like an addict. It was my only vice, and I rationalized eating mole every Friday in a thousand different ways. It was the one pleasure I allowed myself, despite the fact that it was awful for me.

You may have a food you love in your life as well. You know the old song, "Breaking up is hard to do." Well, it's true for food as well. You will find crazy ways to justify your eating habits, just like I did. Every time you are tempted to eat your version of mole, think about it for a few minutes. Are five or ten minutes of food heaven worth tossing out a whole week of work? Is one meal worth negating the twenty other meals you worked so hard on? Do you want to die younger? Do you want to be sicker? Ask yourself what you want out of life. Do you want to be swollen and feel sick, or do you want to look like a million bucks? I had to remind myself constantly what I wanted out of life to beat my mole addiction.

It is easier to kick a food habit if you are feeling upbeat and positive about the future. Why make life harder than it has to be? Getting help from a healthcare professional will assist you with your dietary compliance and your treatment plan. It will smooth out the inevitable bumps along the way.

Getting help and support is logical. Science even proves it. I am trying to make a point here, and it needs to be made. It doesn't make any sense not to get extra help. Your family, spouse, children, parents, and friends all want you to feel better and live longer. Passing on the support is a huge mistake and will increase your odds of dying and getting sick. You might make lifelong friends, do better for your family or job, feel better, and you will likely live longer.

Nothing wrong can come from getting help.

Don't make the same mistake I did. If you are not taking the steps needed to get better, improve your odds, and live longer, something is wrong. It's as good a diagnosis as you can get. Imagine meeting a cancer patient who elected to pass on life-saving treatments like chemotharpy or surgery. You might say to yourself "What the hell is wrong with that person? Do they want to die"?

Our situation is not any different, except death is many years away and painless today. They call kidney disease the "Silent Killer" for a reason. If you could cure or slow your disease enough that you get an extra high quality ten or twenty years of life, would you? You will tell me "yes" to my face, but you might not mean it when presented with a dietary choice later in the day. It's kind of a sickness when you think about it. It's not logical, it's emotional.

Every time you eat a bacon cheeseburger, pepperoni pizza, etc. after reading this book and the science behind it, you know something is wrong. To err is human, but to keep doing it over and over again is a sign your thinking is screwed up. If you are not making right decisions for yourself, something is wrong. A predialysis patient told me they would never give up certain foods. This person said it proudly and defiantly, as if some badge or medal is given to those who do their best to speed their disease and die the fastest. This same person recanted and wished they would have made better decisions when their illness took a turn for the worse.

Be smarter and more self-aware than I was. Looking back, I see that I spent years being completely lost. I don't want that for you or your family.

Check the website: stoppingkidneydisease.com for support group information. It will take some time, but we will get one up and running.

Getting help shows you are thinking logically and have a normal mindset. Refusing help is the best sign that you really need it. Get help, don't be an idiot like me.

References

1. Loosman WL, Rottier MA, Honig A, Siegert CE. Association of depressive and anxiety symptoms with adverse events in Dutch chronic kidney disease patients: a prospective cohort study. *BMC Nephrology.* 2015;16(1):155.

2. Tsai Y-C, Chiu Y-W, Hung C-C, et al. Association of symptoms of depression with progression of CKD. *American Journal of Kidney Diseases.* 2012;60(1):54-61.

3. Andrade SV, Sesso R, Diniz DHdMP. Hopelessness, suicide ideation, and depression in chronic kidney disease patients on hemodialysis or transplant recipients. *Jornal Brasileiro de Nefrologia.* 2015;37(1):55-63.

4. Bautovich A, Katz I, Smith M, Loo CK, Harvey SB. Depression and chronic kidney disease: A review for clinicians. *Australian & New Zealand Journal of Psychiatry.* 2014;48(6):530-541.

5. Lee YJ, Kim M, Cho S, Kim S. Association of depression and anxiety with reduced quality of life in patients with predialysis chronic kidney disease. *International Journal of Clinical Practice.* 2013;67(4):363-368.

6. Hsu H-J, Yen C-H, Chen C-K, et al. Association between uremic toxins and depression in patients with chronic kidney disease undergoing maintenance hemodialysis. *General Hospital Psychiatry.* 2013;35(1):23-27.

7. Duarte PS, Miyazaki MC, Blay SL, Sesso R. Cognitive–behavioral group therapy is an effective treatment for major depression in hemodialysis patients. *Kidney International.* 2009;76(4):414-421.

CHAPTER 20

Obesity and Underweight

Obesity is now considered a worldwide pandemic. Obesity has left behind smoking and has emerged as the number one cause of death. Despite the well-known hazards of being overweight, many of us struggle with our weight. Depending on the study, up to 35% of residents in the U.S. are considered obese.

One thing I wondered is how much weight is too much? Is being underweight a real risk? Can we be too thin? Does carrying a few extra pounds really impact your health?

A standard measurement is body mass index (BMI), which is a calculation based on your current height and weight. I am 5 ft, 10 inches and I weigh 165 lbs. This gives me a BMI of 23.7. The average BMI range is 18.5 to 24.9. 25 to 30 is considered overweight, and over 30 is considered obese. I have to go down to 126 lbs to be called underweight. 126 to 174 lbs is a pretty big range, almost 50 lbs.

I mention this because something known as the BMI paradox, or obesity paradox, exists for people with kidney disease. Studies have shown that kidney patients with higher BMI (overweight and mildly obese) have a higher survival rate. This is the opposite of what happens in healthy patients.

How could being overweight be good for us, but bad for everyone else? Thus the name "BMI paradox."

Using myself as an example, I can't imagine dropping to 126 lbs. It seems to me that 126 lbs would indicate something else is going on with me.

Let's see what the studies say.

Note: It is widely accepted that a BMI between 22 and 25 is considered the healthiest for the normal population.

Study 20.1	Body-mass index and cause-specific mortality in 900 000 adults: collaborative analyses of 57 prospective studies

INTERPRETATION:

Although other anthropometric measures (e.g. waist circumference, waist-to-hip ratio) could well add extra information to BMI, and BMI to them, <u>BMI is in itself a strong predictor of overall mortality both above and below the apparent optimum of about 22·5–25 kg/m^2</u>. The progressive excess mortality above this range is due mainly to vascular disease and is probably largely causal. At 30–35 kg/m^2, median survival is reduced by 2–4 years; at 40–45 kg/m^2, it is reduced by 8–10 years (which is comparable with the effects of smoking). The definite excess mortality below 22·5 kg/m^2 is due mainly to smoking-related diseases and is not fully explained.

This is what is expected. Heart disease and diabetes are associated with higher BMIs. However, when we start adding comorbid conditions or diseases, things begin to change. Some answers:

Study 20.2 — Body mass index has no effect on rate of progression of chronic kidney disease in non-diabetic subjects

CONCLUSIONS:

Neither BMI as a continuous variable nor obesity (BMI > 30) as a categorical variable were associated with an increased rate of progression of existing CKD in this predominantly white population.

Study 20.3 — Association of Body Mass Index with Outcomes in Patients with CKD

ABSTRACT:

Obesity is associated with higher mortality in the general population, but this association is reversed in patients on dialysis. The nature of the relationship of obesity with adverse clinical outcomes in nondialysis-dependent CKD and the putative interaction of the severity of disease with this association is unclear. We analyzed data from a nationally representative cohort of 453,946 United States veterans with eGFR<60 ml/min per 1.73 m^2. The associations of body mass index categories (<20, 20 to <25, 25 to <30, 30 to <35, 35 to <40, 40 to <45, 45 to <50, and $_{\geq}$50 kg/m^2) with all-cause mortality and disease progression (using multiple definitions, including incidence of ESRD, doubling of serum creatinine, and the slopes of eGFR) were examined in Cox proportional hazards models and logistic regression models. Multivariable adjustments were made for age, race, comorbidities and medications, and baseline eGFR. Body mass index levels showed a relatively consistent U-shaped association with clinical outcomes, with the best outcomes observed in overweight and mildly obese patients. Body mass index levels ≤25 kg/m^2 were associated with worse outcomes in all patients, independent of severity of CKD. Body mass index levels ≥35 kg/m^2 were associated with worse outcomes in patients with earlier stages of CKD, but this association was attenuated in those patients with eGFR<30 ml/min per 1.73 m^2. Thus, until clinical trials establish the ideal body mass index, a cautious approach to weight management is warranted in this patient population.

Study 20.4 — The Body Mass Index Paradox and Obesity, Inflammation, and Atherosclerosis Syndrome in Chronic Kidney Disease

ABSTRACT:

The association of high body mass index (BMI) with better survival in chronic kidney disease (CKD) is considered a "risk factor paradox" or "reverse epidemiology." Since malnutrition is a powerful predictor of death and cardiovascular disease is its leading cause, it has been suggested that malnutrition and atherosclerosis must be associated. Thus the current paradigm is that malnutrition is a risk factor for atherosclerosis and obesity is protective in CKD patients. We recently showed that high-BMI patients with inferred high body fat have an increased prevalence of atherosclerosis and subsequent cardiovascular and all-cause mortality. Prior cross-sectional studies also showed that high BMI in CKD is associated with higher C-reactive protein (CRP) levels and increased coronary calcification on electron beam computed tomography (CT) scan. These apparently conflicting data on better survival but increased inflammation and atherosclerosis in high-BMI CKD patients could be explained as follows. It is hypothesized that nutrition exerts a much stronger influence on survival than atherosclerosis in CKD. Malnutrition strongly augments the hazard of death from coexistent diseases, while better nutrition has the opposite effect. Thus the risk of death is highest in malnourished patients (low muscle and low fat mass) and lowest in well nourished patients (high BMI, high muscle mass). Obesity (high BMI, high fat mass) is associated with inflammation and atherosclerosis. The risk of death from obesity and atherosclerosis is increased, but not so much as occurs with malnutrition. Therefore high body fat patients have intermediate survival. Thus it is postulated that an association of obesity, inflammation, and atherosclerosis (OIA syndrome) might exist in CKD.

Study 20.5 Association of anthropometric measures with kidney disease progression and mortality: a retrospective cohort study of pre-dialysis chronic kidney disease patients referred to a specialist renal service

CONCLUSION:

BMI in the overweight range is associated with reduced risks of kidney disease progression and all-cause mortality in stage 3–4 CKD.

This is very surprising to me. How can weight have no impact on kidney disease progression when weight is associated with high blood pressure? Extra weight is also associated with heart disease. So what exactly happens?

It turns out, being underweight is a much bigger risk than being overweight for patients with kidney disease. Underweight is a sign of inadequate nutrition and calories. It could also be the sign of other health problems or comorbid conditions. If you can gain weight, you are likely healthier than someone who cannot gain weight.

Study 20.6 Underweight Is an Independent Risk Factor for Renal Function Deterioration in Patients with IgA Nephropathy

In this study, we found that underweight was associated with increased risk of renal function progression in IgAN by under-nutrition status. It was also reasonable that additional protein wasting caused by chronic disease progression might be worse tolerated in the underweight group due to their low protein reserves.

Study 20.7   Underweight rather than overweight is associated with higher prevalence of hypertension: BP vs BMI in hemodialysis population

CONCLUSIONS:

<u>We demonstrate for the first time that, unlike the general population, no positive correlation exists between BP and increasing BMI in hemodialysis patients.</u> Further analysis is necessary to verify our observation and to test the possibility of whether nutritional improvement would aid in the better control of hypertension in dialysis patients.

The Bottom Line

The truth is not known, from what I can tell. The idea that we should all be overweight seems hard to believe, but that is what the studies suggest.

Restricting calories has been shown to slow down kidney disease progression, but you can't put on extra weight if you are restricting calories. This is a problematic aspect from my point of view. How can we reconcile this conflicting data?

The BMI paradox, i.e., extra pounds equaling a better outcome, is likely explained by the following:

1. You are currently healthy enough to gain weight.

2. You have probably not been critically ill or suffered a long-term illness recently.

3. Your calorie intake is adequate.

4. You are likely to have fewer comorbid conditions or other illnesses.

5. You are getting the proper nutrients and are not malnourished.

If you are underweight:

1. Your health prohibits you from gaining weight.

2. You may have been critically ill or recently had a severe illness.

3. Your calorie intake is not sufficient.

4. You may be suffering from malnutrition.

5. You have other comorbid conditions or illnesses.

These issues likely explain the BMI paradox, but this has not been proven. If you are sick or extremely ill, you are more likely to be underweight. Extra weight may merely mean you are healthier than someone who is underweight. It is likely that simple.

Caloric restriction may slow kidney and heart disease progression, so we are left with more questions than answers. Despite the data on the BMI paradox, I don't think anyone can advocate being overweight.

What Should Our Weight Be

This is also a guess. We don't know the ideal weight for kidney patients. A good guess would be near the top end of a healthy BMI. If 24.9 is the highest BMI considered healthy, we can round it to 25 to make it easy. If we are running about 25 or 26, we might be in the sweet spot. With that number, we would be carrying a few extra pounds, but no so much as to negatively impact our health. However, this is a guess. That number is low enough to prevent future problems, but high enough to be getting adequate nutrition.

I don't feel like we can ignore the statistics for healthy adults and assume we can pack on the pounds in the name of the kidney disease. Your current health most likely explains the BMI paradox, and survival advantage of being overweight is a result of current health and nutrition.

We do know that being underweight is higher risk than being overweight. I wish I had more definitive answers for you on this subject. On the one hand, caloric restriction slows our progression; on the other, having a few extra pounds may be beneficial.

I think the primary message for us is getting adequate nutrition and calories is one of the most important things you can do for yourself.

CHAPTER 21

Renal Hypoxia

Kidneys are highly vascular organs. They are a dense network of tiny vessels that are so small, they allow the smallest particles in our blood to be filtered. Kidneys receive the most blood flow per weight of any organ. The chapter on endothelial dysfunction is also related to renal hypoxia, but I have broken these into two chapters.

Hypoxia is a lack of oxygen. Reduced blood flow is the likely culprit. The kidneys get about 20% of the heart's blood flow, and now hypoxia is being recognized as one of the driving forces of kidney disease progression. What appears to drive lack of oxygen or hypoxia in our kidneys? You guessed it: inflammation, or should I say long-term systemic inflammation? Remember, I said: "Inflammation is killing us."

Could it be that inflammation in densely packed vessels causes blood flow to be restricted to other vessels? We are talking about microscopic size vessels here. If the vessel or surrounding tissue becomes inflamed, then blood flow may be restricted. A little inflammation may have a big impact on the tiniest vessels.

Let's find out.

Study 21.1   Hypoxia: The Force that Drives Chronic Kidney Disease[1]

ABSTRACT:

In the United States, the prevalence of end-stage renal disease (ESRD) reached epidemic proportions in 2012, with over 600,000 patients being treated. The rates of ESRD among the elderly are disproportionally high. Consequently, as life expectancy increases and the babyboom generation reaches retirement age, the alreadyheavy burden imposed by ESRD on the U.S. health care system is set to increase dramatically. ESRD represents the terminal stage of chronic kidney disease (CKD). A large body of evidence indicating that CKD is driven by renal tissue hypoxia has led to the development of therapeutic strategies that increase kidney oxygenation and the contention that chronic hypoxia is the final common pathway to end-stage renal failure. Numerous studies have demonstrated that one of the most potent means by which hypoxic conditions within the kidney produce CKD is by inducing a sustained inflammatory attack by infiltrating leukocytes. Indispensable to this attack is the acquisition by leukocytes of an adhesive phenotype. It was thought that this process resulted exclusively from leukocytes responding to cytokines released from ischemic renal endothelium. However, recently it has been demonstrated that leukocytes also become activated independent of the hypoxic response of endothelial cells. It was found that this endothelium-independent mechanism involves leukocytes directly sensing hypoxia and responding by transcriptional induction of the genes that encode the β2-integrin family of adhe-sion molecules. <u>This induction likely maintains the long-term inflammation by which hypoxia drives the pathogenesis of CKD.</u> Consequently, targeting these transcriptional mechanisms would appear to represent a promising new therapeutic strategy.

Note: Damn, inflammation again!

Study 21.2   Renal hypoxia in kidney disease: Cause or consequence?[2]

ABSTRACT:

Tissue hypoxia has been proposed as an important factor in the pathophysiology of both chronic kidney disease (CKD) and acute kidney injury (AKI), initiating and propagating a vicious cycle of tubular injury, vascular rarefaction and fibrosis and thus exacerbation of hypoxia. Here, we critically evaluate this proposition by systematically reviewing the literature relevant to the following six questions: (i) Is kidney disease always associated with tissue hypoxia? (ii) Does tissue hypoxia drive signaling cascades that lead to tissue damage and dysfunction? (iii) Does tissue hypoxia per se lead to kidney disease? (iv) Does tissue hypoxia precede pathology? (v) Does tissue hypoxia colocalize with pathology? (vi) Does prevention of tissue hypoxia prevent kidney disease? <u>We conclude that tissue hypoxia is a common feature of both AKI and CKD. Furthermore, at least under in vitro conditions, renal tissue hypoxia drives signaling cascades that lead to tissue damage and dysfunction. Tissue hypoxia itself can lead to renal pathology, independent of other known risk factors for kidney disease. There is also some evidence that tissue hypoxia precedes renal pathology, at least in some forms of kidney disease.</u> However, we have made relatively little prog-ress in determining the spatial relationships between tissue hypoxia and pathological processes (i.e. colocalization) or whether therapies targeted to reduce tissue hypoxia can prevent or delay the progression of renal disease. Thus, the hypothesis that tissue hypoxia is a "common pathway" to both AKI and CKD remains to be adequately tested.

Note: Another suggestion that inflammation and/or hypoxia were present before the disease was present.

Study 21.3   Propensity to calcification as a pathway to renal hypoxia in chronic kidney disease and in hypertension[3]

Arterial rigidity is a hallmark of chronic kidney disease (CKD). Arterial calcification recapitulates normal bone formation, and this process is considered central-to-arterial stiffness in CKD and predicts major clinical outcomes including death, cardiovascular events and progression to kidney failure in these patients. <u>Renal hypoxia measured in vivo by blood oxygenation level dependent MRI (BOLD-MRI) goes along with the severity of renal dysfunction and the risk of progression of CKD. In theory arterial stiffness by vascular calcification may explain renal hypoxia in CKD and in essential hypertension, another condition typically associated with arterial stiffness.</u>

Note: Are you noticing a theme? Inflammation and calcification show up over and over in many different ways. Calcification may reduce blood flow.

Study 21.4 **Serum calcification propensity is associated with renal tissue oxygenation and resistive index in patients with arterial hypertension or chronic kidney disease.[4]**

CONCLUSION:

The current study shows that hypertensive patients with preserved renal function, as well as CKD patients, have a higher risk of calcification than controls. <u>High arterial stiffness and calcification propensity are linked to low renal tissue oxygenation and perfusion in hypertensive and CKD patients.</u> These results provide new insights on the relationships among arterial stiffness, renal tissue oxygenation and the risk of developing CKD.

Study 21.5 **Determinants of renal tissue oxygenation as measured with BOLD-MRI in chronic kidney disease and hypertension in humans.[5]**

ABSTRACT:

Experimentally renal tissue hypoxia appears to play an important role in the pathogenesis of chronic kidney disease (CKD) and arterial hypertension (AHT). In this study, we measured renal tissue oxygenation and its determinants in humans using blood oxygenation level dependent magnetic resonance imaging (BOLD-MRI) under standardized hydration conditions. Four coronal slices were selected, and a multi-gradient echo sequence was used to acquire T2* weighted images. The mean cortical and medullary R2* values (=1/T2*) were calculated before and after administration of IV furosemide, a low R2* indicating a high tissue oxygenation. We studied 195 subjects (95 CKD, 58 treated AHT, and 42 healthy controls). Mean cortical R2 and medullary R2* were not significantly different between the groups at baseline. In stimulated conditions (furosemide injection), the decrease in R2* was significantly blunted in patients with CKD and AHT. In multivariate linear regression analyses, neither cortical nor medullary R2* were associated with eGFR or blood pressure, but cortical R2* correlated positively with male gender, blood glucose and uric acid levels. In conclusion, our data show that kidney oxygenation is tightly regulated in CKD and hypertensive patients at rest. However, the metabolic response to acute changes in sodium transport is altered in CKD and in AHT, despite preserved renal function in the latter group. <u>This suggests the presence of early renal metabolic alterations in hypertension. The correlations between cortical R2* values, male gender, glycemia and uric acid levels suggest that these factors interfere with the regulation of renal tissue oxygenation.</u>

Study 21.6 **Glycative Stress and Its Defense Machinery Glyoxalase 1 in Renal Pathogenesis[6]**

ABSTRACT:

Chronic kidney disease is a major public health problem around the world. <u>Because the kidney plays a role in reducing glycative stress, renal dysfunction results in increased glycative stress. In turn, glycative stress, especially that due to advanced glycated end products (AGEs) and their</u>

precursors such as reactive carbonyl compounds, exacerbates chronic kidney disease and is related to premature aging in chronic kidney disease, whether caused by diabetes mellitus or otherwise. Factors which hinder a sufficient reduction in glycative stress include the inhibition of anti-glycation enzymes (e.g., GLO-1), as well as pathogenically activated endoplasmic reticulum (ER) stress and hypoxia in the kidney. Promising strategies aimed at halting the vicious cycle between chronic kidney disease and increases in glycative stress include the suppression of AGE accumulation in the body and the enhancement of GLO-1 to strengthen the host defense machinery against glycative stress.

Renal hypoxia, just like protein energy wasting, appears to be one of the cumulative effects of inflammation, uremia, AGEs, and oxidative stress. We don't know for sure if hypoxia is the cause or a side effect of kidney disease. However, what we do know is that it appears to be a factor.

Remember "renal resistive index" from earlier chapters? It is a measure of blood flow in the kidneys. A high resistive index is an indicator of rapid kidney disease progression. What happens if we can improve the blood flow in our kidneys?

Study 21.7   **Dietary nitrate load lowers blood pressure and renal resistive index in patients with chronic kidney disease: A pilot study.[7]**

ABSTRACT:

Beetroot has a high concentration of inorganic nitrate, which can be serially reduced to form nitrite and nitric oxide (NO) after oral ingestion. Increased renal resistive index (RRI) measured by Doppler ultrasonography is associated with higher cardiovascular mortality in hypertensive patients with reduced renal function over time defined as chronic kidney disease (CKD). Our aim was to investigate whether the supplementation of dietary nitrate by administration of beetroot juice is able to reduce blood pressure and renal resistive index (RRI) as prognostic markers for cardiovascular mortality in CKD patients. In a cross-over study design, 17 CKD patients were randomized to either a dietary nitrate load (300 mg) by highly concentrated beetroot juice (BJ) or placebo (water). Hemodynamic parameters as well as plasma nitrate concentration and RRI were measured before and 4 h after treatment. In this cohort, CKD was mainly caused by hypertensive or diabetic nephropathy. The mean eGFR was 41.6 ± 12.0 ml/min/m2. Plasma nitrate concentrations were significantly increased after ingestion of BJ compared to control. Peripheral systolic and diastolic blood pressure as well as mean arterial pressure (MAP) were significantly reduced secondary to the dietary nitrate load compared to control (e.g. $\Delta MAP_{BJ} = -8.2 \pm 7.6$ mmHg vs. $\Delta MAP_{control} = -2.2 \pm 6.0$ mmHg, $p = 0.012$). BJ also led to significantly reduced RRI values

($\Delta RRI_{BJ} = -0.03 \pm 0.04$ versus $\Delta RRI_{control} = 0.01 \pm 0.04$; $p = 0.017$). Serum potassium levels were not altered secondary to the treatment. In this study, administration of the nitrate donor BJ led to significantly reduced RRI values and peripheral blood pressure, which might be explained by release of the vasodilatator NO after oral intake. Whether supplementation of dietary nitrate in addition to routine pharmacologic therapy is able to decelerate progression of cardiovascular and renal disease in CKD, remains to be investigated.

A widely-accepted treatment for renal hypoxia does not exist at this time. However, nitrates found in beets, watermelon, arugula, cilantro, and other foods may increase blood flow and reduce blood pressure. Nitrate-rich foods may decrease the renal resistive index, which suggests these foods increase blood flow in our kidneys.

Antioxidants may also mitigate hypoxia, but this has not been proven. Antioxidants may have two effects on nitric oxide. First, a surplus of antioxidants ensures vessels perform normally and are not subject to oxidative stress. Second, antioxidants may protect existing nitric oxide by protecting them from free radicals. Some studies suggest nitric oxide may be fragile and easily reduced by oxidative stress.

It is likely (but not proven) that aggressively treating factors like inflammation, oxidative stress, AGEs, etc. might reduce renal hypoxia, since these factors are implicated in renal hypoxia. The same things that are heart-healthy are also kidney-healthy in most cases, because the kidney is a highly vascular organ.

Increasing blood flow to our kidneys should be a part of our treatment goal.

References

1. Fu Q, Colgan SP, Shelley CS. Hypoxia: the force that drives chronic kidney disease. *Clinical Medicine & Research*. 2016;14(1):15-39.

2. Ow CP, Ngo JP, Ullah MM, Hilliard LM, Evans RG. Renal Hypoxia in Kidney Disease: Cause or Consequence? *Acta Physiologica*. 2017;00(e12999).

3. Zoccali C, Mallamaci F. Propensity to calcification as a pathway to renal hypoxia in chronic kidney disease and in hypertension. *Journal of Hypertension*. 2017;35(10):1963-1965.

4. Pruijm M, Lu Y, Megdiche F, et al. Serum calcification propensity is associated with renal tissue oxygenation and resistive index in patients with arterial hypertension or chronic kidney disease. *Journal of Hypertension*. 2017;35(10):2044-2052.

5. Pruijm M, Hofmann L, Piskunowicz M, et al. Determinants of renal tissue oxygenation as measured with BOLD-MRI in chronic kidney disease and hypertension in humans. *PloS one*. 2014;9(4):e95895.

6. Hirakawa Y, Inagi R. Glycative stress and its defense machinery glyoxalase 1 in renal pathogenesis. *International Journal of Molecular Sciences*. 2017;18(1):174.

7. Kemmner S, Lorenz G, Wobst J, et al. Dietary nitrate load lowers blood pressure and renal resistive index in patients with chronic kidney disease: A pilot study. *Nitric Oxide*. 2017;64:7-15.

CHAPTER 22

Endothelial Dysfunction

Endothelial dysfunction (ED) is getting a separate chapter because it seems to be everywhere in kidney and heart disease research.

<u>Here is why: The kidneys have the largest amount of endothelial surface area of any organ. Again, your kidneys have more endothelial cells and membranes than any other part of your body.</u>

"Endothelial" refers to the lining of your blood vessels. This lining is basically an organ, just like skin. The lining of your blood vessels can secrete hormones that increase inflammation and cause your vessels to become less flexible. The cells that line your blood vessels also cause your blood vessels to relax and contract. Think about the combination of your blood vessel walls contracting while they are inflamed. This could be the 1-2 punch that causes renal hypoxia and increases the speed of kidney and heart disease progression.

Think about the smallest blood vessels you can imagine. A tiny amount of inflammation could have a big effect on blood flow when the vessels are this small.

We normally think of ED as related to heart disease, not kidney disease. While ED is certainly a big risk factor for heart disease, it may be just as big of a risk factor for kidney disease. Renal hypoxia may be caused by endothelial dysfunction.

We know that people with kidney disease are in the highest risk group ever studied for heart disease. It may be that endothelial dysfunction over many years or decades is a primary cause. When the lining of your heart and blood vessels become inflamed and/or hard, your vessels loose elasticity, which may cause a stroke or heart attack. We have all heard of the phrase "hardening of the arteries" used to describe arteriosclerosis, or plaque building up in our arteries.

Endothelial cells produce nitric oxide to relax or expand vessels to increase blood flow. Nitric oxide also prevents cells from sticking to the artery walls. A fundamental feature of endothelial dysfunction is impaired or reduced nitric oxide availability. This leads to cells sticking to the walls of our blood vessels and inflammation of vessel walls, which, when combined, accelerate damage to your blood vessels.

This means that blood flow may be reduced, or in some cases, completely stopped, in the smallest vessels in our kidneys, even if there is good blood flow in major vessels. The result may be renal hypoxia, which we discussed in the last chapter.

Therefore, a heart-healthy diet and lifestyle is as important as a healthy lifestyle for our kidneys. In many ways, they are the same.

Research shows several risk factors for endothelial dysfunction relevant to kidney patients.

Risks

> Fluid/Volume overload

> Proteinuria

> Increased parathyroid hormone

> Increased calcium/phosphate levels or intake

> Increased fibroblast growth factor 23

> Reduced vitamin D

> Acidosis

> Anemia

> Hypoalbuminemia

> Reduced fetuin A and other inhibitors of calcification

> Increased asymmetric dimethylarginine and other endogenous NO inhibitors

> Increased high-sensitivity C-reactive protein and other inflammatory markers

> Oxidative stress/increased production of reactive oxygen species

> Increased susceptibility to infections

> Increased homocysteine

> Increased advanced glycation end products (AGE's)

While this seems like a long list (and it is), most of these risks are treatable or manageable.

Let's see what the research says.

Study 22.1 Endothelin antagonism in patients with nondiabetic chronic kidney disease.[2]

ABSTRACT:

The incidence of chronic kidney disease (CKD) is increasing worldwide. Cardiovascular disease is strongly associated with CKD and constitutes one of its major causes of morbidity and mortality. Although current treatments for CKD focus on blood pressure and proteinuria reduction, many CKD patients have ongoing hypertension and residual proteinuria. Newer treatments are needed that not only act on these parameters, but also slow the progression of CKD and improve the cardiovascular risk profile of CKD patients. The endothelins (ETs) are a family of related peptides of which ET-1 is the most powerful endogenous vasoconstrictor and the predominant isoform in the cardiovascular and renal systems. The ET system has been widely implicated in both cardiovascular disease and CKD. ET-1 contributes to the pathogenesis and maintenance of hypertension and arterial stiffness, as well endothelial dysfunction and atherosclerosis. By reversal of these effects, ET antagonists may reduce cardiovascular risk. In CKD patients, antagonism of the ET system may be of benefit in improving renal hemodynamics and reducing proteinuria. ET is likely also involved in the progression of renal disease, and data are emerging that suggest a synergistic role for ET receptor antagonists with angiotensin-converting enzyme inhibitors in slowing CKD progression.

Study 22.2 | The Determinants of Endothelial Dysfunction in CKD: Oxidative Stress and Asymmetric Dimethylarginine[3]

In conclusion, the present study shows that: (1) oxidative stress and increased ADMA levels accompany the deterioration in kidney function, and (2) the main determinants of endothelial function in patients with CKD are oxidative stress and increased ADMA levels. These results encourage implementation of new antioxidant or endogenous nitric oxide synthase sensitizing treatment strategies for patients with CKD.

> **Note:** ADMA is asymmetric dimethylarginine. ADMA interferes with or lowers production of nitric oxide. ADMA levels are elevated by LDL cholesterol. Remember, in the chapter on cholesterol, LDL was indicated in disease progression. This may be why.

Study 22.3 | Endothelial Dysfunction and the Kidney: Emerging Risk Factors for Renal Insufficiency and Cardiovascular Outcomes in Essential Hypertension[4]

CONCLUSION:

A dysfunctional endothelium seems to be a key factor in the risk for renal insufficiency in individuals with essential hypertension. The inverse links between CRP and the GFR and the vasodilatory response to ACh coherently suggest that inflammation is a likely mechanism explaining this association. The endothelium seems to be at the crossroads of the risk for renal impairment and cardiovascular complications in individuals with essential hypertension.

Study 22.4 | Endothelial Dysfunction Contributes to Renal Function-Associated Cardiovascular Mortality in a Population with Mild Renal Insufficiency: The Hoorn Study[5]

Renal function was mildly impaired (mean eGFR 68 ± 12 ml/min per 1.73 m^2) and independently associated with von Willebrand factor (standardized $_\beta$ -0.09; 95% confidence interval [CI] -0.18 to -0.002; $P < 0.05$), soluble vascular cell adhesion molecule-1 (standardized β -0.14; 95% CI -0.22 to -0.05; $P < 0.01$), and albumin creatinine ratio (standardized $_\beta$ -0.15; 95% CI -0.23 to -0.08; $P < 0.001$), but not with markers of inflammatory activity. Renal function was inversely associated with cardiovascular and all-cause mortality. The relative risk for cardiovascular mortality, but not all cause mortality associated with renal function, decreased from 1.22 to 1.12 per 5 ml/min per 1.73 m^2 decrease of eGFR after adjustment for markers of endothelial dysfunction. In conclusion, endothelial dysfunction was related to renal function and contributed to the excess in cardiovascular mortality in this population-based cohort with mild renal insufficiency.

Note: A GFR of 68 is stage 2 kidney disease. Another study confirming early treatment is mandatory.

Study 22.5 Endothelial damage and vascular calcification in patients with chronic kidney disease.[6]

ABSTRACT:

Vascular calcification (VC) is a frequent complication of chronic kidney disease (CKD) and is a predictor of cardiovascular morbidity and mortality. In the present study, we investigated the potential involvement of endothelial microparticles (MPs) and endothelial progenitor cells (EPCs) in the generation of VC in CKD patients. The number of circulating EMPs is greater in patients with VC than without VC (307 ± 167 vs. 99 ± 75 EMPs/$_\mu$l, $P < 0.001$). The percentage of EPCs is significantly lower in patient with VC than in patients without VC ($0.14 \pm 0.11\%$ vs. $0.25 \pm 0.18\%$, $P = 0.002$). The number of EPCs expressing osteocalcin (OCN) was higher in VC patients (349 ± 63 cells/100,000) than in non-VC patients (139 ± 75 cells/100,000, $P < 0.01$). In vitro, MPs obtained from CKD patients were able to induce OCN expression in EPCs from healthy donors; the increase in OCN expression was more accentuated if MPs were obtained from CKD patients with VC. MPs from CKD patients also induced OCN expression in vascular smooth muscle cells and fibroblasts. In CKD patients, the rise in endothelial MPs associated with a decrease in the number of EPCs, suggesting an imbalance in the processes of endothelial damage and repair in CKD patients, mainly those with VC. Our results suggest that EPCs, through OCN expression, may directly participate in the process of vascular calcification.

Note: Calcification is mentioned in yet another study.

Study 22.6 Inflammation, endothelial dysfunction, and platelet activation in patients with chronic kidney disease: the chronic renal impairment in Birmingham (CRIB) study[7]

RESULTS:

There was evidence of low-grade inflammation in the chronic renal impairment group compared with healthy controls, with higher concentrations of C-reactive protein (3.70 versus 2.18 mg/L, $P < 0.01$) and fibrinogen (3.48 versus 2.67 g/L, $P < 0.001$) and lower serum albumin concentration (41.8 versus 44.0 g/dL [418 versus 440 g/L], $P < 0.001$). More severe renal impairment was associated with a trend towards higher fibrinogen and lower albumin concentrations (both $P < 0.001$), although there was no association with higher C-reactive protein level. As compared to healthy controls, plasma von Willebrand factor (142 versus 108 IU/dL, $P < 0.001$) and soluble P-selectin concentrations (57.0 versus 43.3 ng/mL, $P < 0.001$) were also higher in the chronic renal impairment group. More severe renal impairment was associated with a trend towards higher levels of von Willebrand factor ($P < 0.001$) and of soluble P selectin ($P < 0.05$).

CONCLUSION:

This cross-sectional analysis demonstrates that chronic kidney disease is associated with low grade inflammation, endothelial dysfunction and platelet activation, even among patients with moderate renal impairment.

Study 22.7   Endothelial Dysfunction: The Secret Agent Driving Kidney Disease[8]

Two take-home messages come out of this work. First, although we like to categorize TMAs into either clinical categories (such as HUS and TTP) or entities with specific etiologies, the actual disease may involve a variety of factors that alter endothelial function or integrity, and perhaps, this may explain why we frequently see overlap in presentations. Thus, distinction between various entities of TMAs may be lost depending on the relative contribution of the various factors involved. Treatments may, therefore, need to focus on the specific factors involved more than simply treating a disease category.

Second, it is important to maintain a healthy endothelium, because the healthier that it is, the better it can fend off endothelial insults. This may not carry over simply to preventing TMAs but also, many metabolic and kidney diseases. For example, endothelial dysfunction associated with reduce endothelial nitric oxide production may play a key role in the development of primary hypertension, metabolic syndrome, diabetic nephropathy, and even progression of CKD. Thus, more focus needs to be placed on improving endothelial cell health. One important aspect is improving the diet, because some foods, particularly those with fructose from added sugars, such as sucrose and high-fructose corn syrup, can impair endothelial function, partly by their ability to induce uric acid.15 Soft drink intake is known to be a risk factor for preeclampsia.16 Thus, one needs to think about how one might improve endothelial function as a general mea-sure for reducing TMAs and other kidney diseases. For example, endothelial protectants, such as dextran sulfate, have been reported to provide protection in an animal model of HUS.

The last decade can be rightfully claimed as the era of the podocyte. The large numbers of scientific contributions on the nature of the slit diaphragm and how alterations in these proteins can lead to proteinuria have represented some of the greatest breakthroughs in nephrology. However, it is increasingly evident that the health of the vascular endothelium is also key to both the prevention and the treatment of kidney diseases. Activation of the endothelium is key to initiating innate immunity and inflammation, complement activation, coagulation, platelet dysfunction and vaso-constriction. Capillary loss, which is also induced by endothelial injury, can lead to downstream ischemia, which can cause fibrosis and inflammation and impair function. Thus, the secret agent driving many kidney diseases may be endothelial dysfunction, which is defined broadly as alter-ation in any mechanism leading to impaired endothelial function and integrity. Finding ways to improve endothelial health may be a stealth way for both preventing and slowing kidney diseases.

Note: TMAs are thrombotic microangiopathies, HUS stands for hemolytic uremic syndrome, and TTP is short for thrombotic thrombocytopenic purpura. These are all forms of blood clots, aka thrombosis.

Okay, so we can say with certainty that the health of the linings of our blood vessels is critical to the health of our kidneys. We can go a step further and assume that ED plays a role in kidney disease progression. Inflammation of these linings may be the cause of renal hypoxia.

What can we do about this?

Again, this may be the reason that blood-lowering medication works so well for kidney patients. Relaxing and expanding blood vessels is needed, as we may be deficient in nitric oxide production.

Statins lower bad cholesterol, which may also increase nitric oxide production.

Magnesium is also associated with endothelial health.

Study 22.8 — The Relationship between Magnesium and Endothelial Function in End-Stage Renal Disease Patients on Hemodialysis[9]

RESULTS:

In the univariate analysis, When the participants were divided into two groups according to the median magnesium level (3.47 mg/dL), there was a significant difference in EDV of FMD (less than 3.47 mg/dL, 2.8±1.7%; more than 3.47 mg/dL, 5.1±2.0%, p=0.004). In the multivariate analysis, magnesium and albumin were identified as independent factors for FMD (β=1.794, p=0.030 for serum magnesium; β=3.642, p=0.012 for albumin).

CONCLUSION:

This study demonstrated that higher serum magnesium level may be associated with better endothelial function in ESRD patients on HD. In the future, a large, prospective study is needed to elucidate optimal range of serum magnesium levels in ESRD on HD patients.

Study 22.9 — Low magnesium promotes endothelial cell dysfunction: implications for atherosclerosis, inflammation and thrombosis[10]

In conclusion, our results demonstrate a direct role of low magnesium in promoting endothelial dysfunction by generating a pro-inflammatory, pro-thrombotic and proatherogenic environment that could play a role in the pathogenesis cardiovascular disease.

So, high magnesium levels may help as well.

What else can we do?

Exercise

Study 22.10 | The Vascular Endothelium in Chronic Kidney Disease:

A Novel Target For Aerobic Exercise[11]

SUMMARY

Exercise reverses impairments in endothelial L-arginine transport and improves endothelial function in chronic kidney disease by increasing nitric oxide bioavailability.

Extra info from this study:

The mechanisms of endothelial dysfunction appear to change throughout the progression of CKD resulting in endothelial dysfunction that is increasingly less reversible. Competition for L-arginine by the enzyme arginase may play a limited role in early CKD but appears to play less of a role through-out disease progression. Oxidative stress and increased levels of ADMA are important contributors to endothelial dysfunction in mild-to-moderate CKD. The accumulation of uremic toxins that occurs through-out the progression of CKD contributes to impaired transport of L-arginine into the endothelium. During advanced stages of CKD, this uremic toxin burden becomes so severe that a "uremic switch" occurs in which reduced L-arginine transport becomes the rate limiting step for NO production.

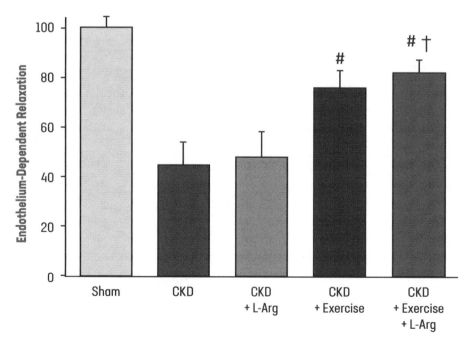

Chart info

Endothelial function is impaired in rats with CKD relative to sham control rats. Supplementation with L-arginine alone does not improve endothelium-dependent relaxation (EDR); however, four weeks of aerobic exercise (through voluntary wheel running) improves EDR in rats with CKD and the greatest benefit is observed when aerobic exercise and L-arginine supplementation are performed in combination. Data represent the area under the dose response curve of EDR in response to increasing doses of the endothelium-dependent vasodilator acetylcholine.

Uremia or uremic toxins reduce the amount of nitric oxide our bodies can make. This study suggests that exercise causes our bodies to adapt and produce an increased amount of nitric oxide. Taking a supplement did not work unless it was combined with exercise. The lesson for us is that good nutrition combined with exercise is needed. We must do both to get the benefits.

How About Diet

Study 22.11 — Association between Dietary Intakes of Nitrate and Nitrite and the Risk of Hypertension and Chronic Kidney Disease: Tehran Lipid and Glucose Study[12]

ABSTRACT:

Conclusion: Our findings indicated that higher intakes of NO2– might be an independent dietary protective factor against the development of HTN and CKD, which are major risk factors for adverse cardiovascular events.

Study 22.12 — The effect of dietary nitrates on vascular function and exercise capacity in chronic kidney disease[13]

Together, these data suggest that acute dietary nitrate ingestion improves BP and microvascular function as well as ventilatory threshold, total exercise time and work performed in individuals with moderate to severe CKD.

Improvements in microvascular function and BP are most likely due to nitrate-derived NO-induced vasodilation and/or decreases in oxidative stress. The improvements in ventilatory thresh-old, work performed and total exercise time may be a result of enhanced vasodilation of the muscle microvasculature, thus improving muscle microvascular oxygenation and tissue diffusion capacity to maintain ATP generation via oxidative metabolism.

Foods high in nitrates and antioxidants may improve the health of our vessel walls as well.

What can we do to improve our blood vessel walls and blood flow in our kidneys?

1. Take blood pressure medication like ACE inhibitors.

2. Take statins to lower LDL cholesterol.

3. Keep your magnesium levels at the high end of the normal range.

4. Eat a diet high in plant-based nitrates and antioxidants.

5. Exercise regularly.

6. Eliminate uremia or uremic toxins, if possible.

As one study suggested, the heath of the vessels in our most vascular organ will become the next big area for kidney disease research. The health of the lining of our blood vessels is almost number one in our treatment plan.

It must be, for us to get better and stay healthy longer.

The focus has always been on uremia via a low-protein diet to slow kidney disease progression but, as I have said from the beginning, we can't ignore the heart. Eating foods that are low in protein to decrease uremia is needed, but we can't eat low-protein foods that cause problems for our blood vessel walls. We also can't eat high-protein foods that will contribute to uremia.

Think again about the health of the smallest blood vessels in your body and kidneys. Your kidneys depend on the smallest vessels getting good blood flow and oxygen. This may also be why reducing inflammation can reduce the amount of protein in your urine. These tiny vessels have several jobs, and inflammation and endothelial dysfunction affect all of these jobs.

References

1. Malyszko J. Mechanism of endothelial dysfunction in chronic kidney disease. *Clinica Chimica Acta*. 2010;411(19-20):1412-1420.

2. Dhaun N, Goddard J, Webb DJ. Endothelin antagonism in patients with nondiabetic chronic kidney disease. In: Barton M, Kohan DE, eds. *Endothelin in Renal Physiology and Disease*. Vol 172: Karger Publishers; 2011:243-254.

3. Yilmaz MI, Saglam M, Caglar K, et al. The determinants of endothelial dysfunction in CKD: oxidative stress and asymmetric dimethylarginine. *American Journal of Kidney Diseases*. 2006;47(1):42-50.

4. Zoccali C, Mallamaci F. Propensity to calcification as a pathway to renal hypoxia in chronic kidney disease and in hypertension. *Journal of Hypertension*. 2017;35(10):1963-1965.

5. Stam F, van Guldener C, Becker A, et al. Endothelial dysfunction contributes to renal function-associated cardiovascular mortality in a population with mild renal insufficiency: the Hoorn Study. *Journal of the American Society of Nephrology*. 2006;17(2):537545.

6. Soriano S, Carmona A, Triviño F, et al. Endothelial damage and vascular calcification in patients with chronic kidney disease. *American Journal of Physiology-Renal Physiology*. 2014;307(11):F1302-F1311.

7. Landray MJ, Wheeler DC, Lip GY, et al. Inflammation, endothelial dysfunction and platelet activation in patients with chronic kidney disease: the chronic renal impairment in Birmingham (CRIB) study. *American Journal of Kidney Diseases*. 2004;43(2):244-253.

8. Johnson RJ, Nangaku M. Endothelial dysfunction: the secret agent driving kidney disease. *Journal of the American Society of Nephrology*. 2015;27.

9. Lee S, Ryu J-H, Kim S-J, Ryu D-R, Kang D-H, Choi KB. The Relationship between Magnesium and Endothelial Function in End-Stage Renal Disease Patients on Hemodialysis. *Yonsei Medical Journal*. 2016;57(6):1446-1453.

10. Maier JA, Malpuech-Brugère C, Zimowska W, Rayssiguier Y, Mazur A. Low magnesium promotes endothelial cell dysfunction: implications for atherosclerosis, inflammation and thrombosis. *Biochimica et Biophysica Acta (BBA)-Molecular Basis of Disease*. 2004;1689(1):13-21.

11. Martens CR, Kirkman DL, Edwards DG. The vascular endothelium in chronic kidney disease: a novel target for aerobic exercise. *Exercise and Sport Sciences Reviews*. 2016;44(1):12.

12. Bahadoran Z, Mirmiran P, Ghasemi A, Carlström M, Azizi F, Hadaegh F. Association between dietary intakes of nitrate and nitrite and the risk of hypertension and chronic kidney disease: Tehran Lipid and Glucose Study. *Nutrients*. 2016;8(12):811.

13. Ramick MG. The effect of dietary nitrates on vascular function and exercise capacity in chronic kidney disease, University of Delaware; 2017.

CHAPTER 23

Caloric and Methionine Restriction

I thought this chapter would simply say that reducing calories was helpful, but I was wrong. The chapter turned into something a little different than expected. We will start with caloric restriction and finish with methionine restriction. Calories first.

I know no one wants to hear about reducing calories, but I am compelled to report the facts.

Any time we eat or drink, we are putting demands on our kidneys. In fact, we put a workload on our kidneys by just living and breathing, regardless of food or drink intake. We can certainly put a monstrous workload on our kidneys when we combine large amounts and bad foods.

It certainly makes sense that, if we eat less, our kidneys have less to process. Overnutrition is a term used to describe excess calories: The amount of nutrients and related calories are more than what is required for healthy growth and development. It is not polite to say overeating. So, using the term overnutrition is more acceptable, I suppose.

Caloric restriction can be defined as eating the minimum amount of foods to meet your nutritional needs for healthy development and growth. Caloric restriction or "CR "has been very successful in animal trials.[1] CR has significantly extended the lives of many animals, but does it work in humans?[2]

Kidney disease disproportionately affects overweight people.[3] Could it be that consuming more calories than we need causes kidney disease, or is it the high blood pressure associated with obesity that causes the disease? It really doesn't matter; the result is the same. Overeating accelerates our illness.

Not only do the kinds of foods we eat speed or slow kidney disease progression, but the amount of food may also be a factor. Dr. Walser writes in his book, *Coping with Kidney Disease*, that caloric restriction is effective in slowing kidney disease.[4]

I asked Dr. Walser why the low-protein or low-calorie diet might work. I am paraphrasing his response: "Maybe we weren't built or designed to eat three high-calorie meals a day, especially high calories and high protein with every meal."

Think of a car driven full throttle for years or decades. How long would the car last? Another car that drives slowly for the same amount of time will have less wear and tear and will likely need fewer repairs. Our kidneys may not be much different. The problem is few studies on humans exist, so we must look at animals and other forms of reducing calories like fasting. It makes sense that eating less puts a lower workload on your kidneys. Nothing mysterious here.

Study 23.1 Acute caloric restriction improves the glomerular filtration rate in patients with morbid obesity and type 2 diabetes.[5]

RESULTS:

After the VLCD(very low calorie diet), both GFR and overall glucose disposal (M value) significantly increased from 72.6 ± 3.8 mL/min/1.73 m(-2) BSA to 86.9 ± 6.1 mL/min/1.73 m(-2) BSA (P=0.026) and from 979 ± 107 moll/min(1)/m(2) BSA to 1205 ± 94 μmol/min(1)/m(2) BSA (P=0.008), respectively. A significant correlation was observed between the increase in GFR and the rise in M value (r=0.625, P=0.017).

CONCLUSION:

Our observation of improved renal function following acute caloric restriction before weight loss became relevant suggesting that calorie restriction per se can affect renal function.

Study 23.2 Calorie Restriction in Obesity: Prevention of Kidney Disease in Rodents.[6]

It has long been known that food restriction, more so than a limitation of any particular dietary component, can significantly enhance longevity in laboratory rodents. These findings are being extended into a variety of other mammals, including nonhuman primates. These studies have indicated that caloric restriction in non-obese laboratory animals does not primarily affect specific disease processes but rather nonspecifically slows the aging process. In contrast, a growing body of evidence suggests that in genetically obese animals, food restriction can prevent or substantially delay the onset of specific degenerative lesions, in particular glomerulonephritis associated with obesity and diabetes.

Study 23.3 Caloric Restriction Delays Disease Onset and Mortality in Rhesus Monkeys.[7]

ABSTRACT:

Caloric restriction (CR), without malnutrition, delays aging and extends life span in diverse species; however, its effect on resistance to illness and mortality in primates has not been clearly established. We report findings of a 20-year longitudinal adult-onset CR study in rhesus monkeys aimed at filling this critical gap in aging research. In a population of rhesus macaques maintained at the Wisconsin National Primate Research Center, moderate CR lowered the inci-dence of aging-related deaths. At the time point reported, 50% of control fed animals survived as compared with 80% of the CR animals. Furthermore, CR delayed the onset of age-associated patholo-gies. Specifically, CR reduced the incidence of diabetes, cancer, cardiovascular disease, and brain atrophy. These data demonstrate that CR slows aging in a primate species.

Study 23.4 Caloric restriction ameliorates kidney ischemia/ reperfusion injury through the PGC-1α-eNOS pathway and enhanced autophagy.[8]

CONCLUSIONS:

Caloric restriction ameliorates acute kidney I/R injury through enhanced autophagy and coun-teraction of I/R induced decreases in the renal expression of eNOS and PGC-1α.

Study 23.5 Caloric restriction confers persistent antioxidative, pro-angiogenic, and anti-inflammatory effects and promotes anti-aging miRNA expression profile in Cerebro- microvascular endothelial cells of aged rats.[9]

Characterization of CR-induced changes in miRNA expression suggests that they likely affect sev-eral critical functions in endothelial cell homeostasis. The predicted regulatory effects of CR-related differentially expressed miRNAs in aged CMVECs are consistent with the anti-aging endothelial effects of CR observed in vivo. Collectively, we find that CR confers persisting antiox-idative, pro-angiogenic, and cellular anti-inflammatory effects, preserving a youthful phenotype in rat Cerebro-microvascular endothelial cells, suggesting that through these effects CR may improve cerebrovascular function and prevent vascular cognitive impairment.

What these studies have in common is the concept that lower caloric intake reduces oxidative stress and inflammation. Remember that eating is one of the greatest causes of oxidative stress and inflammation. Eating less of everything reduces oxidative stress and inflammation. This is a positive for already overworked kidneys that cannot keep up with the body's demands. If we are trying to reduce oxidative stress and inflammation, the easiest way is to reduce the amount we eat.

We typically don't think of foods causing stress and inflammation, but that is what the science tells us. We generally think of food as maybe a little unhealthy, or maybe bad for our waistlines. Think of a bag of potato chips, a cheeseburger, or other processed and fast foods. It may be that our bodies just cannot handle the work these foods put on us, especially our kidneys. They cause inflammation, oxidative stress, extra phosphorus, excess sodium, and the list goes on. It is just too much for our kidneys to handle.

Fasting is another way of looking at restricting calories. Many versions of fasting exist, but the common theme is restricting calories for a finite period of time in an attempt to reduce overall calories. Fasting could be once a month for a few days, every other day, daily fasts for a certain number of hours, and so on.

Alternate-day fasting became popular after a PBS special showing the beneficial effects of fasting. Eat what you want one day, then no calories or low calories the next day (500 calories). The overall reduction in calories accumulates over time. Subjects' blood tests all improved, and they lost weight.

But how about kidney disease?

Study 23.6   Food Restriction Ameliorates the Development of Polycystic Kidney Disease.[10]

Multiple studies have focused on pharmacological approaches to slow the development of the cystic disease; however, little is known about the role of nutrition and dietary manipulation in PKD. Here, we show that food restriction (FR) effectively slows the course of the disease in mouse models of ADPKD. Mild to moderate (10%–40%) FR reduced cyst area, renal fibrosis, inflammation, and injury in a dose-dependent manner. Molecular and biochemical studies in these mice indicate that FR ameliorates ADPKD through a mechanism involving suppression of the mammalian target of the rapamycin pathway and activation of the liver kinase B1/ AMP-activated protein kinase pathway. Our data suggest that dietary interventions such as FR, or treatment that mimics the effects of such interventions, may be potential and novel preventive and therapeutic options for patients with ADPKD.

That's about it for real studies on kidney patients when it comes to fasting. Several studies on fasting during Ramadan exist and are mixed. During Ramadan, no food or drink is consumed between sunup and sundown. The reduction in fluid intake may increase many markers for kidney disease over the short term. However, short-term fasting appears to have few long-term effects.

For a big picture view, we can look at the following study:

Study 23.7   Impact of caloric and dietary restriction regimens on markers of health and longevity in humans and animals: a summary of available findings.[11]

OVERALL SUMMARY AND CONCLUSIONS:

CR has been demonstrated to extend the maximal lifespan of a diverse group of species. This extension of life is maximized when: 1) the magnitude of CR is elevated to the highest possible value before inducing malnutrition and 2) the duration of CR is maximized. Animals on CR regimens exhibit a variety of improvements in overall health in general and cardiovascular health in particular. Unfortunately, the likelihood of discovering whether CR extends human life is rather remote due to the ethical and logistical limitations of research design. The optimal magnitude and duration of CR for humans will also likely never be known for the same reason. Nonetheless, many human CR studies have noted favorable changes in biomarkers related to cardiovascular and glucoregulatory functions, which probably relates to the quality of life and may relate to longevity.

Due to the austerity of following a CR regimen of sufficient magnitude and duration, alternatives such as CE, ADF, and DR may prove to be more appealing. The most pertinent consideration to make when evaluating these options is if they elicit benefits that are comparable to CR. ADF has been demonstrated to extend life and improve both cardiovascular and glucoregulatory function in animals. Human trials have noted heterogeneous findings and sex-specific differences regarding ADF's effects on glucoregulatory function. Unfortunately, it's hard to compare the effects of ADF and CR regimens across different studies due to an enormous number of confounding variables. Future studies should feature an ADF group and a CR group so that direct comparisons can be made. Regarding DR, neither carbohydrate restriction nor lipid restriction extends life. However, protein restriction appears to extend maximum lifespan by 20%. Recent findings suggest that methionine restriction may be the single cause of life extension observed in protein restriction studies. Future studies should examine the effects of different magnitudes of methionine restriction for life extension.

Two issues stand out from this paper:

> "The optimal magnitude and duration of Caloric restriction (CR) will also likely never be known."

> "However, protein restriction appears to extend maximum lifespan by 20%. Recent findings suggest that methionine restriction may be the single cause of life extension observed in protein restriction studies."

The idea is that we will never know about caloric restriction because it takes decades and many dozens, if not hundreds, of different forms of CR could be tested or used. This is troubling to me in some ways. It's hard to know how well caloric restriction works or even if it works in humans. However, the next excerpt is one of those light bulb moments:

> "Protein restriction of amino acid methionine may be the single cause of life extension."

What?

Why is methionine the bad guy when it is an essential amino acid? We need methionine to live. But methionine and the related amino acid cysteine contain the highest amounts of sulfur, which contributes to renal acid load. Another reason to think renal acid load is a much bigger factor than anyone else thinks. Again, everything is connected with kidney disease. The amino acid methionine is necessary because our bodies can't produce it.

It doesn't make sense that an essential amino acid reduces our life span. Let's look at little deeper:

Study 23.8   **Methionine restriction fundamentally supports health by tightening epithelial barriers.[12]**

ABSTRACT:

Dietary methionine restriction (MR) has been found to affect one of the most primary tissue-level functions of an organism: the efficiency with which the epithelial linings of major organs separate the fluid compartments that they border. This process, epithelial barrier function, is basic for proper function of all organs, including the lung, liver, gastrointestinal tract, reproductive tract, blood-brain barrier, and kidney. Specifically, MR has been found to modify the protein composition of tight junctional complexes surrounding individual epithelial cells in a manner that renders the complexes less leaky. This has been observed in both a renal epithelial cell culture model and in gastrointestinal tissue. In both cases, MR increased the transepithelial electrical resistance across the epithelium, while decreasing passive leak of small nonelectrolytes. However, the specific target protein modifications involved were unique to each case. Overall, this provides an example of the primary level on which MR functions to modify, and improve, an organism.

Study 23.9   **Restriction of sulfur-containing amino acids alters claudin composition and improves tight junction barrier function.**[13]

ABSTRACT:

Restriction of sulfur-containing amino acids (SCAA) has been shown to elicit a similar increase in life span and decrease in age-related morbidity as caloric restriction. The singular importance of epithelial barrier function in both physiological homeostasis and prevention of inflammation raised the issue of examining the effect of SCAA restriction on epithelial tight junction structure and permeability.

Study 23.10   **Transcriptional impact of dietary methionine restriction on systemic inflammation: relevance to biomarkers of metabolic disease during aging.**[14]

Dietary methionine restriction (MR) has emerged as an effective CR mimetic because it produces a comparable extension in lifespan. MR also reduces adiposity through a compensatory increase in energy expenditure that effectively limits fat accumulation, but essentially nothing is known about the effects of MR on systemic inflammation. Here, we review the relationships between these two interventions and discuss their transcriptional impact. Also, using tissues from rats after long-term consumption of CR or MR diets, transcriptional profiling was used to examine retrospectively the systems biology of 59 networks of molecules annotated to inflammation. Transcriptional effects of both diets occurred primarily in white adipose tissue and liver, and the responses to MR were far more robust than those to CR. The primary transcriptional targets of MR in both liver and white adipose tissue were phagocytes and macrophages, where expression of genes associated with immune cell infiltration and quantity was reduced.

Note: Methionine restriction was more effective than calorie restriction.

Study 23.11   **Mitochondrial oxidative stress, aging and caloric restriction: the protein and methionine connection.**[15]

Recently it was observed that 40% protein restriction without strong CR also decreases MitROS generation and oxidative stress. This is interesting because protein restriction also increases maximum longevity (although to a lower extent than CR) and is a much more possible intervention in humans than CR. Moreover, recently it was discovered 80% methionine restriction, substituting it for l-glutamate in the diet also decreases MitROS generation in rat liver. Thus, methionine restriction seems to be responsible for the decrease in ROS production observed in caloric restriction. This is interesting because it is known that precisely that methionine restriction procedure also increases maximum longevity. Moreover, recent data show that methionine levels in tissue proteins negatively correlate with the greatest longevity in mammals and birds. All these suggest that the lowering of methionine levels is involved in the control of mitochondrial oxidative stress and vertebrate longevity using at least two different mechanisms: decreasing the sensitivity of proteins to oxidative damage and lowering the rate of ROS generation at mitochondria.

Study 23.12 Lowered methionine ingestion as responsible for the decrease in rodent mitochondrial oxidative stress in protein and dietary restriction possible implications for humans.[16]

ABSTRACT:

Available information indicates that long-lived mammals have low rates of reactive oxygen species (ROS) generation and oxidative damage of their mitochondria. On the other hand, many studies have consistently shown that dietary restriction (DR) in rodents also decreases mitochondrial ROS (mtROS) production and oxidative damage to mitochondrial DNA and proteins. It has been observed that protein restriction also decreases mtROS generation and oxidative stress in rat liver, whereas neither carbohydrate nor lipid restriction changes these parameters. This is interesting because protein restriction also increases maximum longevity in rodents (although to a lower extent than DR) and is a much more practical intervention for humans than DR, whereas neither carbohydrate nor lipid restriction seems to change rodent longevity. Moreover, it has been found that isocaloric methionine restriction also decreases mtROS generation and oxidative stress in rodent tissues, and this manipulation also increases maximum longevity in rats and mice. Also, excessive dietary methionine also increases mtROS production in rat liver. These studies suggest that the reduced intake of dietary methionine can be responsible for the decrease in mitochondrial ROS generation and the ensuing oxidative damage that occurs during DR, as well as for part of the increase in maximum longevity induced by this dietary manipulation. Also, the mean intake of proteins (and thus methionine) of Western human populations is much higher than needed. Therefore, decreasing such levels to the recommended ones has a great potential to lower tissue oxidative stress and to increase healthy life span in humans while avoiding the possible undesirable effects of DR diets.

Study 23.13 Carbohydrate restriction does not change mitochondrial free radical generation and oxidative DNA damage.[17]

ABSTRACT:

Many previous investigations have consistently reported that caloric restriction (40%), which increases maximum longevity, decreases mitochondrial reactive species (ROS) generation and oxidative damage to mitochondrial DNA (mtDNA) in laboratory rodents. These reductions take place in rat liver after only seven weeks of caloric restriction. Moreover, it has been discovered that seven weeks of 40% protein restriction, independent of caloric restriction, also decreases these two parameters, whereas they do not change after seven weeks of 40% lipid restriction. This is interesting since we know that protein restriction can extend longevity in rodents, whereas lipid restriction does not have such effect. However, before concluding that the ameliorating effects of caloric restriction on mitochondrial oxidative stress are due to restriction in protein intake, studies on the third energetic component of the diet, carbohydrates, are needed. In the present study, using semi-purified diets, the carbohydrate ingestion of male Wistar rats was decreased by 40% below controls without changing the level of intake of the other dietary components. After seven weeks of treatment, the liver mitochondria of the carbohydrate restricted animals did not show changes in the rate of mitochondrial ROS production, mitochondrial oxygen consumption or percent free radical leak with any substrate (complex I- or complex II-linked) studied. In agreement with this, the levels of oxidative damage in hepatic mtDNA and nuclear DNA were not modified in carbo-hydrate restricted animals. Oxidative damage in mtDNA was one order of magnitude higher than that in nuclear DNA in both dietary groups. These results, together with previous ones, discard lipids and carbohydrates and indicate that the lowered ingestion of dietary proteins is respon-sible for the decrease in mitochondrial ROS production and oxidative damage in mtDNA that occurs during caloric restriction.

The last study shows that restricting carbohydrates did not change oxidative stress; only limited protein reduces oxidative stress and damage. To all those people who say carbs are bad: you are wrong, dead wrong. I have heard dozens of times that protein is better than carbs for certain things. I could not find any science to support this nutrition myth when it comes to kidney and heart health. Carbohydrates did not increase oxidative stress, but protein did.

In today's protein-obsessed marketplace, are we eating ourselves into an early grave? Are we speeding the aging process? Is the incredible rise in autoimmune diseases caused by protein overnutrition?

Could it be that too much methionine could cause our kidneys to "leak"? Claudins are the proteins that keep our cells watertight, or let them transfer the right amount of fluids. Methionine may cause these cells to "leak," including cells in our kidneys. A related condition is referred as "Leaky Gut" and is related to endotoxemia. Endotoxemia is a driver of kidney disease progression. Bacteria normally contained in our gut leak into our bloodstream, wreaking havoc as they go.

Study 23.14 Claudins and the Kidney.[18]

ABSTRACT:

Claudins are tight-junction membrane proteins that function as both pores and barriers in the paracellular pathway in epithelial cells. In the kidney, claudins determine the permeability and selectivity of different nephron segments along the renal tubule. In the proximal tubule, claudins have a role in the bulk reabsorption of salt and water. In the thick ascending limb, claudins are essential for the reabsorption of calcium and magnesium and are tightly regulated by the calci-um-sensing receptor. In the distal nephron, claudins need to form cation barriers and chloride pores to facilitate electrogenic sodium reabsorption and potassium and acid secretion. Aldosterone and the with-no-lysine (WNK) proteins likely regulate claudins to fine-tune distal nephron salt transport. Genetic mutations in claudin-16 and -19 cause familial hypomagnesemic hypercal-ciuria with nephrocalcinosis, whereas polymorphisms in claudin-14 are associated with kidney stone risk. It is likely that additional roles for claudins in the pathogenesis of other types of kidney diseases have yet to be uncovered.

Note: Methionine restriction improves claudins performance. We see that salt, calcium, and magnesium metabolism may be affected by methionine intake. It could be that reducing methionine intake improves management of salt, calcium, and magnesium. We don't know yet.

Study 23.15 **Tight junction claudins and the kidney in sickness and health.[19]**

CONCLUSION:

The recent discovery of the claudin family of tight junction associated membrane proteins represents a major breakthrough in our understanding of the structure and function of tight junctions in epithelial organs such as the kidney. We are only in the infancy of understanding how claudins work in the mammalian nephron tight junction. Important clues into the role of a few of the claudin family members are emerging from human genetic diseases of the tight junction, animal knockout models, and epithelial cell culture models. It is becoming increasingly apparent that the family of claudin molecules is of critical importance in renal function during normal and diseased physiological conditions. However, much more work will be required to fully understand how these claudins function normally within the tight junction as well as how abnormal claudin operates in the kidney relates to human disease processes.

Study 23.16 **Targeted colonic claudin-2 expression renders resistance to epithelial injury, induces immune suppression, and protects from colitis.[21]**

Expression of claudin-2, a tight junction protein, is highly upregulated during inflammatory bowel disease (IBD) and, due to its association with epithelial permeability, has been postulated to promote inflammation. Notably, claudin-2 has also been implicated in the regulation of intestinal epithelial proliferation. However, the precise role of claudin-2 in regulating colonic homeostasis remains unclear.

Taken together, our findings reveal a critical, albeit complex role of claudin-2 in intestinal homeostasis by regulating epithelial permeability, inflammation, and proliferation and suggest novel therapeutic opportunities.

A convincing amount of evidence suggests (but doesn't prove) methionine and the related impact on our body and kidneys could be an essential part of our disease. If the renal tubules are inflamed, or the barrier is weak, they may "leak," and the result is protein in our urine and loss of control of normal things like calcium and magnesium. Albumin is one of the smallest proteins floating around in our bloodstream. If we have inflammation or leaking renal tubules, it makes sense that the smallest component of our bloodstream would be the first to "leak" through in our urine.

Remember, the studies that showed soybeans did not affect kidney function like tuna. The studies showed no reaction after eating soybeans and suggested that soybeans may even have protected the kidneys. Guess what amino acid is very low in soybeans? Methionine. Methionine is so low in soybeans that methionine supplements are used if soy protein is someone's only source of protein. However, methionine is highest in fish. Tuna has 600%+ more methionine than an equal serving of soybeans.

Methionine may be responsible, or I should say a methionine overload may be the culprit, in some chronic diseases, including ours. It has already been proven to be a factor in other autoimmune diseases like inflammatory bowel disease.

Methionine restriction may even slow cancer.

Study 23.17 **A review of methionine dependency and the role of methionine restriction in cancer growth control and lifespan extension.[22]**

ABSTRACT:

Methionine is an essential amino acid with many key roles in mammalian metabolism, such as protein synthesis, methylation of DNA and polyamine synthesis. Restriction of methionine may be an important strategy in cancer growth control, particularly in cancers that exhibit dependence on methionine for survival and proliferation. Methionine dependence in cancer may be due to one or a combination of deletions, polymorphisms or alterations in expression of genes in the methionine de novo and salvage pathways. Cancer cells with these defects are unable to regenerate methionine via these pathways. Defects in the metabolism of folate may also contribute to the methionine dependence phenotype in cancer. Selective killing of methionine dependent cancer cells in coculture with normal cells has been demonstrated using culture media deficient in methionine. Several animal studies utilizing a methionine restricted diet have reported inhibition of cancer growth and extension of a healthy lifespan. In humans, vegan diets, which can be low in methionine, may prove to be a useful nutritional strategy in cancer growth control. The development of methioninase, which depletes circulating levels of methionine, may be another useful approach in limiting cancer growth. The application of nutritional methionine restriction and methioninase in combination with chemotherapeutic regimens is the current focus of clinical studies.

Ok, what about the fountain of youth? Can methionine restriction help us live longer, or take off a few pounds?

Study 23.18 **The Impact of Dietary Methionine Restriction on Biomarkers of Metabolic Health.[23]**

Over the last 20 years, dietary methionine restriction (MR) has emerged as a promising DR mimetic because it produces a comparable extension in life span, but surprisingly, does not require food restriction. Dietary MR also reduces adiposity but does so through a paradoxical increase in both energy intake and expenditure. The increase in energy expenditure completely compensates for greater energy intake and efficiently limits fat deposition. Perhaps more importantly, the diet increases metabolic flexibility and overall insulin sensitivity and improves lipid metabolism while decreasing systemic inflammation.

| Study 23.19 | Dietary methionine restriction increases fat oxidation in obese adults with metabolic syndrome.[24] |

CONCLUSIONS:

Sixteen weeks of dietary MR in subjects with metabolic syndrome produced a shift in fuel oxidation that was independent of weight loss, decreased adiposity, and improved insulin sensitivity that was common to both diets.

| Study 23.20 | Methionine restriction slows down senescence in human diploid fibroblasts.[25] |

Abstract

Methionine restriction (MetR) extends lifespan in animal models including rodents. Using human diploid fibroblasts (HDF), we report here that MetR significantly extends their replicative lifespan, thereby postponing cellular senescence. MetR significantly decreased the activity of mitochondrial complex IV and diminished the accumulation of reactive oxygen species. Lifespan extension was accompanied by a significant reduction in the levels of subunits of mitochondrial complex IV, but also complex I, which was due to a reduced translation rate of several mtDNA-encoded subunits. Together, these findings indicate that meteor slows down aging in human cells by modulating the mitochondrial protein synthesis and respiratory chain assembly.

Senescence is a process of cell deterioration with age. Cells may age faster with higher methionine levels and age slower with lower levels. Remember from earlier chapters that kidney disease is an accelerated form of aging in many ways. Could it be that methionine and its related compounds are responsible for the accelerated aging in people with kidney disease?

Did you also catch the studies that suggest methionine restriction increases fat burning and reduces adiposity (body fat)? Might methionine restrictions slow aging and decrease fat? Sign me up.

Homocysteine is produced in the body from dietary methionine intake. Homocysteine leads to inflammation and is associated with increased heart disease risk. Plasma homocysteine levels are strongly correlated with GFR. Hyperhomocysteinemia occurs when plasma homocysteine levels are too high. This starts happening at GFR around 60 and keeps increasing as our GFR declines.

This provides another big clue. We may need to limit methionine intake as our GFR starts to fall. Homocysteine is a cause of inflammation, which we are trying to limit or stop. This is more evidence that we must change our diets when we get a kidney disease diagnosis. Our bodies and kidneys cannot get rid of homocysteine fast enough, and that causes levels to rise.

In healthy adults, high methionine or protein intake does not lead to high homocysteine levels. However, our kidneys are not healthy and cannot keep up with the workload.

Study 23.21 **Folic Acid and Homocysteine in Chronic Kidney Disease and Cardiovascular Disease Progression: Which Comes First.**[26]

ABSTRACT:

Background: Hyperhomocysteinemia (Hhcy) occurs in about 85% of chronic kidney disease (CKD) patients because of impaired renal metabolism and reduced renal excretion. Folic acid (FA), the synthetic form of vitamin B_9, is critical in the conversion of homocysteine (Hcy) to methi-onine. If there is not enough intake of FA, there is not enough conversion, and Hcy levels increase.

Summary: Hhcy is regarded as an independent predictor of cardiovascular morbidity and mortality in end-stage renal disease. Hhcy exerts its pathogenic action on the primary processes involved in the progression of vascular damage. Research has shown Hhcy suggests enhanced risks for inflammation and endothelial injury which lead to cardiovascular disease (CVD), stroke, and CKD. FA has also been shown to improve endothelial function without lowering Hcy, suggesting an alternative explanation for the effect of FA on endothelial function. Recently, interest in the role of FA and Hhcy in CVD and CKD progression was renewed in some randomized trials.

Key Messages: In the general population and CKD patients, it remains a topic of discussion whether any beneficial effects of FA therapy are related to its direct effect or a reduction of Hhcy. While waiting for the results of confirmatory trials, it is reasonable to consider FA with or without methylcobalamin supplementation as appropriate adjunctive therapy in patients with CKD.

Study 23.22 **The Kidney and Homocysteine Metabolism.**[27]

ABSTRACT:

Homocysteine (Hcy) is an intermediate of methionine metabolism that, at elevated levels, is an independent risk factor for vascular disease and atherothrombosis. Patients with renal disease, who exhibit unusually high rates of cardiovascular morbidity and death, tend to have hyperhomocysteinemia, especially as renal function declines. This observation and the inverse relationship between Hcy levels and GFR implicate the kidney as an important participant in Hcy handling. The healthy kidney plays a significant role in plasma amino acid clearance and metabolism. The existence of distinct Hcy uptake mechanisms and Hcy-metabolizing enzymes in the kidney suggests that this role extends to Hcy. Dietary protein intake may affect renal Hcy handling and must be considered when measuring Hcy plasma flux and renal clearance. The underlying cause of hyperhomocysteinemia in renal disease is not entirely understood; but, it seems to involve reduced clearance of plasma Hcy. This reduction may be attributable to defective renal clearance and/or extrarenal clearance and metabolism, the latter possibly resulting from retained uremic inhibitory substances. Although the currently available evidence is not conclusive, it seems more likely that a reduction in renal Hcy clearance and metabolism is the cause of the hyperhomocysteinemic state. Efforts to resolve this important issue will advance the search for effective Hcy-lowering therapies in patients with renal disease.

Study 23.23 Association between serum homocysteine and markers of impaired kidney function in adults in the United States.[28]

CONCLUSION:

In the general population, renal insufficiency is strongly associated with an increased risk of elevated circulating homocysteine, independent of B vitamin status. These results raise the possibility that elevated homocysteine may be a significant risk factor to explain the heavy burden of CVD associated with kidney disease.

These studies, however, do not point to an exact conclusion about dietary methionine intake and homocysteine levels. Other studies indicate that folic acid and vitamin B12 may be helpful in reducing homocysteine levels.

A lot of conflicting data exists regarding homocysteine. Homocysteine levels have been correlated with kidney and heart disease progression. We know homocysteine metabolism is impaired or slowed with kidney disease. In many studies, increasing or decreasing methionine intake appears not to impact homocysteine levels. When intake is low, the body conserves, and when intake is high, the body excretes the excess.

Cysteine is an amino acid made from methionine in our bodies. Cysteine is also a sulphur amino acid. Sulphur equals high renal acid load. Let's see what we can find out about cysteine.

Study 23.24 A Close relationship between redox state of human serum albumin and serum cysteine levels in nondiabetic CKD patients with various degrees of renal function.[29]

RESULTS:

Total cysteine and homocysteine plasma levels increased with decreasing renal function and showed a significant negative correlation with glomerular filtration rate. The protein-bound ratio of serum cysteine also changed with the degree of renal dysfunction. The HPLC fraction of human mercapto albumin (HMA) (%) was significantly lower in nondiabetic CKD patients than in healthy subjects. The redox state of human serum albumin (i.e., HMA %) correlated significantly with the total serum cysteine level.

CONCLUSION:

The HPLC fraction of HMA (%) closely correlated with the serum cysteine level in nondiabetic CKD patients. An increase in oxidized cysteine with impaired renal function and a reduced plasma redox capacity associated with a decrease in the reduced form of serum albumin (HMA %) may be important risk factors for promoting long-term complications in patients with renal dysfunction.

Study 23.25 **Plasma cysteine/cystine reduction potential correlates with plasma creatinine levels in chronic kidney disease.[30]**

Healthy plasma presented Eh(Cyss/2Cys) of -123 ± 7 mV. Plasma Eh(Cyss/2Cys) correlated significantly with creatinine levels ($p < 0.0001$, $r = 0.62$).

CONCLUSION:

Plasma Eh(Cyss/2Cys) correlated with increased levels of plasma creatinine, supporting the view that uremia triggers oxidative stress. Additionally, it may be used as a quantitative oxidative stress biomarker in uremic conditions.

As with methionine, higher cysteine levels accumulate, leading to oxidative stress.

Study 23.26 **Dietary proteins with high isoflavone content or low methionine-glycine and lysine-arginine ratios are hypocholesterolemic and lower the plasma homocysteine level in male Zucker fa/fa rats.[31]**

It was previously demonstrated that soy protein, which contains isoflavones and low methionine-glycine and lysine–arginine ratios, has a hypocholesterolemic effect. In the present study, the hypocholesterolemic consequences of an isoflavone-enriched casein diet (HDI) and a single-cell protein-based diet (SCP), devoid of isoflavones but with low methionine–glycine and lysine–arginine ratios, was investigated in obese Zucker rats after six weeks of feeding. The control diet contained casein, which has high rates of methionine–glycine, and lysine–arginine. HDI and SCP feeding reduced the concentrations of total cholesterol and cholesteryl esters in plasma and liver and changed the fatty acid composition of the hepatic cholesteryl esters. Fecal cholesterol and bile acid levels were markedly higher in SCP-fed rats than in controls, whereas HDI feeding had only minor effects. However, both HDI and SCP feeding increased the hepatic gene expression of cholesterol 7α hydroxylase. In contrast, the hepatic acyl-CoA synthetase and acyl-CoA: cholesterol acyltransferase activities and the gene expression of the LDL receptor were increased by HDI, but not by SCP feeding. The present results suggested that the cholesterol-lowering effect of SCP was related to the enterohepatic circulation, whereas HDI seemed to lower the plasma cholesterol via the circulation. Plasma homocysteine level was reduced in rats fed HDI and SCP compared to rats fed casein. In summary, diets enriched in isoflavones or containing proteins with low methionine–glycine and lysine–arginine ratios lowered the plasma cholesterol and homocysteine levels, changing the plasma profile from atherogenic to cardioprotective.

85% of kidney patients have hyperhomocysteinemia. 85% is a pretty significant number, and hyperhomocysteinemia is a mortality and morbidity indicator. Clearly, we must reduce these numbers.

Let's see what we know at this point:

Methionine is an essential amino acid that our bodies cannot make.

Excess or higher than needed methionine or related compounds like cysteine and homocysteine are implicated in the following diseases and conditions:

> Cancer

> Autoimmune diseases

> Aging

> Weight gain

> Inflammation

> Oxidative stress

> Heart disease

> Kidney disease

The data is both compelling and confusing, from my point of view. We need methionine, but too much or impaired methionine metabolism can cause all manner of health problems.

The foods highest in methionine are fish, chicken, beef, eggs, and pork. As an error check, maybe we can look at vegans and vegetarians to see if they have lower methionine levels. And if they do, does it hurt them?

Study 23.27 The low-methionine content of vegan diets may make methionine restriction feasible as a life extension strategy.32

ABSTRACT:

Recent studies confirm that dietary methionine restriction increases both mean and maximal lifespan in rats and mice, achieving "aging retardant" effects very similar to those of caloric restriction, including a suppression of mitochondrial superoxide generation. Although voluntary caloric restriction is never likely to gain much popularity as a pro-longevity strategy for humans, it may be more feasible to achieve moderate methionine restriction, because vegan diets tend to be relatively low in this amino acid. Plant proteins—especially those derived from legumes or nuts—tend to be lower in methionine than animal proteins. Furthermore, the total protein content of vegan diets, as a function of calorie content, tends to be lower than that of omnivore diets, and plant protein has a somewhat lower bioavailability than animal protein. Whole-food vegan diets that moderate bean and soy intake, while including ample amounts of fruit and wine or beer, can be quite low in methionine, while supplying sufficient nutrition for health (assuming concurrent B12 supplementation). Furthermore, low-fat vegan diets, coupled with exercise training, can be expected to promote longevity by decreasing systemic levels of insulin and free IGF-I; the latter effect would be amplified by methionine restriction—though it is not clear whether IGF-I down-regulation is the sole basis for the impact of low-methionine diets on longevity in rodents.

Plasma concentrations and intakes of amino acids in male meat-eaters, fish-eaters, vegetarians, and vegans: a cross-sectional analysis in the EPICOxford cohort.[33]

Intakes of amino acids by habitual diet group:

> Geometric mean intake (95% confidence interval), g/d

> % mean difference compared with meat-eaters

Pdifferenceb				
	Meat-eaters	Fish-eaters	Vegetarians	Vegans
Methionine	(1.60)	(1.33)	(1.20)	(0.84)

As you can see, methionine is much lower for vegans; not so much for vegetarians. This will be important later.

Summary

Vegans have lower levels of methionine by a measurable amount, but vegetarians don't.

Lowering our intake of methionine will likely lower methionine in our bodies as well.

Consuming more methionine than needed is just extra work for our kidneys with no benefit. In fact, it could be harmful. We don't know for sure, but the evidence points in that direction.

Eating less methionine should lower the load on our kidneys and reduce the amount of homocysteine (which is a problem for 85% of us). It should also decrease acidosis. If lowering methionine can also help with aging and reducing fat, that may be too much to ask. However, we will take it if we can get it.

For our purposes, we are going to focus on methionine restriction and not caloric restriction. We need to make things as easy as possible. Caloric restriction is tough to follow and it is hard to get adequate nutrients without a lot of planning. CR is almost impossible when you add the restrictions for a kidney diet.

Restricting methionine is pretty easy when you limit fish, chicken, beef, pork, eggs, and dairy. The calculation for food in the Total Kidney Workload Diet considers the amount of methionine.

I wish we had several studies about restricting methionine in people with kidney disease, but they don't exist. However, where there is smoke, there is usually fire. Dozens of studies point us in this direction. Restricting methionine is a common-sense idea based on the information we have today.

I could not find any data that suggests that consuming a high amount of methionine is beneficial to kidney patients.

If we don't restrict methionine, we are putting our foot on the gas of kidney disease progression and increasing renal acid load, in my opinion.

References

1. Heilbronn LK, Ravussin E. Calorie restriction and aging: review of the literature and implications for studies in humans. *The American Journal of Clinical Nutrition.* 2003;78(3):361-369.

2. Most J, Tosti V, Redman LM, Fontana L. Calorie restriction in humans: an update. *Ageing Research Reviews.* 2017;39:36-45.

3. Kopple JD, Feroze U. The effect of obesity on chronic kidney disease. *Journal of Renal Nutrition.* 2011;21(1):66-71.

4. Walser M, Thorpe B. *Coping with kidney disease: A 12-step treatment program to help you avoid dialysis.* John Wiley & Sons; 2010.

5. Giordani I, Malandrucco I, Donno S, et al. Acute caloric restriction improves glomerular filtration rate in patients with morbid obesity and type 2 diabetes. *Diabetes & Metabolism.* 2014;40(2):158-160.

6. Stern JS, Gades MD, Wheeldon CM, Borchers AT. Calorie restriction in obesity: prevention of kidney disease in rodents. *The Journal of nutrition.* 2001;131(3):913S-917S.

7. Colman RJ, Anderson RM, Johnson SC, et al. Caloric restriction delays disease onset and mortality in rhesus monkeys. *Science.* 2009;325(5937):201-204.

8. Lempiäinen J, Finckenberg P, Mervaala E, Sankari S, Levijoki J, Mervaala E. Caloric restriction ameliorates kidney ischaemia/ reperfusion injury through PGC-1α–eNOS pathway and enhanced autophagy. *Acta Physiologica.* 2013;208(4):410-421.

9. Csiszar A, Gautam T, Sosnowska D, et al. Caloric restriction confers persistent anti-oxidative, pro-angiogenic, and antiinflammatory effects and promotes anti-aging miRNA expression profile in cerebromicrovascular endothelial cells of aged rats. *American Journal of Physiology-Heart and Circulatory Physiology.* 2014;307(3):H292-H306.

10. Warner G, Hein KZ, Nin V, et al. Food restriction ameliorates the development of polycystic kidney disease. *Journal of the American Society of Nephrology.* 2015:ASN. 2015020132.

11. Trepanowski JF, Canale RE, Marshall KE, Kabir MM, Bloomer RJ. Impact of caloric and dietary restriction regimens on markers of health and longevity in humans and animals: a summary of available findings. *Nutrition Journal.* 2011;10(1):107.

12. Mullin JM, Skrovanek SM, Ramalingam A, DiGuilio KM, Valenzano MC. Methionine restriction fundamentally supports health by tightening epithelial barriers. *Annals of the New York Academy of Sciences.* 2016;1363(1):59-67.

13. Skrovanek S, Valenzano M, Mullin JM. Restriction of sulfur-containing amino acids alters claudin composition and improves tight junction barrier function. *American Journal of Physiology-Regulatory, Integrative and Comparative Physiology.* 2007;293(3):R1046-R1055.

14. Wanders D, Ghosh S, Stone KP, Van NT, Gettys TW. Transcriptional impact of dietary methionine restriction on systemic inflammation: relevance to biomarkers of metabolic disease during aging. *Biofactors.* 2014;40(1):13-26.

15. Pamplona R, Barja G. Mitochondrial oxidative stress, aging and caloric restriction: the protein and methionine connection. *Biochimica Et Biophysica Acta (BBA)-Bioenergetics.* 2006;1757(5):496-508.

16. López-Torres M, Barja G. Lowered methionine ingestion as responsible for the decrease in rodent mitochondrial oxidative stress in protein and dietary restriction: possible implications for humans. *Biochimica et Biophysica Acta (BBA)-General Subjects.* 2008;1780(11):1337-1347.

17. Sanz A, Gomez J, Caro P, Barja G. Carbohydrate restriction does not change mitochondrial free radical generation and oxidative DNA damage. *Journal of Bioenergetics and Biomembranes.* 2006;38(5):327-333.

18. Alan S. Claudins and the kidney. *Journal of the American Society of Nephrology.* 2014:ASN. 2014030284.

19. Balkovetz DF. Tight junction claudins and the kidney in sickness and in health. *Biochimica et Biophysica Acta (BBA)Biomembranes.* 2009;1788(4):858-863.

20. Enck AH, Berger UV, Alan S. Claudin-2 is selectively expressed in proximal nephron in mouse kidney. *American Journal of Physiology-Renal Physiology.* 2001;281(5):F966-F974.

21. Ahmad R, Chaturvedi R, Olivares-Villagómez D, et al. Targeted Colonic Claudin-2 Expression Renders Resistance to Epithelial Injury, Induces Immune Suppression and Protects from Colitis. *Mucosal Immunology.* 2014;7(6):1340.

22. Cavuoto P, Fenech MF. A review of methionine dependency and the role of methionine restriction in cancer growth control and lifespan extension. *Cancer Treatment Reviews.* 2012;38(6):726-736.

23. Orgeron ML, Stone KP, Wanders D, Cortez CC, Van NT, Gettys TW. The impact of dietary methionine restriction on biomarkers of metabolic health. *Progress in Molecular Biology and Translational Science.* 2014;121:351.

24. Plaisance EP, Greenway FL, Boudreau A, et al. Dietary methionine restriction increases fat oxidation in obese adults with metabolic syndrome. *The Journal of Clinical Endocrinology & Metabolism.* 2011;96(5):E836-E840.

25. Kozieł R, Ruckenstuhl C, Albertini E, et al. Methionine restriction slows down senescence in human diploid fibroblasts. *Aging Cell.* 2014;13(6):1038-1048.

26. Cianciolo G, De Pascalis A, Di Lullo L, Ronco C, Zannini C, La Manna G. Folic Acid and Homocysteine in Chronic Kidney Disease and Cardiovascular Disease Progression: Which Comes First. *Cardiorenal Medicine.* 2017;7(4):255-266.

27. Friedman AN, Bostom AG, Selhub J, Levey AS, Rosenberg IH. The kidney and homocysteine metabolism. *Journal of the American Society of Nephrology.* 2001;12(10):2181-2189.

28. Francis ME, Eggers PW, Hostetter TH, Briggs JP. Association between serum homocysteine and markers of impaired kidney function in adults in the United States. *Kidney international.* 2004;66(1):303-312.

29. Suzuki Y, Suda K, Matsuyama Y, Era S, Soejima A. Close relationship between redox state of human serum albumin and serum cysteine levels in non-diabetic CKD patients with various degrees of renal function. *Clinical Nephrology.* 2014;82(5):320-325.

30. Rodrigues SD, Batista GB, Ingberman M, Pecoits-Filho R, Nakao LS. Plasma cysteine/cystine reduction potential correlates with plasma creatinine levels in chronic kidney disease. *Blood purification.* 2012;34(3-4):231-237.

31. Gudbrandsen OA, Wergedahl H, Liaset B, Espe M, Berge RK. Dietary proteins with high isoflavone content or low methionine– glycine and lysine–arginine ratios are hypocholesterolaemic and lower the plasma homocysteine level in male Zucker fa/fa rats. *British Journal of Nutrition.* 2005;94(3):321-330.

32. McCarty MF, Barroso-Aranda J, Contreras F. The low-methionine content of vegan diets may make methionine restriction feasible as a life extension strategy. *Medical Hypotheses.* 2009;72(2): 125-128.

33. Schmidt JA, Rinaldi S, Scalbert A, et al. Plasma concentrations and intakes of amino acids in male meat-eaters, fish-eaters, vegetarians and vegans: a cross-sectional analysis in the EPIC-Oxford cohort. *European Journal of Clinical Nutrition.* 2016;70(3):306.

CHAPTER 24

Endotoxemia: The Unknown Driver of Heart and Kidney Disease Progression

Endotoxemia was unknown to me before writing this book. However, it may be a potent driver of heart and kidney disease progression. Research on endotoxemia is still in its infancy, but it is mandatory for us to at least think about it.

The research is so new that one doctor told me endotoxemia was not related to kidney disease (he has since recanted) and another said he has never ordered an endotoxemia test in his thirty-year career. For me, this makes endotoxemia more dangerous for us because it is unlikely we will ever get tested or know about it.

Endotoxemia is caused by bacteria, specifically gram-negative bacteria. Many gram-negative bacteria are pathogenic, or cause disease. These bacteria are harder to kill and more resistant to antibiotics. Gram-negative bacteria are more resistant to treatment. Gram-positive bacteria are easier to kill than gram-negative bacteria.

The bacteria in our gut are collectively called a "microbiome." The newest research shows that kidney disease affects the health of our microbiome. Evidence is mounting that, as kidney disease progresses, the health of our gut bacteria appears to decline as well, resulting in endotoxemia.

Over 100 million bacteria in our body help with digestion and immune response, and generate healthy things like short chain fatty acids. However, when the bad bacteria normally contained in our stomach run loose in our bloodstream, then bad things happen. Scientists are starting to think about your microbiome as another organ.

Endotoxemia is indicated in many diseases including septic shock, atherosclerosis, obesity, chronic fatigue, metabolic syndrome, and many other conditions. The research is sobering.

In the following chart, notice how higher levels of endotoxins, aka bad bacteria, dramatically increase mortality rates. You will see the term "lipopolysaccharide." This is the medical term for gram-negative bacteria.

FIGURE 24.1: **Circulating Endotoxemia: a Novel Factor in Systemic Inflammation and Cardiovascular Disease in Chronic Kidney Disease[1]**

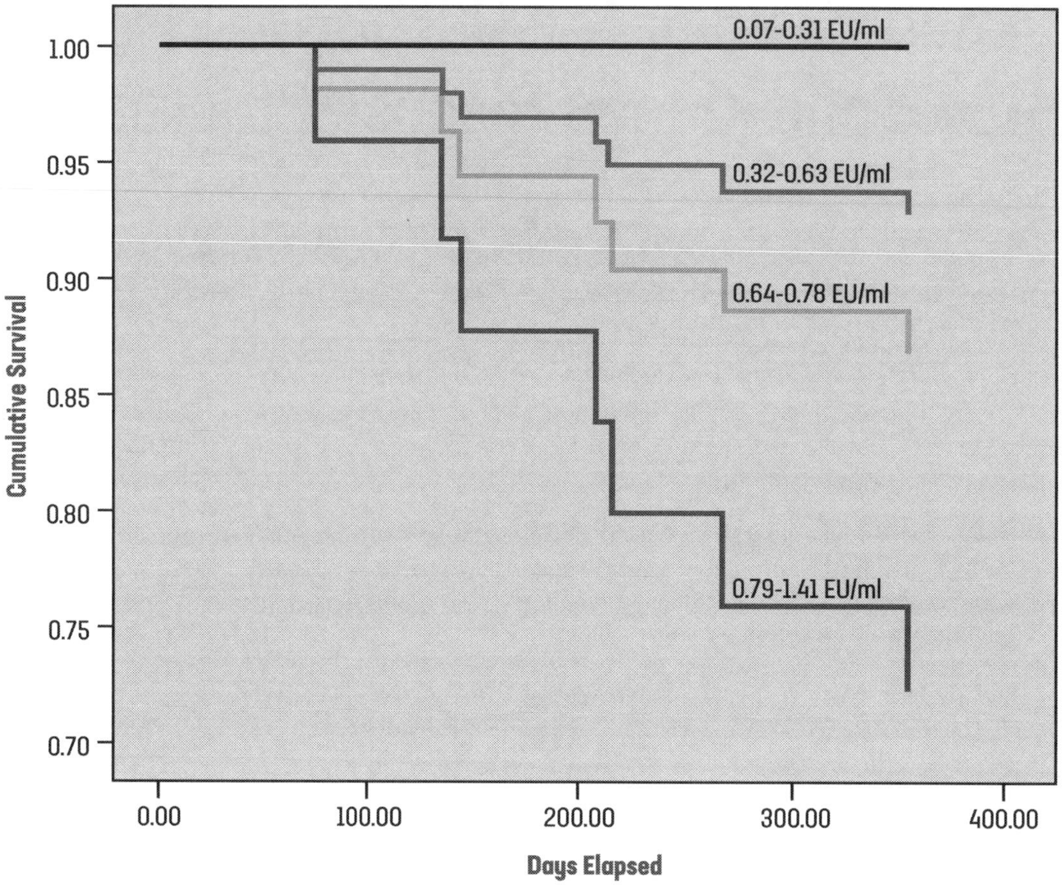

Data from same study:

Study 24.1

RESULTS:

Circulating endotoxemia was most notable in those with the highest CV disease burden (increasing with CKD stage), and a sharp increase was observed after initiation of HD. In HD patients, predialysis endotoxin correlated with dialysis-induced hemodynamic stress (ultrafiltration volume, relative hypotension), myocardial stunning, serum cardiac troponin T and high-sensitivity C-reactive protein. Endotoxemia was associated with risk of mortality.

CONCLUSIONS:

CKD patients are characteristically exposed to significant endotoxemia. In particular, HD-induced systemic circulatory stress and recurrent regional ischemia may lead to increased endotoxin translocation from the gut. Resultant endotoxemia is associated with systemic inflammation, markers of malnutrition, cardiac injury and reduced survival. This represents a crucial missing link in understanding the pathophysiology of the grossly elevated CV disease risk in CKD patients, highlighting the potential toxicity of conventional HD and providing a novel set of potential therapeutic strategies to reduce CV mortality in CKD patients.

Note: Ok, we have an idea now that endotoxins are a strong mortality indicator, but what about kidney disease progression? Reminder, LPS stands for serum lipopolysaccharide, which is the standard reference name for gram-negative bacteria.

Study 24.2 | **Serum Lipopolysaccharide Activity Is Associated with the Progression of Kidney Disease in Finnish Patients with Type 1 Diabetes[2]**

RESULTS:

Serum LPS activity was significantly higher in the macroalbuminuric group than in the normoalbuminuric group (P 0.001). Notably, normoalbuminuric progressor patients had a significantly higher LPS activity at baseline than normoalbuminuric nonprogressor patients (median 49 [interquartile range 34–87] vs. 39 [29–54] EU/ml; P 0.001). The normoalbuminuric progressor patients exhibited features of the metabolic syndrome with higher triglyceride concentrations and lower estimated glucose disposal rate. A high LPS-to-HDL ratio was associated with the progression of kidney disease in both groups. Insulin resistance (P 0.001) and serum LPS activity (P 0.026) were independent risk factors of disease development, when A1C was removed from the regression analysis.

CONCLUSIONS:

High serum LPS activity is associated with the development of diabetic nephropathy in Finnish patients with type 1 diabetes.

Study 24.3 | **Endotoxemia is Related to Systemic Inflammation and Atherosclerosis in Peritoneal Dialysis (PD) Patients[3]**

In summary, we found that endotoxemia was common in PD patients, and the degree of circulating endotoxemia was related to the severity of systemic inflammation and features of atherosclerosis. Our result suggests that endotoxemia may contribute to the systemic inflammatory state and accelerated atherosclerosis in PD patients.

Study 24.4   A Gut Feeling on Endotoxemia: Causes and Consequences in Chronic Kidney Disease[4]

ABSTRACT:

Chronic inflammation is closely linked to several complications of chronic kidney disease (CKD), such as vascular calcification, accelerated atherosclerosis, loss of appetite, insulin resistance, increased muscle catabolism and anemia. As a consequence, inflammation is a predictor of mortality in this group of patients. Specific causes of the activation of the immune system in CKD are largely unknown. Endotoxin (ET) release to the circulation represents a potentially important target for interventions aiming to reduce mortality in CKD patients. In this mini review, we propose that there are several potential sources of endotoxemia in CKD and that gut translocation, leading to the generation of ligands of the innate immune response, represents a potentially reversible cause. Prevention of endotoxemia, through treating foci of ET (periodontal disease, catheters, vascular access) or reducing translocation from the gut, will potentially reduce the inflammatory response.

Study 24.5   The Associations of Endotoxemia with Systemic Inflammation, Endothelial Activation and Cardiovascular Outcome in Kidney Transplantation (KTR)[5]

CONCLUSIONS:

Endotoxemia in KTRs(Transplant) contributes to inflammation, endothelial activation and increased cardiovascular events. This study highlights the clinical relevance of endotoxemia in KTRs, suggesting future interventional targets.

As you can see, kidney disease progression may be directly related to what is going on in our guts.

Kidney disease appears to directly change our gut microbiomes. As our disease progresses, it is likely that our microbiomes have a harder time staying in balance. Uremia may be a factor.

Study 24.6   Chronic kidney disease alters intestinal microbial flora[6]

In conclusion, ESRD significantly modifies the composition of gut microbiome in humans. The presence of an equally significant difference in the intestinal microbial flora between the uremic and control rats, which were otherwise identical, helped to substantiate the impact of uremia *per se* on the composition of the gut microbial flora. In addition to uremia, the strict dietary restrictions that ESRD patients were under must have contributed to the observed changes in their microbial flora. Further studies are needed to dissect the effect of the dietary restrictions from those of uremia, *per se*, in this population.

Study 24.7   The Gut Microbiome, Kidney Disease and Targeted Interventions[7]

PARTIAL ABSTRACT:

Endotoxin derived from gut bacteria incites a powerful inflammatory response in the host organism. Furthermore, protein fermentation by gut microbiota generates myriad toxic metabolites, including p-cresol and indoxyl sulfate. Disruption of gut barrier function in CKD allows translocation of endotoxin and bacterial metabolites to the systemic circulation, which contributes to uremic toxicity, inflammation, progression of CKD and associated cardiovascular disease.

Note: Lowering protein consumption may have the unexpected benefit of improving the health of our gut microbiomes.

Study 24.8   Gut microbiome in chronic kidney disease[8]

A myriad of factors contribute to dysbiosis in patients with CKD, such as slowing of intestinal transit, decreases in digestive capacity and secretion of ammonia and urea into the gut (Ramezani & Raj, 2014; Fig. 1). The cause of slow colonic transit time and frequent constipation observed in CKD and particularly haemodialysis patients seems to be multifactorial. Dietary restriction and low fiber consumption, lack of activity, use of phosphate binders and comorbidities, such as diabetes and heart disease, might all contribute to the greater prevalence of constipation in these patients (Wu *et al.* 2004). Slowing of the intestinal transit permits proliferation of bacteria. Impaired protein digestion results in undigested protein being delivered to the colon, which also causes proliferation of proteolytic bacteria.

Note: The term dysbiosis is used to describe a gut microbiome that is out of balance, damaged, or out of normal ranges. Notice, ammonia and urea may also be causes.

Study 24.9   Gut microbiome and kidney disease: a bidirectional relationship[9]

CONCLUSION:

The relationship between the human microbiome and kidney disease is bidirectional. Recent studies have described how kidney disease contributes to dysbiosis and how dysbiosis contributes to progression of kidney disease. Clinicians must be aware of the potential, unintended effects of treatments that may alter the gut microbiome, exercise self-discipline, and weigh risks and benefits when prescribing prophylactic antibiotics to patients with recurrent urinary tract infections, vesicoureteral reflux and other infections. There is a pressing need for more studies that characterize the microbiome profile in children with CKD and explore the relationship between different pediatric kidney disease parameters and the microbiome of the growing child. This is not only needed to estab-lish relationships by association, but to examine the interaction between certain early-life microbial and antibiotic exposure on the pathogenesis of kidney disease. Multiple promising interventions have been described to restore a more balanced microbiome and possibly slow the progression of CKD; such interventions need to be further examined in large, controlled trials before they can become part of our mainstream management.

Study 24.10 | Role of the Gut Microbiome in Uremia: A Potential Therapeutic Target[10]

ABSTRACT:

Also known as the "second human genome," the gut microbiome plays important roles in both the maintenance of health and the pathogenesis of disease. The symbiotic relationship between host and microbiome is disturbed due to proliferation of dysbiotic bacteria in patients with chronic kidney disease (CKD). Fermentation of protein and amino acids by gut bacteria generate excess amounts of potentially toxic compounds such as ammonia, amines, thiols, phenols and indoles, but generation of short chain fatty acids is reduced. Impaired intestinal barrier function in CKD permits translocation of gut-derived uremic toxins into the systemic circulation, contributing to progression of CKD, cardiovascular disease, insulin resistance, and protein energy wasting. The field of microbiome research is still nascent, but evolving rapidly. Establishing symbiosis to treat uremic syndrome is a novel concept, but if proven effective, will have significant impact on the management of patients with CKD.

Study 24.11 | The gut as a source of inflammation in chronic kidney disease[11]

ABSTRACT:

Chronic inflammation is a non-traditional risk factor for cardiovascular mortality in the chronic kidney disease (CKD) population. In recent years, the gastrointestinal tract has emerged as a major instigator of systemic inflammation in CKD. Post-mortem studies previously discovered gut wall inflammation present throughout the digestive tract in chronic dialysis patients. In CKD animals, colon wall inflammation is associated with breakdown of the epithelial tight junction barrier ("leaky gut") and translocation of bacterial DNA and endotoxin into the bloodstream. Gut bacterial DNA and endotoxin have also been detected in the serum from CKD and dialysis patients, whereby endotoxin levels increase with CKD stage and correlate with severity of systemic inflammation in the dialysis population. The CKD diet that is low in plant fiber and symbiotic organisms (in adherence with low potassium, low phosphorus intake) can alter the normal gut microbiome, leading to overgrowth of bacteria that produce uremic toxins such as cresyl and indoxyl molecules. The translocation of these toxins from the "leaky gut" into the bloodstream further promotes systemic inflammation, adverse cardiovascular outcomes and CKD progression. Data is lacking on optimal fiber and yogurt consumption in CKD that would favor growth of a more symbiotic microbiome while avoiding potassium and phosphorus overload. Prebiotic and probiotic formulations have shown promise in small clinical trials, in terms of lowering serum levels of uremic toxins and improving quality of life. The evidence points to a strong relationship between intestinal inflammation and adverse outcomes in CKD, and more trials investigating gut-targeted therapeutics are needed.

> **Note:** More evidence that traditional kidney diets may be making this worse due to the potassium and phosphorus restrictions. Again, we are getting 1950s diet advice.

We see some common themes here again. Uremic toxins like indoxyl sulfate come from the amino acid tryptophan, and p-cresol sulfate comes from tyrosine. Ammonia, urea, malnutrition from diet, lack of fiber, inflammation, and so on are also common themes.

What about certain diets? Can diet increase or decrease endotoxemia?

FIGURE 24.1: **A High-Fat Diet Is Associated With Endotoxemia That Originates from the Gut[12]**

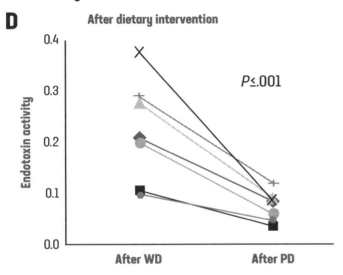

This chart shows how endotoxins levels dropped after just one month on a healthier diet. Diet changes alone cause a net difference of 102%, a 71% increase on a Western-style high-fat diet, and a 31% drop in endotoxins by eating a healthy diet. This is remarkable, as endotoxemia has no proven treatment. It should be noted that saturated fats were the bad guy, not healthy fats.

| Study 24.12 | ABSTRACT FROM SAME STUDY: |

Endotoxemia, characterized by an excess of circulating bacterial wall lipopolysaccharide, is associated with systemic inflammation and the metabolic syndrome. Placing eight healthy subjects on a Western-style diet for one month induced a 71% increase in plasma levels of endotoxin activity (endotoxemia), whereas a prudent-style diet reduced levels by 31%. The Western-style diet might, therefore, contribute to endotoxemia by causing changes in gastrointestinal barrier function or the composition of the microbiota. Endotoxemia might also develop in individuals with gastrointestinal barrier impairment. Therapeutic reagents that reduce endotoxemia might reduce systemic inflammation in patients with gastrointestinal diseases or metabolic syndrome.

Note: The prudent diet is a heart-healthy diet with no eggs, milk, liver, shellfish, or flour products like pastries, and a higher intake of fruits, vegetables, and grains.

| Study 24.13 | Effect of Dietary Lipids on Endotoxemia Influences Postprandial Inflammatory Response.[13] |

ABSTRACT:

Metabolic syndrome (MetS) results in postprandial metabolic alterations that predisposes one to a state of chronic low-grade inflammation and increased oxidative stress. We aimed to assess the effect of the consumption of the quantity and quality of dietary fat on fasting and postprandial plasma lipopolysaccharides (LPS). A subgroup of 75 subjects with metabolic syndrome was randomized to receive one of four diets: HSFA, rich in saturated fat; HMUFA, rich in mono-unsaturated fat; LFHCC n-3, low-fat, rich in complex carbohydrate diet supplemented with n-3 polyunsaturated fatty acids; LFHCC low-fat, rich in complex carbohydrate diet supplemented with placebo, for 12 weeks each. We administered a fat challenge reflecting the fatty acid composition of the diets at post-intervention. We determined the plasma lipoproteins and glucose and gene expression in peripheral blood mononuclear cells (PBMC) and adipose tissue. LPS and LPS binding protein (LBP) plasma levels were determined by ELISA, at fasting and postprandial (four hours after a fat challenge) states. We observed a postprandial increase in LPS levels after the intake of the HSFA meal, whereas we did not find any postprandial changes after the intake of the other three diets. Moreover, we found a positive relationship between the LPS plasma levels and the gene expression of IkBa and MIF1 in PBMC. No statistically significant differences in the LBP plasma levels at fasting or postprandial states were observed. Our results suggest that the consumption of HSFA diet increases the intestinal absorption of LPS, which, in turn, increases postprandial endotoxemia levels and the postprandial inflammatory response.

Note: We see gene expression again in relation to diet and saturated fats.

The evidence is compelling, especially when you look at how new the science of gut bacteria is. It also makes sense that the bacteria in our stomach would be affected by increased levels of urea, ammonia, and pH.

Treatments and Testing

It appears that testing for endotoxemia is very rare. The correct medical test is "LAL," which is an assay for "limulus amoebocyte lysate." Ideally, we would be tested to find out if endotoxemia is an issue for us. However, these tests are not done in local labs and your doctor may resist due to costs or lack of evidence. In addition, the test may not pick up all forms of gram-negative bacteria.

Treatments may be available to slow or reduce endotoxins. None of these treatments can be considered definitive, but they bear mentioning in an attempt to be thorough.

1. Diet appears to have the most impact.

2. Probiotics: Intestinal bacteria to seed or increase good bacteria may help. Studies differ in results, so it's hard to tell.

3. Prebiotics: Usually a starch that is not digestible, which acts as food for good bacteria. As with probiotics, there is some proof that it increases good bacteria, but it is not conclusive.

4. AST-120: Charcoal in a capsule. Conflicting studies exist on AST-120, so we don't really know if it works or not.

I am always suspect of the claims of probiotics, and any other supplement claim. Probiotics appear to have little, if any, benefit in healthy patients. It is unknown at this time if probiotics would help kidney patients in a meaningful way. It is likely that a specialized version of probiotics or prebiotics would be required to get a benefit that is measurable in blood or urine tests. A clinical trial would be needed to determine real benefits.

I found that most (if not all) probiotics purchased in stores are a strain or type that is easy to grow in labs. Strains that are easy to grow in labs may not be the ones that will survive in highly acidic stomach conditions. Remember the section on supplements when it comes to probiotic or prebiotic claims.

Now let's apply some common sense to what we have learned about endotoxemia. How can we effectively reduce or limit endotoxemia as people with kidney disease?

1. Reduce our intake of protein, especially tyrosine and tryptophan.

2. Restrict our dietary methionine intake, which may improve bowel and gut barriers.

3. Eat a healthy diet low in saturated fats, similar to the "prudent diet."

4. Consume more than the RDA of fiber each day.

5. Treat constipation so bad bacteria doesn't have time to grow.

6. If you have taken antibiotics, you may need to take probiotics to help establish good bacteria for a period of time. However, diet is a better option over the long term.

I hope to add to this chapter in the future, and to raise awareness of this potential issue for kidney patients. An effective treatment for endotoxemia might help slow the progression of kidney disease.

This is another reason to stay on a heart- and kidney-healthy diet. It may help build the good bacteria in our bodies and reduce yet another driver of disease progression.

References

1. McIntyre CW, Harrison LE, Eldehni MT, et al. Circulating endotoxemia: a novel factor in systemic inflammation and cardiovascular disease in chronic kidney disease. Clinical *Journal of the American Society of Nephrology.* 2011;6(1):133-141.

2. Nymark M, Pussinen PJ, Tuomainen AM, et al. Serum lipopolysaccharide activity is associated with the progression of kidney disease in finnish patients with type 1 diabetes. *Diabetes Care.* 2009;32(9):1689-1693.

3. Szeto C-C, Kwan BC-H, Chow K-M, et al. Endotoxemia is related to systemic inflammation and atherosclerosis in peritoneal dialysis patients. *Clinical Journal of the American Society of Nephrology.* 2008;3(2):431-436.

4. Hauser AB, Stinghen AE, Gonçalves SM, Bucharles S, Pecoits-Filho R. A gut feeling on endotoxemia: causes and consequences in chronic kidney disease. *Nephron Clinical Practice.* 2011;118(2):c165-c172.

5. Chan W, Bosch JA, Phillips AC, et al. The associations of endotoxemia with systemic inflammation, endothelial activation, and cardiovascular outcome in kidney transplantation. *Journal of Renal Nutrition.* 2018;28(1):13-27.

6. Vaziri ND, Wong J, Pahl M, et al. Chronic kidney disease alters intestinal microbial flora. *Kidney International.* 2013;83(2):308-315.

7. Ramezani A, Raj DS. The gut microbiome, kidney disease, and targeted interventions. *Journal of the American Society of Nephrology.* 2014;25(4):657-670.

8. Armani R, Ramezani A, Yasir A, Sharama S, Canziani M, Raj D. Gut microbiome in chronic kidney disease. *Current hypertension reports.* 2017;19(4):29.

9. Al Khodor S, Shatat IF. Gut microbiome and kidney disease: a bidirectional relationship. *Pediatric Nephrology.* 2017;32(6):921-931.

10. Ramezani A, Massy ZA, Meijers B, Evenepoel P, Vanholder R, Raj DS. Role of the gut microbiome in uremia: a potential therapeutic target. *American Journal of Kidney Diseases.* 2016;67(3):483-498.

11. Lau WL, Kalantar-Zadeh K, Vaziri ND. The gut as a source of inflammation in chronic kidney disease. *Nephron.* 2015;130(2):92-98.

12. Pendyala S, Walker JM, Holt PR. A high-fat diet is associated with endotoxemia that originates from the gut. *Gastroenterology.* 2012;142(5):1100-1101. e1102.

13. Lopez-Moreno J, García-Carpintero S, Jimenez-Lucena R, et al. Effect of dietary lipids on endotoxemia influences postprandial inflammatory response. *Journal of Agricultural and Food Chemistry.* 2017;65(35):7756-7763.

CHAPTER 25

Anemia

Anemia is a common problem for people with kidney disease. When our kidney function is failing, our kidneys do not produce enough of the hormone that tells our bodies to make more red blood cells. The hormone is called erythropoietin, also referred to as EPO.

EPO is the same substance that is banned from sporting competitions. It increases the number of red blood cells, which increase the ability of our blood to carry oxygen.[1]

Anemia could also be related to diet. A diet low in iron, vitamin B12, or folic acid may also contribute to anemia.[2]

Synthetic EPO and iron supplements are the most common ways to address anemia. However, in my case, as inflammation dropped, my red blood cell counts came back into the normal range. We find that inflammation is related to anemia as well as many other things we struggle with.[3]

We find that inflammation and nutrition are key drivers of anemia.

Let's see what the research says.

Study 25.1 **Association of inflammation with anemia in patients with chronic kidney disease not requiring chronic dialysis[4]**

RESULTS:

Of the 7389 participants included in the analytic cohort 2221 (30.1%) participants had eGFR ≥90 mL/min/m^2, 4310 (58.3%) 60–89 mL/min/m 2 and 858 (11.6%) <60 mL/min/m^2. There were significant, graded, increases in high sensitivity C-reactive protein (hs-CRP) and haemoglobin concentrations across eGFR categories independent of age, gender, plasma glucose and lipids (P < 0.0001 for trends). In the multivariable regression analysis, increased hs-CRP concentrations were independently associated with lower haemoglobin concentrations at different stages of eGFR (P < 0.0001 for all). Other independent predictors of lower haemoglobin were older age, female gender and lower eGFR.

CONCLUSIONS:

Our findings suggest that increased plasma hs-CRP concentrations are independently associated with anaemia in the setting of decreased kidney function in a large cohort of unselected adult outpatients.

Study 25.2 Inflammation and its impact on anemia in chronic kidney disease: from hemoglobin variability to hyporesponsiveness[5]

ABSTRACT:

The availability of erythropoiesis-stimulating agents (ESAs) has revolutionized the treatment of anaemia in patients with chronic kidney disease. However, maintaining patients at haemoglobin (Hb) levels that are both safe and provide maximal benefit is a continuing challenge in the field. Based on emerging data on the potential risks of Hb treatment targets >13 g/dL, treatment targets have recently been lowered. In the latest revision (March 2008) of the European product labelling for the ESA class of drugs, the target treatment range was lowered to 10–12 g/dL. Fluctuation of Hb levels or 'Hb variability' during treatment with ESAs is a well-documented phenomenon. Hb levels that are either too high or too low may have an adverse effect on patient outcomes; thus, it is important to understand the causes of Hb variability in order to achieve optimal treatment. Several factors are believed to contribute to variation in the Hb level, including patient comorbidities and intercurrent events. Inflammation is also an important factor associated with Hb variability, and the consequences of persistent inflammatory activity are far-reaching in affected patients. This review addresses the complex role of inflammation in chronic kidney disease, as evidenced by the apparent state of deranged inflammatory markers. The mechanisms by which inflammatory cytokines may affect the response to ESAs, the development of anaemia and poor treatment outcomes are also examined. In addition, various options for intervention to enhance the response to ESAs in haemodialysis patients with inflammation are considered.

Study 25.3 Renal Anemia of Inflammation: The Name Is Self-Explanatory[6]

ABSTRACT:

Results: The discovery of hepcidin as the major controller of iron metabolism in anemia of inflammation answered many questions regarding the interaction of erythropoietin, iron and bone marrow. Hepcidin production in the liver is driven by three major factors: inflammation, iron overload and anemia/hypoxia. Hepcidin levels are increased in patients with CKD due to the interaction of many factors; a comprehensive understanding of these pathways is thus critical in the effort to alleviate anemia of inflammation and ESA resistance.

> **Note:** Increased hepcidin levels lead to low iron in red blood cells. C-reactive protein (CRP) is used as a marker for inflammation as hepcidin is not tested. If C-reactive protein (CRP) is high, then it is likely hepcidin levels are high.

Study 25.4 Anemia Is Correlated with Malnutrition and Inflammation in Croatian Peritoneal Dialysis Patients: A Multicenter Nationwide Study.[7]

ABSTRACT:

Malnutrition, inflammation, and anemia are common in peritoneal dialysis (PD) patients. In this study, correlations between Malnutrition Inflammation Score (MIS), laboratory and anthropometric parameters, and anemia indices in Croatian PD patients were analyzed. One hundred and one PD patients (males/females 54/47, age 58.71 ± 14.68 years, mean PD duration 21.82 ± 21.71 months) were included. Clinical, laboratory, and anthropometric parameters were measured. Statistically significant correlations between MIS and erythropoietin weekly dose per kg of body weight (ESA weekly dose), hemoglobin (Hb), and erythrocytes were found (r = 0.439, p < 0.001; r = -0.032, p < 0.001; r = -0.435, p < 0.001), respectively. Also, statistically significant correlations were found between MIS and mean corpuscular volume (r= 0.344, p < 0.001), iron (r = -0.229, p = 0.021), and total iron binding capacity (TIBC) (r = -0.362, p < 0.001), respectively. Furthermore, statistically significant correlations between ESA weekly dose and serum albumin level and body mass index (BMI) were found (r = -0.272, p= 0.006; r = -0.269, p = 0.006), respectively. When we divided PD patients into 2 groups according Hb level (Hb ≥ 110 [N = 60, 59.41 %]) and Hb < 110 [N = 41, 40.59%]), statistically significant differences were found in MIS score (3.02 ± 2.54 vs 4.54 ± 3.54, p = 0.014), C-reactive protein (CRP) (3.52 ± 6.36 vs 7.85 ± 7.96, p = 0.005), and serum albumin level (44.22 ± 8.54 vs 39.94 ± 8.56, p = 0.003), respectively. Our findings suggest that anemia is correlated with malnutrition and inflammation in Croatian PD patients. Further studies are needed to assess whether modulating inflammatory or nutritional processes can improve anemia management in PD patients.

Note: If inflammation and malnutrition are severe, then our bodies may not respond to EPO treatments. The same is true for albumin and prealbumin.

Study 25.5   **Effect of malnutrition-inflammation complex syndrome on EPO hyporesponsiveness in maintenance hemodialysis patients.[8]**

RESULTS:

A total of 339 maintenance hemodialysis (MHD) outpatients, including 181 men, who were aged 54.7 +/- 14.5 years (mean +/- SD), who had undergone dialysis for 36.3 +/- 33.2 months, were selected randomly from 7 DaVita dialysis units in Los Angeles South/East Bay area. The average weekly dose of administered recombinant human EPO within a 13-week interval was 217 +/- 187 U/kg. Patients were receiving intravenous iron supplementation (iron gluconate or dextran) averaging 39.5 +/- 47.5 mg/wk. The MIS and serum concentrations of high-sensitivity C-reactive protein, interleukin 6 (IL-6), tumor necrosis factor-alpha, and lactate dehydrogenase had positive correlation with required EPO dose and EPO responsiveness index (EPO divided by hemoglobin), whereas serum total iron binding capacity (TIBC), prealbumin and total cholesterol, as well as blood lymphocyte count had statistically significant but negative correlations with indices of refractory anemia. Most correlations remained significant even after multivariate adjustment for case-mix and anemia factors and other relevant covariates. Similar associations were noticed across EPO per body weight tertiles via analysis of variance and after estimating odds ratio for higher versus lower tertile via logistic regression after same case-mix adjustment.

CONCLUSION:

The existence of elements of MICS as indicated by a high MIS and increased levels of proinflammatory cytokines such as IL-6 as well as decreased nutritional values such as low serum concentrations of total cholesterol, prealbumin, and TIBC correlates with EPO hyporesponsiveness in MHD patients.

Study 25.6   **Effect of protein-energy malnutrition on erythropoietin requirement in maintenance hemodialysis patients.[9]**

ABSTRACT:

Possible interactions between inflammatory and nutritional markers and their impact on recombinant human erythropoietin (rHuEPO) hyporesponsiveness are not well understood. We investigated the role of nutritional status in rHuEPO requirement in maintenance hemodialysis (MHD) patients without evidence of inflammation. This cross-sectional study included 88 MHD patients. The associations between required rHuEPO dose and malnutrition-inflammation score (MIS) and several laboratory values known to be related to nutrition and/or inflammation were analyzed. Anthropometric measures including body mass index, triceps skinfold thickness, and midarm circumferences were also measured. Twenty-three patients with serum C-reactive protein levels >10 mg/L were excluded from the analysis. The remaining 65 patients (male/female, 41/24; age 49.1+/-11.4 years; dialysis duration 99.7+/-63.0 months) were studied. These patients had moderate malnutrition and the average MIS was 7.4 (range 3-17). The average weekly dose of administered rHuEPO was 69.1+/-63.1 U/kg. Malnutrition-inflammation score had a positive correlation with the serum concentration of tumor necrosis factor-alpha, whereas it had a negative correlation with anthropometric measures, total iron-binding capacity, prealbumin, phosphorus, creatinine, and triglyceride. According to Pearson's correlation analysis, significant relationships of increased MIS with increased required rHuEPO dose and rHuEPO responsiveness index (EPO divided by hematocrit) were observed (p=0.008, r=-0.326; p=0.017, r=-0.306, respectively). Recombinant human erythropoietin dose requirement is correlated with MIS and adverse nutritional status in MHD patients without evidence of inflammation. Further research should focus on reversing the undergoing microinflammation for a better outcome in dialysis patients.

Note: Anemia is a mortality indictor for people with kidney disease.

Study 25.7   **Risk Factors for Heart Failure in Patients with Chronic Kidney Disease: The CRIC (Chronic Renal Insufficiency Cohort) Study.[10]**

CONCLUSIONS:

Our study indicates that cystatin C-based eGFR and albuminuria are better predictors for risk of heart failure compared to creatinine-based eGFR. Furthermore, anemia, insulin resistance, inflammation, and poor glycemic control are independent risk factors for the development of heart failure among patients with chronic kidney disease.

Anemia: A significant cardiovascular mortality risk after ST-segment elevation myocardial infarc-tion complicated by the comorbidities of hypertension and kidney disease.[11]

METHODS AND RESULTS:

From January 2005 to December 2014, 1751 patients experienced STEMI checked serum hemo-globin initially before any administration of fluids or IV medications. 1751 patients then received primary percutaneous intervention immediately. A total of 1388 patients were enrolled in the non-anemia group because their serum hemoglobin level was more than 13 g/L in males, and 12 g/L in females. A total of 363 patients were enrolled in the anemia group because their serum hemoglo-bin level was less than 13 g/L in males, and 12 g/L in females. Higher incidences of major adverse cerebral cardiac events (22.9% vs. 33.8%; p<0.001) were also noted in the anemia group, and these were related to higher incidence of cardiovascular mortality (6.5% vs. 20.4%; p<0.001). A higher incidence of all-cause mortality (8.6% vs. 27.7%; p<0.001) was also noted in the anemia group. A Kaplan-Meier curve of one-year cardiovascular mortality showed significant differences between the non-anemia and anemia group in all patients (P<0.001), and the patients with hypertension (P<0.001), and chronic kidney disease (CKD) (P = 0.011).

CONCLUSION:

Anemia is a marker of an increased risk in one-year cardiovascular mortality in patients with STEMI. If the patients have comorbidities such as hypertension, or CKD, the effect of anemia is very significant.

So, we know a few things about anemia:

1. Anemia is a mortality indictor.
2. Inflammation is a factor.
3. Nutrition or malnutrition is a factor.
4. Uremic toxins are also a factor.
5. Iron levels matter.

The treatment of anemia is traditionally focused on iron levels, and then EPO injections if iron supplementation does not raise red blood cell counts. We know from the data in this book that anemia should also be treated by reducing inflammation, ensuring adequate nutrition and calories, and reducing uremic toxins.

Treatment of anemia looks something like this:

1. Ensure adequate iron levels.
2. Treat inflammation.
3. Address malnutrition and calorie intake.

4.   Reduce protein intake to reduce uremic toxins.

5.   Use EPO to further increase red blood cell counts as needed.

EPO treatment may not work well, or may not work at all if inflammation, malnutrition, or uremic toxins are severe enough. These are all low-risk strategies to reduce or eliminate anemia.

Again, we come back to inflammation and uremic toxins as primary drivers of our disease. I don't know how many times we have to read this to get the message. Inflammation and uremic toxins are indicated in almost every ailment we have as people with kidney disease.

In my case, white and red blood cell counts improved as inflammation markers started dropping. I was able to get back in the normal range.

References

1. Hughes D. The World Anti-Doping Code in sport: Update for 2015. *Australian prescriber.* 2015;38(5):167.

2. Scholl TO, Hediger ML. Anemia and iron-deficiency anemia: compilation of data on pregnancy outcome. *The American journal of clinical nutrition.* 1994;59(2):492S-501S.

3. Jurado RL. Iron, infections, and anemia of inflammation. *Clinical Infectious Diseases.* 1997;25(4):888-895.

4. Chonchol M, Lippi G, Montagnana M, Muggeo M, Targher G. Association of inflammation with anaemia in patients with chronic kidney disease not requiring chronic dialysis. *Nephrology Dialysis Transplantation.* 2008;23(9):2879-2883.

5. de Francisco AL, Stenvinkel P, Vaulont S. Inflammation and its impact on anaemia in chronic kidney disease: from haemoglobin variability to hyporesponsiveness. *NDT plus.* 2009;2(suppl_1):i18-i26.

6. Yilmaz MI, Solak Y, Covic A, Goldsmith D, Kanbay M. Renal anemia of inflammation: the name is self-explanatory. *Blood Purification.* 2011;32(3):220-225.

7. Radić J, Bašić-Jukić N, Vujičić B, et al. Anemia Is Correlated with Malnutrition and Inflammation in Croatian Peritoneal Dialysis Patients: A Multicenter Nationwide Study. *Peritoneal Dialysis International.* 2017;37(4):472-475.

8. Kalantar-Zadeh K, McAllister CJ, Lehn RS, Lee GH, Nissenson AR, Kopple JD. Effect of malnutrition-inflammation complex syndrome on EPO hyporesponsiveness in maintenance hemodialysis patients. *American Journal of Kidney Diseases.* 2003;42(4):761-773.

9. Akgul A, Bilgic A, Sezer S, et al. Effect of protein-energy malnutrition on erythropoietin requirement in maintenance hemodialysis patients. *Hemodialysis International.* 2007;11(2):198-203.

10. He J, Shlipak M, Anderson A, et al. Risk factors for heart failure in patients with chronic kidney disease: The CRIC (Chronic Renal Insufficiency Cohort) study. *Journal of the American Heart Association.* 2017;6(5):e005336.

11. Lee W-C, Fang H-Y, Chen H-C, et al. Anemia: A significant cardiovascular mortality risk after ST-segment elevation myocardial infarction complicated by the comorbidities of hypertension and kidney disease. *PLoS One.* 2017;12(7):e0180165.

CHAPTER 26

Grip Strength

Grip strength has long been a tool to assess current health. Grip strength is also an accurate predictor of mortality and kidney disease progression.[1] What is grip strength telling us?

Declining grip strength is a sign we are not healthy enough to maintain muscle mass. This can be for several reasons. We need enough calories and protein, and need to have inflammation under control in order to maintain muscle mass. In this chapter, grip strength overlaps with exercise, but covering some important points twice maybe helpful.

Weightlifters know you have to consume excess calories to build muscle.[2] Assume you need 2,000 calories a day to maintain your weight. In order to grow or build increased muscle mass, you need excess calories. In this example, you would need 2,100 or 2,200 calories so you could meet your nutritional needs and have enough calories (aka energy) to increase strength.

If you are not active, your muscles may also atrophy, reducing grip strength. A healthy active person consuming enough calories should maintain or even build grip strength.

Other factors such as protein or amino acid catabolism can be factors. Our bodies may not effectively metabolize amino acids or protein. Some studies suggest we may become 20% to 30% less efficient at using amino acids as we age, and that inflammation and oxidative stress may be factors. This may be why older adults have higher protein requirements.

Studies on handgrip strength:

Study 26.1   **Handgrip strength is an independent predictor of renal outcomes in patients with chronic kidney diseases[3]**

CONCLUSIONS:

This is the first study demonstrating that HGS is an independent predictor of composite renal outcomes in CKD-ND patients. HGS can be incorporated to clinical practice for assessing nutritional status and renal prognosis in patients with CKD-ND.

Study 26.2   **Association of physical activity with cardiovascular and renal outcomes and quality of life in chronic kidney disease[4]**

CONCLUSIONS:

In conclusion, upper and lower extremity endurance was positively correlated with QOL (quality of life) in CKD patients. Impaired lower extremity endurance was significantly associated with increased risks for MACEs and first hospitalization, and the relationship between poor upper extremity endurance and entering commencing dialysis was mentioned. Impaired physical activity might be a potential predictor of adverse clinical outcomes in CKD. Further studies are needed to evaluate the effect of trained exercise program on improvement of clinical outcomes in CKD patients.

Note: MACEs are major adverse cardiac events.

Study 26.3 Evaluation of handgrip strength as a nutritional marker and prognostic indicator in peritoneal dialysis patients[5]

CONCLUSIONS:

Handgrip strength not only is a marker of body lean muscle mass but also provides important prognostic information independent of other covariates, including CRP and serum albumin. Our data suggest that handgrip strength may be used in conjunction with serum albumin as a nutrition-monitoring tool in patients undergoing PD.

Study 26.4 Association between Physical Performance and All-Cause Mortality in CKD[6]

In conclusion, our study demonstrates that lower extremity physical performance is substantially impaired in persons with CKD not treated with dialysis and is associated with all-cause mortality after adjustment. Associations with mortality were similar in magnitude to kidney function and were stronger than traditionally measured biomarkers of CKD. Measurements of lower extremity function are relatively easy to perform and may capture a complex set of skeletal muscle and neurologic impairments that develop in CKD patients and substantially affect their survival. These results argue for further investigation into the principle biologic mechanisms underlying decreased physical performance in CKD patients and evaluating whether interventions improving physical performance in CKD translate to improvements in overall comorbid burden and clinical outcomes.

Study 26.5 Handgrip strength is an independent predictor of all-cause mortality in maintenance dialysis patients.[7]

CONCLUSIONS:

HGS (hand grip strength) cut-offs that predict mortality were 22.5 kg for men and 7 kg for women. HGS was associated with mortality independent of dialysis modality.

Study 26.6 Hand grip strength: outcome predictor and marker of nutritional status[8]

RESULTS AND CONCLUSIONS:

Numerous clinical and epidemiological studies have shown the predictive potential of hand grip strength regarding short and long-term mortality and morbidity. In patients, impaired grip strength is an indicator of increased postoperative complications, increased length of hospitalization, higher rehospitalization rate and decreased physical status. In elderly in particular, loss of grip strength implies loss of independence. Epidemiological studies have moreover demonstrated that low grip strength in healthy adults predicts increased risk of functional limitations and disability in higher age as well as all-cause mortality. As muscle function reacts early to nutritional deprivation, hand grip strength has also become a popular marker of nutritional status and is increasingly being employed as outcome variable in nutritional intervention studies.

Note: This study is on healthy adults.

Studies related to exercise, but not specifically handgrip strength.

Study 26.7 — Effects of exercise in the whole spectrum of chronic kidney disease: a systematic review[9]

ABSTRACT:

Chronic kidney disease (CKD) is a public health problem. Although physical activity is essential for the prevention and treatment of most chronic diseases, exercise is rarely prescribed for CKD patients. The objective of the study was to search for and appraise evidence on the effectiveness of exercise interventions on health endpoints in CKD patients. A systematic review was performed of randomized clinical trials (RCTs) designed to compare exercise with usual care regarding effects on the health of CKD patients. MEDLINE, EMBASE, Cochrane Central, Clinical Trials registry, and proceedings of major nephrology conference databases were searched, using terms defined according to the PICO (Patient, Intervention, Comparison and Outcome) methodology. RCTs were independently evaluated by two reviewers. A total of 5489 studies were assessed for eligibility, of which 59 fulfilled inclusion criteria. Most of them included small samples, lasted from 8 to 24 weeks and applied aerobic exercises. Three studies included only kidney transplant patients, and nine included pre-dialysis patients. The remaining RCTs allocated hemodialysis patients. The out-come measures included quality of life, physical fitness, muscular strength, heart rate variability, inflammatory and nutritional markers and progression of CKD. Most of the trials had high risk of bias. The strongest evidence is for the effects of aerobic exercise on improving physical fitness, muscular strength and quality of life in dialysis patients. The benefits of exercise in dialysis patients are well established, supporting the prescription of physical activity in their regular treatment. RCTs including patients in earlier stages of CKD and after kidney transplantation are urgently required, as well as studies assessing long-term outcomes. The best exercise protocol for CKD patients also remains to be established

Study 26.8 — Physical function was related to mortality in patients with chronic kidney disease and dialysis.[10]

ABSTRACT:

Previous studies have shown that exercise improves aerobic capacity, muscular functioning, cardiovascular function, walking capacity, and health-related quality of life (QOL) in patients with chronic kidney disease (CKD) and dialysis. Recently, additional studies have shown that higher physical activity contributes to survival and decreased mortality as well as physical function and QOL in patients with CKD and dialysis. Herein, we review the evidence that physical function and physical activity play an important role in mortality for patients with CKD and dialysis. During November 2016, Medline and Web of Science databases were searched for published English medical reports (without a time limit) using the terms "CKD" or "dialysis" and "mortality" in conjunction with "exercise capacity," "muscle strength," "activities of daily living (ADL)," "physical activity," and "exercise." Numerous studies suggest that higher exercise capacity, muscle strength, ADL, and physical activity contribute to lower mortality in patients with CKD and dialysis. Physical function is associated with mortality in patients with CKD and dialysis. Increasing physical function may decrease the mortality rate of patients with CKD and dialysis. Physicians and medical staff should recognize the importance of physical function in CKD and dialysis. In addition, exercise is associated with reduced mortality among patients with CKD and dialysis.

Study 26.9 — Physical working capacity and muscle strength in chronic renal failure are improved by exercise.[11]

ABSTRACT:

Patients with chronic kidney disease (CKD) show a decline in maximal exercise capacity and muscle strength as renal function decreases. Renal anaemia, skeletal muscle dysfunction, tiredness and increasing inactivity are the major causes of this deterioration. Exercise training improves maximal exercise capacity, muscle strength and endurance in young, middle-aged and elderly patients at all stages of CKD. Preferably exercise training should be started during the pre dialysis stage, however, it is equally effective in dialysis patients and after renal transplantation. It has a positive effect on muscle catabolism and counteracts weight loss and malnutrition. Moreover, exercise training has positive effects on functional capacity and health related quality of life. Exercise training should be prescribed by a nephrologist and administered by a trained neurological physiotherapist. Exercise training is an integral part of care of the CKD patient. It not only reduces suffering but also costs, resulting in major potential benefits for the patient, the healthcare system and society.

Study 26.10 — A comparison of aerobic exercise and resistance training in patients with and without chronic kidney disease.[12]

ABSTRACT:

The morbidity and mortality associated with chronic kidney disease (CKD) are primarily caused by atherosclerosis and cardiovascular disease, which may be in part caused by inflammation and oxidative stress. Aerobic exercise and resistance training have been proposed as measures to combat obesity, inflammation, endothelial dysfunction, oxidative stress, insulin resistance, and progression of CKD. In non-CKD patients, aerobic exercise reduces inflammation, increases insulin sensitivity, decreases microalbuminuria, facilitates weight loss, decreases leptins, and protects against oxidative injury. In nondialysis CKD, aerobic exercise decreases microalbuminuria, protects from oxidative stress, and may increase the glomerular filtration rate (GFR). Aerobic exercise in hemodialysis patients has been reported to enhance insulin sensitivity, improve lipid profile, increase hemoglobin, increase strength, decrease blood pressure, and improve quality of life. Resistance training, in the general population, decreases C-reactive protein, increases insulin sensitivity, decreases body fat content, increases insulin-like growth factor-1 (IGF-1), and decreases microalbuminuria. In the nondialysis CKD population, resistance training has been reported to reduce inflammation, increase serum albumin, maintain body weight, increase muscle strength, increase IGF-1, and increase GFR. Resistance training in hemodialysis increases muscle strength, increases physical functionality, and improves IGF-1 status. Combined aerobic exercise and resistance training during dialysis improves muscle strength, work output, cardiac fitness, and possibly dialysis adequacy. There is a need for more investigation on the role of exercise in CKD. If the benefits of aerobic exercise and strength training in non-CKD populations can be shown to apply to CKD patients as well, renal rehabilitation will begin to play an important role in the approach to the treatment, prevention, and slowed progression of CKD.

Study 26.11   Regular exercise during haemodialysis promotes an anti-inflammatory leucocyte profile.[13]

CONCLUSIONS:

These findings suggest that regular intradialytic exercise is associated with an anti-inflammatory effect at a circulating cellular level but not in circulating cytokines. This may be protective against the increased risk of cardiovascular disease and mortality that is associated with chronic inflammation and elevated numbers of intermediate monocytes.

Study 26.12   Inflammatory Factors and Exercise in Chronic Kidney Disease[14]

ABSTRACT:

Patients with chronic kidney disease frequently present with chronic elevations in markers of inflammation, a condition that appears to be exacerbated by disease progression and onset of haemodialysis. Systemic inflammation is interlinked with malnutrition and muscle protein wasting and is implicated in a number of morbidities including cardiovascular disease: the most common cause of mortality in this population. Research in the general population and other chronic disease cohorts suggests that an increase in habitual activity levels over a pro-longed period may help redress basal increases in systemic inflammation. Furthermore, those populations with the highest baseline levels of systemic inflammation appear to have the great-est improvements from training. On the whole, the activity levels of the chronic kidney disease population reflect a sedentary lifestyle, indicating the potential for increasing physical activity and observing health benefits. This review explores the current literature investigating exercise and inflammatory factors in the chronic kidney disease population and then attempts to explain the contradictory findings and suggests where future research is required.

What do these studies tell us?

1. Adequate calorie intake is very important.

2. Adequate protein intake is very important.

3. Normal albumin levels are very important.

4. Inflammation is at least a partial cause of muscle-related problems.

5. Oxidative stress is a partial cause.

6. Exercise can reduce inflammation, reduce proteinuria and blood pressure, and increase quality of life.

7. Exercise reduces heart disease risk.

8. If we don't exercise, we may be accelerating the rate of kidney disease progression.

The message here is we have to exercise and if we are not healthy enough to exercise, our goal has to be to get healthy enough to exercise. Exercise is recommended for everyone, but we may have more at risk from sedentary lifestyles than most groups. Accelerated heart disease should be enough of a reason to get us moving.

If we can reduce heart disease progression, reduce inflammation and albuminuria, while at the same time looking and feeling better, why wouldn't we?

I know it's hard to find time to exercise, but it is something we have do to improve our odds of survival in a big way.

References

1. Gale CR, Martyn CN, Cooper C, Sayer AA. Grip strength, body composition, and mortality. *International Journal of Epidemiology*. 2006;36(1):228-235.

2. Metter EJ, Talbot LA, Schrager M, Conwit R. Skeletal muscle strength as a predictor of all-cause mortality in healthy men. *The Journals of Gerontology Series A: Biological Sciences and Medical Sciences*. 2002;57(10):B359-B365.

3. Chang Y-T, Wu H-L, Guo H-R, et al. Handgrip strength is an independent predictor of renal outcomes in patients with chronic kidney diseases. *Nephrology Dialysis Transplantation*. 2011;26(11):3588-3595.

4. Tsai Y-C, Chen H-M, Hsiao S-M, et al. Association of physical activity with cardiovascular and renal outcomes and quality of life in chronic kidney disease. *PloS one*. 2017;12(8):e0183642.

5. Wang AY-M, Sea MM-M, Ho ZS-Y, Lui S-F, Li PK-T, Woo J. Evaluation of handgrip strength as a nutritional marker and prognostic indicator in peritoneal dialysis patients–. *The American Journal of Clinical Nutrition*. 2005;81(1):79-86.

6. Roshanravan B, Robinson-Cohen C, Patel KV, et al. Association between physical performance and all-cause mortality in CKD. *Journal of the American Society of Nephrology*. 2013:ASN. 2012070702.

7. Vogt BP, Borges MCC, de Goés CR, Caramori JCT. Handgrip strength is an independent predictor of all-cause mortality in maintenance dialysis patients. *Clinical Nutrition*. 2016;35(6):1429-1433.

8. Norman K, Stobäus N, Gonzalez MC, Schulzke J-D, Pirlich M. Hand grip strength: outcome predictor and marker of nutritional status. *Clinical Nutrition*. 2011;30(2):135-142.

9. Barcellos FC, Santos IS, Umpierre D, Bohlke M, Hallal PC. Effects of exercise in the whole spectrum of chronic kidney disease: a systematic review. *Clinical Kidney Journal*. 2015;8(6):753-765.

10. Morishita S, Tsubaki A, Shirai N. Physical function was related to mortality in patients with chronic kidney disease and dialysis. *Hemodialysis International*. 2017;21(4):483-489.

11. Clyne N. Physical working capacity and muscle strength in chronic renal failure are improved by exercise. *Lakartidningen*. 2004;101(50):4111-4115.

12. Moinuddin I, Leehey DJ. A comparison of aerobic exercise and resistance training in patients with and without chronic kidney disease. *Advances in Chronic Kidney Disease*. 2008;15(1):83-96.

13. Dungey M, Young HM, Churchward DR, Burton JO, Smith AC, Bishop NC. Regular exercise during haemodialysis promotes an anti-inflammatory leucocyte profile. *Clinical Kidney Journal*. 2017;10(6):813-821.

14. Dungey M, Hull KL, Smith AC, Burton JO, Bishop NC. Inflammatory factors and exercise in chronic kidney disease. *International Journal of Endocrinology*. 2013(Article ID 569831).

Neutral "Factors"

Several "Factors" appear to have little effect on kidney disease progression or the treatment is debatable, not a standard practice.

It's hard to know exactly how to treat these "Factors" or give the best advice. These factors still need to be managed, but I felt they should go in another section.

CHAPTER 27

Potassium: A Constant Struggle

Let me get this off my chest: Potassium frustrates me to no end. I don't understand how potassium levels can be so different from kidney patient to kidney patient. Patients with very low—almost single-digit—GFR may be fine with potassium. Other patients with GFR in the 50s and 60s may have to reduce their potassium intake.

My frustration comes from not having a good answer to hundreds of emails. After keto acids, potassium is the most common topic for questions I get from readers.

So, the first lesson on potassium is that potassium restrictions vary wildly from patient to patient. I still wanted to know why.

Let's start with a real-life story about the dangers of managing potassium. My then 83-year-old father was very sick for a few days and couldn't keep anything down. My wife pleaded with him to go to the doctor, but he resisted. He will always be a stubborn Texan, no matter where he lives today.

My father lives with us and suddenly called out to me to take him to the doctor. He said, "Something is really wrong. I don't feel right." He felt shaky and weak. A visit to his regular doctor ended in the emergency room and three days in the cardiac unit. The reason was his potassium was so high they thought his heart might stop. Dehydration was the cause. The combination of heart disease and high potassium can be a real threat to us. I am not talking about high potassium and kidney disease, but high potassium and heart disease.

As heart disease is the number one killer of kidney patients, the threat of high potassium is real. We need to look at potassium as a heart disease issue caused by our kidneys' inability to manage potas-sium. Yes, our kidneys are the ones screwing up our ability to handle potassium. High potas-sium doesn't stop your kidneys, but it can stop your heart.

Some background and definitions:

You don't have to guess that potassium metabolism is handled by the kidneys. As kidney function drops, so does your ability to get rid of excess potassium. The kidneys have two jobs in terms of potassium handling. One is to excrete excess potassium, and the other is to retain or reabsorb potassium.

Hyperkalemia is high potassium, and hypokalemia is low potassium.

You will see "K" in upcoming studies. "K" is the symbol for potassium.

The normal range is 3.5 to 5.0 mEq/L.

The questions for us as people with kidney disease: Are we better off running high or low in potassium over the long term, and does potassium increase or decrease the rate of kidney disease progression? At what point does potassium increase mortality rates?

I incorrectly assumed that, since high potassium can be a killer, high potassium was much worse than low potassium levels. As you may guess, I was wrong again.

It appears that high potassium levels are lower-risk than low potassium levels. Again, the normal range for potassium is 3.5 to 5.0 mEq/L.

Let see what the research has to tell us.

FIGURE 27.1: **Serum Potassium and Outcomes in CKD: Insights from the RRI-CKD Cohort Study[1]**

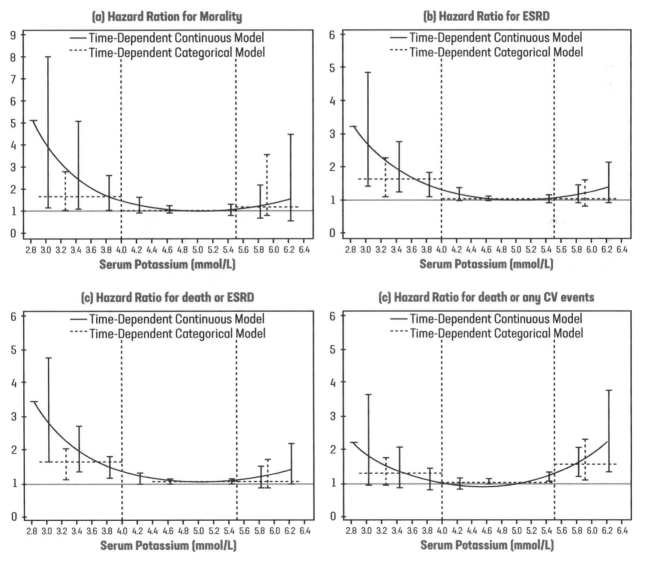

Study 27.1

These charts suggest that the lowest risk is between 4.6 and 5.5 mEq/L. Hold on a second; the normal range is 3.5 to 5.0 mEq/L. Is going below 4.6 really that bad? I can't say for sure, but this study suggests anything below 4.1 is a higher risk than, say, 5.5.

Here is the conclusion to the study:

CONCLUSIONS:

Lower SK (potassium) (even less than or equal to a "normal" level of 4.0 mmol/L) seems to predict mortality to a relatively greater degree compared with the risk associated with SK ≥5.5 mmol/L. This study shows that the levels of SK that are associated with lowest risk for mortality are between 4.1 and 5.5 mmol/L, which suggests that maintaining SK in this range may potentially help optimize survival in patients with CKD. Practice patterns could potentially be adapted to supplement potassium (through dietary modification or pills) and avoid use of loop diuretics whenever possible. The benefits of potassium-sparing diuretics such as aldosterone receptor-blocking agents may be due in part to their ability to "normalize" serum potassium levels. Aldosterone is increasingly recognized to be important in the pathogenesis of CKD (37,38), and mineralocorticoid receptor blockade is an increasingly used strategy in lowering proteinuria with the potential of both slowing renal disease progression and lowering mortality. These issues warrant future studies that specifically address the role of potassium supplementation in determining outcomes and study the deliberate optimization of serum potassium levels by use of specific drugs in randomized trials. Overall, our findings suggest that attention should be paid to patients who have CKD and are at the lower ranges of SK as well as those with elevated serum potassium to prevent adverse outcomes such as mortality, ESRD and cardiovascular events.

Study 27.2   Serum Potassium, End-Stage Renal Disease and Mortality in Chronic Kidney Disease[2]

After adjustment for covariates including kidney function, serum potassium levels <4.0 and >5.0 mmol/l were significantly associated with increased mortality risk, but there was no increased risk for progression to ESRD. Time-dependent repeated measures analysis confirmed these findings. When potassium was examined as a continuous variable, there was a U-shaped association between serum potassium levels and mortality.

CONCLUSION:

In patients with stage 3-4 CKD, serum potassium levels <4.0 and >5.0 mmol/l are associated with higher mortality, but not with ESRD.

Note: This study suggests that anything over 5.0 may increase risk, but does not contribute to end-stage renal disease. This study contradicts the first study in terms of what level of potassium is safe.

Study 27.3 Hyperkalemia and Hypokalemia in CKD: Prevalence, Risk Factors and Clinical Outcomes.[3]

ABSTRACT:

Abnormalities of serum potassium are common in patients with CKD. Although hyperkalemia is a well-recognized complication of CKD, the prevalence rates of hyperkalemia (14%-20%) and hypokalemia (12%-18%) are similar. CKD severity, use of medications such as renin-angiotensin aldosterone system inhibitors and diuretics, and dietary potassium intake are major determinants of serum potassium concentration in CKD. Demographic factors, acid-base status, blood glucose, and other comorbidities contribute as well. Both hyperkalemia and hypokalemia are associated with similarly increased risks of death, cardiovascular disease, and hospitalization. On the other hand, limited evidence suggests a link between hypokalemia, but not hyperkalemia and progression of CKD. This article reviews the prevalence rates and risk factors for hyperkalemia and hypokalemia, and their associations with adverse outcomes in CKD.

Note: Both high and low potassium are risky, but low potassium is higher risk. In addition, lower potassium may increase the progression of CKD.

Study 27.4 Low Serum Potassium Concentration is a Predictor of Chronic Kidney Disease[4]

RESULTS:

Compared with the subjects without development of CKD, age, body mass index, fasting plasma glucose, uric acid (UA), creatinine and serum sodium concentration were higher, and serum potassium concentration was lower in subjects with development of CKD. Univariate Cox regression analyses demonstrated that age, body mass index, fasting plasma glucose, UA, creatinine, serum sodium concentration and serum potassium concentration were associated with progression of CKD. Multiple Cox regression analysis revealed that age, gender, creatinine and serum potassium concentration were independent predictors of CKD after adjustment for covariates. When serum potassium concentration was below 4.0 mmol/l at baseline, hazard ratio (95% confidence interval) of developing CKD was 2.65 (2.04-3.44; $p < 0.0001$).

CONCLUSIONS:

Serum potassium concentration could be a clinically relevant risk factor for the progression of CKD, defined as eGFR < 60 ml/min/1.73 m(2), in healthy subjects.

Note: It is interesting that low potassium is a predictor of kidney disease as early as in stage 3 kidney disease.

Study 27.5   Association of Hypo- and Hyperkalemia with Disease Progression and Mortality in Males with Chronic Kidney Disease: the Role of Race[5]

RESULTS:

Both hypo- and hyperkalemia were associated with mortality overall in 933 white patients, but in 294 blacks, hypokalemia was a stronger death predictor. Hypokalemia was associated with loss of kidney function independent of race: a 1 mEq/l lower potassium was associated with an adjusted difference in slopes of eGFR of -0.13 ml/min/1.73 m(2)/year (95% CI: -0.20 to -0.07), p < 0.001.

CONCLUSION:

Hypo- and hyperkalemia are associated with higher mortality in CKD patients. Blacks appear to better tolerate higher potassium than whites. Hypokalemia is associated with faster CKD progression independent of race. Hyperkalemia management may warrant race-specific consideration, and hypokalemia correction may slow CKD progression.

Note: If race is a factor, then genetics must also play a part in potassium disorders.

How Scorpions Changed the Way I Thought About Potassium

Growing up in Texas, scorpions were common. Not the big, dark-colored ones you see on TV and in movies, but small, light brown ones with a stripe on their backs. They were only a few inches long at most. Despite the small size, they feel like the big ones from the movies when you step on one as a kid.

When I came across an article on scorpion venom and potassium, I was fascinated. Scorpion venom attacks the kidneys, and specifically, the kidneys' ability to process potassium. Bioengineered versions of scorpion venom are being used to study how kidneys handle potassium. This fact is crazy to me—that venom can be used to study how our kidneys handle potassium.

The venom causes an inflammatory response, which in turns reduces the victim's ability to manage potassium, almost exactly like kidney disease. Think about it for a minute. A scorpion sting simulates exactly the same response to potassium as kidney disease.

| Study 27.6 | Scorpion Venom, Kidneys and Potassium[6] |

Scorpion venom causes renal injury by the interaction of renal ischemia due to intense renal vasoconstriction and inflammatory reactions due to proinflammatory cytokines and mediators. Renal vasoconstriction is not only induced by catecholamine storm, but also by angiotensin II and the direct action of venom on vascular ion channels. Increased aldosterone also contributes to hypertension. Blocking of renal tubular K channels decreases renal K excretion and increases serum K level, which increases aldosterone release.

Note: Look at the similarities. Vasoconstriction (think endothelial dysfunction, renal hypoxia), inflammation, angiotensin II (increases blood pressure in kidneys), and aldosterone all affect the kidneys' handling of salt and potassium. We have seen these issues over and over again. It sounds exactly like kidney disease. Crazy, right?

| Study 27.7 | Serum electrolyte changes in pediatric patients stung by scorpions[7] |

ABSTRACT

Scorpion sting[s are] a health problem in some places of Mexico. The clinical manifestations of scorpion envenomation are variable and include metabolic alterations. Hyperkalemia is the most frequently reported metabolic alteration.

Note: Read this again. The most frequent symptom (aside from pain and swelling) is high potassium. The fascinating idea for me is that potassium handling can be turned on or off. After the venom has subsided or been treated with antivenom, your kidneys go back to handling potassium just like normal.

If you doubted any concepts in this book like endothelial dysfunction, renal hypoxia, inflammation, or blood pressure, we have proof that these factors affect our kidneys, courtesy of the lowly scorpion. Maybe the reason so many patients have different potassium restrictions is the amount of endothelial dysfunction, hypoxia, inflammation and so on? I want to be clear; I am going out on a limb here, but it would explain the wild swings in potassium restriction from patient to patient.

Could it be that your potassium restriction says a lot about your current health? I don't know, but I would love to study this issue in the future.

I am just one case, but my ability to handle potassium did improve. Could it be that focusing on reducing inflammation and blood flow allowed my kidneys to handle potassium better? I can't say for sure, but the latest research is suggesting that inflammation and blood flow may be factors.

Study 27.8 — Proinflammatory Cytokines and Potassium Channels in the Kidney[8]

CONCLUSION:

Renal K+ channels play important roles in maintaining the normal transport function of renal tubule epithelia. The kidney sometimes suffers from renal ischemia, endotoxemia and diabetic nephropathy, where proinflammatory cytokines are produced. However, it was only during the last decade that the effects of proinflammatory cytokines on renal K+ channels were reported. The effects of cytokines on K+ channels may be involved in alterations of tubular transport or onset of renal cell injury. However, the physiological and pathological significances of proinflammatory cytokines in modulating renal tubular K+ channels are not well understood. To complicate the matters, a variety of cytokines with different actions are produced during inflammatory responses. Some cytokines activate renal K+ channels, while others suppress the same channels. The complexity of cytokine actions gives rise to difficulties in interpreting the final outcome of their effects. Additional studies are required to further clarify the effects of proinflammatory cytokines on renal K+ channels.

> **Note:** This data suggests that lowering inflammation may affect your kidney's ability to handle potassium. Other studies also indicate that the same is true for sodium handling. This is relatively new research, and we don't have dozens of studies on this issue. However, my experience was that as inflammation dropped, potassium handling improved.

Study 27.9 — Effects of Cytokines on Potassium Channels in Renal Tubular Epithelial[9]

Renal tubular potassium (K+) channels play important roles in the formation of cell-negative potential, K+ recycling, K+ secretion and cell volume regulation. In addition to these physiological roles, it was reported that changes in the activity of renal tubular K+ channels were involved in exacerbation of renal cell injury during ischemia and endotoxemia. Because ischemia and endotoxemia stimulate production of cytokines in immune cells and renal tubular cells, it is possible that cytokines would affect K+ channel activity. Although the regulatory mechanisms of renal tubular K+ channels have extensively been studied, little information is available about the effects of cytokines on these K+ channels. The first report was that tumor necrosis factor acutely stimulated the single-channel activity of the 70 pS K+ channel in the rat thick ascending limb through activation of tyrosine phosphatase. Recently, it was also reported that interferon-γ (IFN-γ) and interleukin-1β (IL-1β) modulated the activity of the 40 pS K+ channel in cultured human proximal tubule cells. IFN-γ exhibited a delayed suppression and an acute stimulation of K+ channel activity, whereas IL-1β acutely suppressed the channel activity.

Furthermore, these cytokines suppressed gene expression of the renal outer medullary potassium channel. The renal tubular K+ channels are functionally coupled to the coexisting transporters. Therefore, the effects of cytokines on renal tubular transporter activity should also be taken into account, when interpreting their effects on K+ channel activity.

Note: Cytokines are proinflammatory and include interleukin-1 (IL-1), IL-12, IL-18, tumor necrosis factor (TNF), interferon gamma (IFN-gamma), and more.

In this new research, we see several themes that are familiar to us:

1. Our old friend inflammation shows up again, and so do other inflammation-causing substances like tumor necrosis factor (TNF).

2. Gene expression is suppressed or we turn off genes that may help our kidneys manage potassium.

3. Several factors contribute to postassium handling, not just one.

Can we improve potassium handling by:

> Decreasing inflammation?

> Reducing or eliminating endotoxemia?

> Increasing blood flow to the kidneys?

I don't know yet. There are not enough studies to say this is possible, but I am betting these issues do have an impact on our kidneys' ability to handle potassium.

Potassium restriction is probably the most common diet restriction, and I am sorry that I don't have more concrete answers.

What can you do to lower potassium?

We have a few options:

1. **Lower intake of potassium.**

    This is likely the most common dietary restriction for kidney patients. Lowering your intake of potassium will lower your potassium levels by a corresponding amount. Lower your intake by 10%, and you should expect your potassium levels to drop by about 10% as well.

2. **Diuretics**

    Diuretics increase urine production and therefore increase potassium excretion. Diuretics fall into two broad categories for us: potassium-reducing or potassium-sparing. Your doctor will choose a diuretic based on the desired effect of reducing or increasing potassium.

3. **Potassium binders**

    There are several drugs that work to bind with potassium in the gut to keep potassium from being absorbed. Sodium polystyrene sulfonate is taken several times a day to absorb potassium. Veltassa, generic name Patiromer, is another type of potassium binder. These drugs are usually powders and bind with potassium in gut and bowels. These binders can also bind other drugs and minerals, but they are effective.

The good news is we have a few options. Lowering potassium intake, using potassium reducing diuretics, and using binders allows almost all of us to control potassium, especially if we combine all three. This is almost never needed, but it is nice to know we have a few options.

So what do we know about potassium and kidney disease progression?

1. Both high and low potassium pose a risk.

2. Low potassium appears to be a higher risk than high potassium.

3. Low potassium may increase kidney disease progression.

4. Mildly high potassium does not appear to increase kidney disease progression.

5. Race (genetics) and type of kidney disease are also factors.

6. The normal range for potassium is 3.5 to 5.0 mEq/L, but it appears we need to be above 4.0 and not exceed 5.0 mEq/L for the most benefits.

We also need to consider what other factors may be driving our ability to manage potassium. These are not proven, but it is very likely they play a role as well:

Inflammation

Renal blood flow

Endotoxemia

The diet and treatment plan will help with inflammation and hopefully renal blood flow. Endotoxemia is covered in another chapter.

The range of potassium restrictions from person to person is still a mystery to me. The most likely answer is that potassium-handling issues are related to many issues and not just one. For now, the best solution is managing your daily potassium intake and then using drugs if this is not enough.

References

1. Korgaonkar S, Tilea A, Gillespie BW, et al. Serum potassium and outcomes in CKD: insights from the RRI-CKD cohort study. *Clinical Journal of the American Society of Nephrology.* 2010(CJN. 05850809).

2. Nakhoul GN, Huang H, Arrigain S, et al. Serum potassium, end-stage renal disease and mortality in chronic kidney disease. *American Journal of Nephrology.* 2015;41(6):456-463.

3. Gilligan S, Raphael KL. Hyperkalemia and hypokalemia in CKD: prevalence, risk factors, and clinical outcomes. *Advances in Chronic Kidney Disease.* 2017;24(5):315-318.

4. Fukui M, Tanaka M, Toda H, et al. Low serum potassium concentration is a predictor of chronic kidney disease. *International Journal of Clinical Practice.* 2014;68(6):700-704.

5. Hayes J, Kalantar-Zadeh K, Lu JL, Turban S, Anderson JE, Kovesdy CP. Association of hypo-and hyperkalemia with disease progression and mortality in males with chronic kidney disease: the role of race. *Nephron Clinical Practice.* 2012;120(1).

6. Angsanakul J, Sitprija V. Scorpion venoms, kidney and potassium. *Toxicon.* 2013;73:81-87.

7. Osnaya-Romero N, Hernández T, Basurto G, et al. Serum electrolyte changes in pediatric patients stung by scorpions. *Journal of Venomous Animals and Toxins Including Tropical Diseases.* 2008;14(2):372-377.

8. Nakamura K, Hayashi H, Kubokawa M. Proinflammatory cytokines and potassium channels in the kidney. *Mediators of inflammation.* 2015;2015.

9. Nakamura K, Komagiri Y, Kubokawa M. Effects of cytokines on potassium channels in renal tubular epithelia. *Clinical and Experimental Nephrology.* 2012;16(1):55-60.

CHAPTER 28

Vitamin D

Vitamin D issues have frustrated me, just like potassium. There seems to be no consensus on treating vitamin D problems in people with kidney disease. Should we treat, or does it do harm?

No one seems to know.

Vitamin D is the sunshine vitamin. Our bodies make vitamin D when exposed to the sun. Vitamin D helps our bodies absorb calcium and phosphorus, so vitamin D is needed for strong bones. Vitamin D also blocks the parathyroid hormone (PTH). Too much PTH encourages our body to absorb calcium from our bones and results in weak, thin, or brittle bones.

In kidney disease, the hormone calcitriol that is needed to convert vitamin D into a useable form of vitamin D is impaired. We don't produce enough of this hormone, so our vitamin D levels fall. PTH helps us maintain strong bonds. When PTH levels fall, our bodies start rebuilding our bones (a good thing). When PTH levels are too high, we start accumulating too much calcium in our blood (hypercalcemia).

To make things more confusing, magnesium and PTH are related. PTH tells the body how much magnesium to reabsorb, thus controlling magnesium levels. High magnesium levels may inhibit PTH. PTH is also blocked by very low magnesium levels. Magnesium on the low end of the normal range may increase PTH hormone. Science is still working on this complex relationship.

Because vitamin D and PTH are joined at the hip, we will cover these two issues in one chapter.

There are two types of hyperparathyroid issues. Primary is something wrong with your thyroid. Secondary is caused by something other than the thyroid which, in our case, is kidney disease. Secondary hyperthyroidism is what we are concerned about.

Let's see what we can find about vitamin D and kidney disease progression.

Note: I eliminated dozens of studies that reached no conclusion. These studies don't really help us make a decision, but they do point to the debate about vitamin D supplementation.

Study 28.1   Vitamin D in chronic kidney disease.[1]

ABSTRACT:

Vitamin D deficiency is highly prevalent in patients with chronic kidney disease (CKD). The low vitamin D status is, to a large extent, caused by dysregulation of vitamin D metabolism as a result of renal insufficiency. Recent studies indicate that vitamin D-deficiency may promote or accelerate the progression of CKD, whereas treatment with low calcemic vitamin D analogs can reduce proteinuria and ameliorate renal damage in animal models of kidney disease and in patients with CKD. The renoprotective activity of vitamin D regulates multiple signaling path-ways known to play important roles in renal injury. These findings underscore the importance of correcting vitamin D deficiency with vitamin D supplementation or with activated vitamin D analogs in the management of CKD.

Study 28.2 Prevalence and prognostic implications of vitamin D deficiency in chronic kidney disease.[2]

ABSTRACT:

Vitamin D is an important nutrient involved in bone mineral metabolism, and vitamin D status is reflected by serum total 25-hydroxyvitamin D (25[OH]D) concentrations. Vitamin D deficiency is highly prevalent in patients with chronic kidney disease (CKD), and nutritional vitamin D supplementation decreases elevated parathyroid hormone concentrations in subgroups of these patients. Furthermore, vitamin D is supposed to have pleiotropic effects on various diseases such as cardiovascular diseases, malignancies, infectious diseases, diabetes, and autoimmune diseases. Indeed, there is cumulative evidence showing the associations of low vitamin D with the development and progression of CKD, cardiovascular complication, and high mortality. Recently, genetic polymorphisms in vitamin D-binding protein have received great attention because they largely affect bioavailable 25(OH)D concentrations. This finding suggests that the serum total 25(OH)D concentrations would not be comparable among different gene polymorphisms and thus may be inappropriate as an index of vitamin D status. This finding may refute the conventional definition of vitamin D status based solely on serum total 25(OH)D concentrations.

Study 28.3 25 (OH) vitamin D levels and renal disease progression in patients with type 2 diabetic nephropathy and blockade of the renin-angiotensin system.[3]

RESULTS:

Fifty-three patients (51.5%) had 25 (OH) vitamin D deficiency (<15 ng/ml). After a median follow-up of 32 months, the endpoint was reached by 23 patients with deficiency (43.4%) and 8 patients without (16%). Multivariate Cox regression analysis adjusted for urinary protein/creatinine ratio, estimated GFR, and baseline aldosterone showed that 25 (OH) vitamin D deficiency was associated with the primary endpoint (hazard ratio, 2.88; 95% confidence interval, 1.84 to 7.67; P=0.04).

CONCLUSIONS:

These results show that 25 (OH) vitamin D deficiency is independently associated with a higher risk of the composite outcome in patients with type II diabetic nephropathy.

Study 28.4 Role of vitamin D in the pathogenesis of chronic kidney disease.[4]

Chronic kidney disease (CKD) is a relevant health problem due to its worldwide increasing prevalence and the morbidity and mortality linked to its complications. Since the early stages of CKD, although patients are completely asymptomatic, important mineral homeostasis disorders occur.

These disorders, involving serum levels of calcium, phosphorus, parathyroid hormone, and vitamin D, have a striking impact on patient prognosis as they affect the cardiovascular system. The new term of Chronic Kidney Disease-Mineral Bone Disease (CKD-MBD) was intro-duced to label bone disease during CKD as a systemic disorder tightly linked to cardiovascular calcifications and disabilities. Vitamin D deficiency has a main role in the pathogenesis of CKD-MBD, throughout the pleiotropic actions of this hormone. Vitamin D receptors (VDRs) are ubiquitous and their activation has shown protective effects against secondary hyperparathyroidism development and anti-hypertensive, anti-inflammatory, anti-fibrotic, immunomodulating, anti-proliferative, anti-diabetic and anti-proteinuric properties. These mechanisms explain, at least in part, vitamin D status influence in avoiding and delaying cardiovascular disease and CKD progression. These find-ings strongly support the importance of an early diagnosis of mineral homeostasis disorders in CKD and the need for correction of vitamin D deficiency to prevent related disabilities and major events.

Study 28.5 — New insights on the role of vitamin D in the progression of renal damage.[5]

ABSTRACT:

Several studies indicate a relationship between hypovitaminosis D, survival, vascular calcification and inflammation. In addition to its central role in the regulation of bone mineral metabolism, vitamin D also contributes to other systems, including the immune, cardiovascular and endo-crine systems. Vitamin D analogs reduces proteinuria, in particular through suppression of the renin-angiotensin-aldosterone system (RAAS) and exerts anti-inflammatory and immunomod-ulatory effects. In particular vitamin D deficiency contribute to an inappropriately activated RAAS, as a mechanism for progression of chronic kidney disease (CKD) and/or cardiovascular disease. Human and experimental models of CKD showed that vitamin D may interact with B and T lymphocytes and influence the phenotype and function of the antigen presenting cells and dendritic cells, promoting properties that favor the induction of tolerogenic T regulators rather than T effectory. Interstitial fibrosis may be prevented through vitamin D supplementation. Renal myofibroblast, an activated fibroblast with expression of a molecular hallmark α-smooth muscle actin (α-SMA), is generally considered the principal matrix-producing effector cells that are responsible for the excess production of extracellular matrix (ECM) components in the fibrotic tissues. It turns out that calcitriol effectively blocks myofibroblast activation from interstitial fibroblasts, as evidenced by suppression of TGF-β1-mediated α-SMA expression.

Study 28.6 — Vitamin D and the kidney[6]

In the course of chronic kidney disease, alterations in vitamin D metabolism contribute to increases in the levels of parathyroid hormone and the development of skeletal disorders, and in addition, may contribute to hypertension, systemic inflammation and cardiovascular risk. In the course of chronic kidney disease, the production of 1,25-dihydroxyvitamin D from the kidney shows a progressive decline due to several factors, which include a reduction in the ability to convert 25-hydroxyvitamin-D to the active hormone, 1,25-dihydroxyvitamin D. The result-ing 1,25-dihydroxyvitamin D, as well as 25-hydroxyvitamin D deficiency, correlates strongly with accelerated disease progression and mortality. An understanding of the pathophysiology involved leads to therapeutic strategies to correct these abnormalities, with the ultimate view to improve outcomes for patients with CKD.

Study 28.7 The effect of cholecalciferol for lowering albuminuria in chronic kidney disease: a prospective controlled study.[7]

RESULTS:

Cholecalciferol administration led to a rise in mean 25(OH)D levels by 53.0 ± 41.6% (P < 0.001). Urinary albumin-to-creatinine ratio (uACR) decreased from (geometric mean with 95% confidence interval) 284 (189-425) to 167 mg/g (105-266) at 6 months (P < 0.001) in the cholecalciferol group, and there was no change in the control group. Reduction in a uACR was observed in the absence of significant changes in other factors, which could affect proteinuria, like weight, blood pressure (BP) levels or antihypertensive treatment. Six-month changes in 25(OH)D levels were significantly and inversely associated with that in the uACR (Pearson's R = -0.519; P = 0.036), after adjustment by age, sex, body mass index, BP, glomerular filtration rate and antiproteinuric treatment. The mean PTH decreased by -13.8 ± 20.3% (P = 0.039) only in treated patients, with a mild rise in phosphate and calcium-phosphate product [7.0 ± 14.7% (P = 0.002) and 7.2 ± 15.2% (P = 0.003), respectively].

CONCLUSIONS:

In addition to improving hyperparathyroidism, vitamin D supplementation with daily cholecalciferol (vitamin D3) had a beneficial effect in decreasing albuminuria with potential effects on delaying the progression of CKD.

Study 28.8 Active vitamin D treatment for reduction of residual proteinuria: a systematic review[8]

ABSTRACT:

Despite renin-angiotensin-aldosterone system blockade, which retards progression of CKD by reducing proteinuria, many patients with CKD have residual proteinuria, an independent risk factor for disease progression. We aimed to address whether active vitamin D analogs reduce resid-ual proteinuria. We systematically searched for trials published between 1950 and September of 2012 in the Medline, Embase, and Cochrane Library databases. All randomized controlled trials of vitamin D analogs in patients with CKD that reported an effect on proteinuria with sample size ≥50 were selected. Mean differences of proteinuria change over time and odds ratios for reaching ≥15% proteinuria decrease from baseline to last measurement were synthesized under a random effects model. From 907 citations retrieved, six studies (four studies with paricalcitol and two studies with calcitriol) providing data for 688 patients were included in the meta-analysis. Most patients (84%) used an angiotensin-converting enzyme inhibitor or angiotensin receptor blocker throughout the study. Active vitamin D analogs reduced proteinuria (weighted mean difference from baseline to last measurement was -16% [95% CI, -13% to -18%]) compared with controls (+6% [95% CI, 0% to +12%]; P<0.001). Proteinuria reduction was achieved more commonly in patients treated with an active vitamin D analog (204/390 patients) than control patients (86/298 patients; OR, 2.72 [95% CI, 1.82 to 4.07]; P<0.001). Thus, active vitamin D analogs may further reduce proteinuria in CKD patients in addition to current regimens. Future studies should address whether vitamin D therapy also retards progressive renal functional decline.

Study 28.9   Normal 25-Hydroxyvitamin D Levels Are Associated with Less Proteinuria and Attenuate Renal Failure Progression in Children with CKD.[9]

ABSTRACT:

Angiotensin-converting enzyme inhibitors (ACEi) for renin-angiotensin-aldosterone system (RAAS) blockade are routinely used to slow CKD progression. However, vitamin D may also promote renoprotection by suppressing renin transcription through cross-talk between RAAS and vitamin D-fibroblast growth factor-23 (FGF-23)-Klotho pathways. To determine whether vitamin D levels influence proteinuria and CKD progression in children, we performed a post hoc analysis of the Effect of Strict Blood Pressure Control and ACE Inhibition on Progression of CKD in Pediatric Patients (ESCAPE) cohort. In 167 children (median eGFR 51 ml/min per 1.73 m(2)), serum 25-hydroxyvitamin D (25(OH)D), FGF-23, and Klotho levels were measured at baseline and after a median 8 months on ACEi. Children with lower 25(OH)D levels had higher urinary protein/ creatinine ratios at baseline (P=0.03) and at follow-up (P=0.006). Levels of 25(OH)D and serum vitamin D-binding protein were not associated, but 25(OH)D ≤50 nmol/L associated with higher diastolic BP (P=0.004). ACEi therapy also associated with increased Klotho levels (P<0.001). The annualized loss of eGFR was inversely associated with baseline 25(OH)D level (P<0.001, r=0.32). Five-year renal survival was 75% in patients with baseline 25(OH)D ≥50 nmol/L and 50% in those with lower 25(OH)D levels (P<0.001). This renoprotective effect remained significant but attenuated with ACEi therapy (P=0.05). Renal survival increased 8.2% per 10 nmol/L increase in 25(OH) D (P=0.03), independent of eGFR; proteinuria, BP, and FGF-23 levels; and underlying renal diagnosis. In children with CKD, 25(OH)D ≥50 nmol/L was associated with greater preservation of renal function. This effect was present but attenuated with concomitant ACEi therapy.

Study 28.10   Vitamin D deficiency may predict a poorer outcome of IgA nephropathy.[10]

CONCLUSION:

A 25(OH)D deficiency at baseline is significantly correlated with poorer clinical outcomes and more severe renal pathological features, and low levels of 25(OH)D at baseline were strongly associated with increased risk of renal progression in IgAN.

Study 28.11   Therapeutic use of calcitriol.[11]

ABSTRACT:

The synthesis of 1α,25-dihydroxyvitamin D3 (Calcitriol) takes place mostly in the kidneys through the action of 1α-hydroxylase (CYP27B1) which converts 25(OH)D into 1,25(OH)2D3. Renal production of calcitriol is stimulated by PTH, low calcium and low phosphate and it is reduced by high phosphate and FGF23. Binding of 1α,25-dihydroxyvitamin D3 to its receptor (VDR) causes gut absorption of calcium and phosphate, decrease in PTH synthesis, and stimulation of FGF23. At the bone level calcitriol suppresses pre-osteoblasts and activates mature osteoblasts. VDR is present in a large variety of cells that do not have any direct role in the regulation of mineral metabolism. Calcitriol regulates immune and inflammatory response, cell turnover, cell differentiation, renin production, reduces proteinuria and others. In patients with Chronic Kidney Disease (CKD) there is a decrease in calcitriol that is apparent at early stages of renal disease; this is probably due to the elevation of FGF23 which is present since very early stage of CKD. In CKD stage, 3-4 moderate doses of calcitriol are effective to control secondary hyperparathyroidism and observational studies suggest that calcitriol therapy increases survival and slows the progression of renal disease as long as phosphate and calcium levels are controlled. Calcitriol (0.5 µg calcitriol twice per week) has been effective in decreasing proteinuria in patients with IgA nephropathy. In dialysis patients, the administration of calcitriol reduces serum PTH levels but it is also known that high doses of calcitriol are associated with hypercalcemia and worse control of hyperphosphatemia. In kidney transplant patients, the administration of calcitriol, 0.5 µg/48h prevents bone mass loss during the first few months after transplantation.

Note: This study suggests a reduced amount of calcitriol taken just two days a week was beneficial. I point this out because nothing says we have to take any supplement every day. Once or twice a week may be the sweet spot.

So we have some evidence for taking a form of vitamin D, but what about the other side of the argument? Does any evidence exist to suggest that vitamin D is bad for us? For some perspective, I looked at healthy adults first. The following is an analysis of 159 related studies.

Study 28.12 Vitamin D supplementation for prevention of mortality in adults.[12]

AUTHORS' CONCLUSIONS:

Vitamin D3 seemed to decrease mortality in elderly people living independently or in institutional care. Vitamin D2, alfacalcidol and calcitriol had no statistically significant beneficial effects on mortality. Vitamin D3 combined with calcium increased nephrolithiasis. Both alfacalcidol and calcitriol increased hypercalcaemia. Because of risks of attrition bias originating from substantial dropout of participants and of outcome reporting bias due to a number of trials not reporting on mortality, as well as a number of other weaknesses in our evidence, further placebo-controlled randomised trials seem warranted.

Note: Nephrolithiasis is what caught my eye. Nephrolithiasis is calcium buildup in the kidneys. In healthy adults, taking vitamin D3 with calcium or a calcium supplement with vitamin D3 resulted in an increased risk of nephrolithiasis. This may be a warning shot for us to think twice about taking vitamin D3 with calcium.

Study 28.13 Do the benefits of using calcitriol and other vitamin D receptor activators in patients with chronic kidney disease outweigh the harms?[13]

CONCLUSION AND SUGGESTED FUTURE RESEARCH:

Secondary hyperparathyroidism is an inevitable consequence of advanced CKD, and the suppression of PTH levels with calcitriol/VDRA therapy has been a cornerstone of nephrology practice. The effectiveness of calcitriol/VDRA in lowering PTH has been well established in numerous stud-ies, and a mortality benefit of lower PTH levels has been demonstrated in many (but not all) large observational studies. However, there is still no evidence for patient-level outcomes from RCT with the use of calcitriol/VDRA in CKD; the optimal level of PTH in CKD stages 3–5 is not known; and at present, their routine use in stages 3–5 CKD cannot be recommended. Instead, there are concerns about the effects of higher doses of calcitriol/VDRA on mortality outcomes in certain CKD cohorts, with their potential to promote hypercalcaemia and, potentially, vascular calcification. Consequently, the current guidelines remain intentionally vague and are difficult to implement in clinical practice.

Many aspects pertaining to the use of calcitriol/VDRA require further evaluation in clinical trials. These include their use in CKD 3–5, appropriate timing and doses, and use of calcitriol/VDRA in combination with other therapies such as phosphate binders and nutritional vitamin D. The effect of calcitriol/VDRA on the progression of SHPT and on parathyroidectomy rates also needs further investigation; and their effects on bone, fracture and musculoskeletal outcomes remain unclear. Despite the negative results of recent RCT, there is considerable interest in the use of calcitriol/VDRA for extra-renal indications such as improving cardiac outcomes and proteinuria. Future clinical trials need to evaluate clinically significant outcomes, in particular mortality and cardiovascular morbidity, as these will in turn inform revised versions of clinical guidelines pertaining to calcitriol/VDRA use. The withdrawal of reimbursement of cinacalcet therapy in Australia will afford an opportunity to re-evaluate the future use of calcitriol/VDRA in CKD, as well as refining the timing of therapy, their use in combination with other therapies, and their effects on biomarkers (other than PTH) in CKD-MBD.

Study 28.14 The new kidney disease: improving global outcomes (KDIGO) guidelines - expert clinical focus on bone and vascular calcification[14]

ABSTRACT:

Chronic kidney disease-mineral and bone disorder (CKD-MBD) defines a triad of interrelated abnormalities of serum biochemistry, bone and the vasculature associated with chronic kidney disease (CKD). The new kidney disease: improving global outcomes (KDIGO) guidelines define the quality and depth of evidence supporting therapeutic intervention in CKD-MBD. They also highlight where patient management decisions lack a strong evidence base. Expert interpretation of the guidelines, along with informed opinion, where evidence is weak, may help develop effective clinical practice. The body of evidence linking poor bone health and reservoir function (the ability of bone to buffer calcium and phosphorus) with vascular calcification and cardiovascular outcomes is growing. Treating renal bone disease should be one of the primary aims of therapy for CKD. Evaluation of the biochemical parameters of CKD-MBD (primarily phosphorus, calcium, parathyroid hormone and vitamin D levels) as early as CKD Stage 3, and an assessment of bone status (by the best means available), should be used to guide treatment decisions. The adverse effects of high phosphorus intake relative to renal clearance (including stimulation of hyperparathyroidism) precede hyperphosphatemia, which presents late in CKD. Early reduction of phosphorus load may ameliorate these adverse effects. Evidence that calcium load may influence progression of vascular calcification with effects on mortality should also be considered when choosing the type and dose of phosphate binder to be used. The risks, benefits, and strength of evidence for various treatment options for the abnormalities of CKD-MBD are considered.

CONCLUSION:

The evidence-based KDIGO guidelines highlight the gaps in evidence that must be filled to achieve better diagnosis and management of CKD-MBD. This is an extremely complex disorder with interplay between several biochemical parameters, patient demographics and additional comorbidities. As a result, there are no universal treatment algorithms that should be applied to all patients with CKD-MBD. Rather, physicians need to treat patients as individuals and react to changes in the full spectrum of CKD-MBD parameters.

Ok, so vitamin D supplementation practices are clear as mud. We don't really know what to do and our doctors may not know either. "Intentionally vague" guidelines aren't much help, but we can take a look at the existing data and be a little more informed.

First, let's figure out some common sense steps to deal with vitamin D.

1. First, know how your levels change with each season.

I live in a northern climate now. My vitamin D levels are normal in the summer and fall, but below the average range in winter and spring. Those of you who live in warm areas may be able to get some sun every week of the year. This is a clue. You may not need to supplement vitamin D in the summer or fall; maybe you just need supplements in the winter. This would remove some of the risk of vitamin D therapies.

2. Get some sun as often as you can. Thirty minutes of sun exposure three times a week (30x3), should help with your vitamin D levels.

3. A level of 20 nanograms/milliliter, expressed as ng/ml, is the low end and 50 ng/ml is the high end of the normal range. Studies suggest levels of 25 ng/ml or higher are needed to avoid problems. 12 ng/ml or lower is considered deficient. If you do take a vitamin D supplement, take the absolute smallest dose you can.

4. Be careful of fortified foods. Many foods today contain added vitamin D. Many milk alternatives like rice or coconut milk/beverages contain 25% of the RDA of vitamin D. You may be supplementing vitamin D and don't know it. In most cases (but not all), we should not choose unenriched foods and drinks.

5. If you take vitamin D, the type of vitamin D matters. Only take the type of vitamin D your doctor recommends and don't take vitamin D unless your doctor recommends it.

6. As your diet improves and all of your metabolic numbers get better, your vitamin D levels will also likely improve. As your body starts working better, your vitamin D levels should get better as well. Vitamin D will be a moving target just like your other numbers for a while.

References

1. Dusso A, González EA, Martin KJ. Vitamin D in chronic kidney disease. *Best practice & Research Clinical Endocrinology & Metabolism.* 2011;25(4):647-655.

2. Obi Y, Hamano T, Isaka Y. Prevalence and prognostic implications of vitamin D deficiency in chronic kidney disease. *Disease Markers.* 2015;2015(Article ID 868961).

3. Fernández-Juárez G, Luño J, Barrio V, et al. 25 (OH) vitamin D levels and renal disease progression in patients with type 2 diabetic nephropathy and blockade of the renin-angiotensin system. *Clinical Journal of the American Society of Nephrology.* 2013:CJN. 00910113.

4. Cozzolino M, Brunini F, Capone V, et al. Role of vitamin D in the pathogenesis of chronic kidney disease. *Recenti Progressi in Medicina.* 2013;104(1):33-40.

5. Lucisano S, Buemi M, Passantino A, Aloisi C, Cernaro V, Santoro D. New insights on the role of vitamin D in the progression of renal damage. *Kidney and Blood Pressure Research.* 2013;37(6):667-678.

6. Kumar R, Tebben PJ, Thompson JR. Vitamin D and the kidney. *Archives of biochemistry and biophysics.* 2012;523(1):77-86.

7. Molina P, Górriz JL, Molina MD, et al. The effect of cholecalciferol for lowering albuminuria in chronic kidney disease: a prospective controlled study. *Nephrology Dialysis Transplantation.* 2013;29(1):97-109.

8. de Borst MH, Hajhosseiny R, Tamez H, Wenger J, Thadhani R, Goldsmith DJ. Active vitamin D treatment for reduction of residual proteinuria: a systematic review. *Journal of the American Society of Nephrology.* 2013:ASN. 2013030203.

9. Shroff R, Aitkenhead H, Costa N, et al. Normal 25-hydroxyvitamin D levels are associated with less proteinuria and attenuate renal failure progression in children with CKD. *Journal of the American Society of Nephrology.* 2016;27(1):314-322.

10. Li X-H, Huang X-P, Pan L, et al. Vitamin D deficiency may predict a poorer outcome of IgA nephropathy. *BMC nephrology.* 2016;17(1):164.

11. Rodriguez M, R Munoz-Castaneda J, Almaden Y. Therapeutic use of calcitriol. *Current Vascular Pharmacology.* 2014;12(2):294-299.

12. Bjelakovic G, Gluud LL, Nikolova D, et al. Vitamin D supplementation for prevention of mortality in adults. *Cochrane Database Syst Rev.* 2014;1(1).

13. Toussaint ND, Damasiewicz MJ. Do the benefits of using calcitriol and other vitamin D receptor activators in patients with chronic kidney disease outweigh the harms? *Nephrology.* 2017;22:51-56.

14. London G, Coyne D, Hruska K, Malluche H, Martin K. The new kidney disease: improving global outcomes (KDIGO) guidelines–expert clinical focus on bone and vascular calcification. *Clinical Nephrology.* 2010;74(6):423.

CHAPTER 29

Supplements—Friend or Foe

I wanted to have a chapter on supplements that are beneficial or harmful to kidney patients. This turned into a monster for a few reasons. First is the number of supplements requested by patients. I have 30-plus supplements on my list right now to research. I am hesitant to recommend any unregulated supplements at this stage. Any number of problems exist with this market.

Second is lack of testing in the unregulated supplement market, and third is the unregulated nature of the internet.

Just because someone claims something on the internet or on a bottle doesn't make it true. Once you take a look behind the supplement industry curtain, you will find some disturbing facts. I don't want to say that all supplements are bad or not as advertised. I am quite sure many are good, but in many cases, we don't have any way to know.

Over the past three years, I have visited supplement and drug manufacturing facilities in several countries. I have also met with numerous supplement and drug manufacturers. I have a pretty good understanding of this industry now, and it's a little scary, to be honest.

To understand the risks of this market, we first need to understand the hierarchy of drugs and supplements.

Prescription drugs—These require Federal Drug Administration (FDA) approval and are manufactured to high standards to ensure quality. Drug manufacturers are subject to FDA inspections and audits on a routine basis.

Medical foods—These fall under the Orphan Drug Act and are nutritional foods for patients with specific diseases or illnesses. Medical foods are overseen by the FDA and subject to FDA inspections and audits on a routine basis. They may require a prescription, just like a drug.

Supplements—These products are also under the supervision of the FDA, but do not require audits or inspections. The FDA is charged with regulating claims on labels and ensuring that the product in the bottle is the same as the one on the label. The FDA takes action on these products after a problem is reported.

The normal drug standard is 95% and 105%, or a 5% deviation. The product should not vary from the advertised or labeled content by more than 5%. Testing is done throughout the manufacturing process to ensure that this standard is met. If you don't meet the standard, the product cannot be sold. Think about this standard when you read the upcoming paragraphs.

Testing by the state of New York on the supplements sold by major stores like Walmart, Target, Walgreens, and GNC found that four out of five bottles contained none of the herbs on the label.[1] You read that right; most bottles didn't even contain the main ingredient on the label. Seventy-nine percent of supplements tested negative for the main ingredient on the label. Only 4% of Walmart products tested to actually contain the active ingredients.

The FDA has also been busy in 2018 recalling supplements.

Study 29.1   **The FDA has recalled 885 dietary supplements, according to its website, www.fda.gov. The FDA also includes the following warning:**

This list only includes a small fraction of the potentially hazardous products with hidden ingredients marketed to consumers on the internet and in retail establishments. FDA is unable to test and identify all products marketed as dietary supplements on the market that have potentially harmful hidden ingredients. Even if a product is not included in this list, consumers should exercise caution before using certain products. To learn more about how to reduce your risk of encountering a product mar-keted as a dietary supplement with a hidden ingredient, please visit FDA Medication Health Fraud webpage linked above.

The most common recall in 2018 appears to be supplements that claimed to increase testosterone which reduced erectile dysfunction. Multiple supplements in this category were recalled because they contained sildenafil, the active ingredient in Viagra. Sildenafil is a prescription drug, but supplements laced with sildenafil were coming from China. Supplement marketing companies buy these pills already made and don't test for the actual ingredients or contaminants. The U.S. marketers of these products likely never knew sildenafil was in the pills.

Here is a recent comment in the Journal of Sleep Medicine on the poor quality of over-the-counter melatonin. Melatonin is used as an over-the-counter supplement sleep aid. Testing was done on 31 melatonin supplements purchased at grocery stores to determine if melatonin supplements had the advertised amount of melatonin.

"Melatonin content varied from an egregious −83% to +478% of labeled melatonin and 70% had melatonin concentration ≤ 10% of what was claimed. Worse yet, the content of melatonin between lots of the same product varied by as much as 465%."

The most variable sample was a chewable tablet (and most likely to be used by children). It contained almost 9 mg of melatonin when it was supposed to contain 1.5 mg, and also exhibited the greatest variability between lots (465% difference).

These stories and studies can be used to educate us as potential supplement buyers.

Let's see what we can learn:

1. Content as advertised on the bottle may not be reliable.

2. Quality control may not be reliable from bottle to bottle, even from the same manufacturer.

3. Nothing is standing between you buying and taking 70 to 90 times the normal amount of a substance that naturally occurs in your body or taking a prescription drug without knowing it.

The idea that over-the-counter or unregulated supplements are safe for kidney patients has to be questioned. Our kidneys can't process toxins, vitamins, minerals, and waste like normal kidneys can. Some caution is clearly warranted here.

Paying for the lowest-priced supplements may mean that what's on the bottle has little to do with what's in the bottle. Price should likely be our last issue if we take supplements. Keep in mind that the supplement industry is very competitive. This means they have to use the lowest-cost, and most likely the lowest-quality, ingredients to be price competitive. Do we really want to be taking the lowest-quality stuff in the world in a supplement? It's a question that each of us needs to ask.

To be clear, I am not saying all supplements are bad or mislabeled. What I am saying is to be very careful when buying and taking supplements. I found this out firsthand when working on keto acids for kidney patients. I won't go into detail, but I am very suspicious of the supplement industry after meeting with over a dozen companies.

There are several companies that test and certify supplements. The most well-known is USP, or United States Pharmacopeia: www.usp.org. Supplement companies can pay USP to verify the ingredients. The current rate for this service is around $30,000. Large companies like Nature Made and Kirkland (Costco brand) have invested in USP testing for many of their products.

A consumer tip: Costco will carry other brands of supplements that may or may not be USP verified. Always look at the labels. The USP logo will be displayed if they are USP tested.

Study 29.2   Beware of internet claims of miracle cure or untested treatments

I was recently forwarded an herbal tea recipe that is claimed to reverse kidney disease. The tea has three ingredients. The first ingredient may have some merit. However, no research could be found on one ingredient, and the third ingredient had one negative study and no others.

Let's think about this for a minute and ask a few sane questions:

Do we really believe a three-ingredient homemade tea is a treatment for kidney disease?

Do we want to consume a tea or supplement with questionable ingredients?

This patient paid a price seven times higher than a softcover book on Amazon for a PDF download. If this really worked, why aren't they selling this to the world and doing medical studies? Every drug company in the world would be beating down their door offering tens of millions of dollars.

If we pursue a certain treatment plan, it needs to pass the sniff test, if you know what I mean. Reputable books by reputable authors sell for $9.99 on Amazon and in other book stores. Why is the secret treatment priced at $60 or $70? I will let you draw your own conclusion.

Other common terms you should be on guard for are:

Ancient secret or wisdom or healing

Secret formulas

Undiscovered materials or substances

Miracle cures

You get the idea. A California company was fined tens of thousands of dollars recently for these kinds of claims. Take one look at life expectancies throughout history, and you will see that ancient secrets don't hold up to any scrutiny.

I am not the first to think about this.

Study 29.3   Internet claims on dietary and herbal supplements in advanced nephropathy: truth or myth.3

RESULTS:

Of the 184 websites, 28% claimed to decrease CKD progression, 60% did not advise to consult a doctor before taking the supplement, and >90% did not mention any potential drug interaction, disease interaction or caution in use during pregnancy or in children. The 10 common plant ingredients claiming to be beneficial in kidney diseases were uva ursi, dandelion, parsley, corn silk, juniper, celery, buchu, horsetail, marshmallow and stinging nettle. In contrast to their claims, these substances were not adequately studied in humans. The available animal studies showed detrimental effects and potential drug interactions with commonly used medications in the CKD/ESRD population.

CONCLUSIONS:

Nephrologists need to be cognizant of the lack of substantiated proven benefits of these substances and of the potential adverse effects in the animal models that can translate to the patients. Most importantly, the policy needs to change regarding the regulation of these products to prevent patient harm and misinformation.

Note: This was a warning for nephrologists, but the message is clear.

Any website, guide, book, or supplement for kidney disease that does not strongly suggest or require you to be under a doctor's supervision should be viewed with great skepticism. Research on any supplement you take should be exhaustive and based on a double-digit number of studies, not just one random study.

Other over-the-counter amino acids may be harmful to our health if our kidneys cannot get rid of excess toxins. Tyrosine, tryptophan, and ornithine come to mind. The next study has to do with both over-the-counter supplements and endotoxemia.

FIGURE 29.1: **Impact of Altered Intestinal Microbiota on Chronic Kidney Disease Progression**[4]

Over-the-counter food supplements or prescription drugs with the potential to generate uremic toxins with nephrotoxic effects. Information obtained from reference [13]. Putative benefit or indications refers to the reasons sellers use to peddle the supplement. It does not imply that we endorse these benefits or indications.

Supplement	Putative Benefits or Indications	Resulting Uremic Toxins with Nephrotoxicity Potential
L-tyrosine (para-tyrosine, 4-hydroxyphenylalanine)	Enhanced physical performance, enhanced cognitive performance	pCS, pCG
Tryptophan	Antidepressant, anxiolytic, sleep aid	IS, IAA
Choline/phosphatidylcholine/lecithin	Liver health, memory, Alzheimer disease, enhanced physical performance, pregnancy	TMAO
L-carnitine	Enhanced physical performance, haemodialysis	TMAO

pCS: p-cresyl sulphate, pCG: p-cresyl-glucuronide, IS: indoxyl sulphate, IAA: indole-3 acetic acid, TMAO: trimethylamine N-oxide.

A good example for this chart is buying an essential amino acid supplement designed for people with normal kidney function. These supplements may contain relatively high amounts of tryptophan, which may result in increased uremic toxins. In addition, due to the unregulated nature of the supplement market, the amount in one serving or pill may or may not be what is on the label.

Here is a list, from the National Kidney Foundation, of supplements that may have an adverse effect on kidneys.[5]

Herbs from NKF list found in reported dietary supplements and associated adverse renal effects:

Herb	Nephrotoxic	Aggravates CKD risk factor	Risky in CKD
Alfalfa	Triggers lupus	-	-
Aloe	Albuminuria, acute or progressive kidney injury	-	Hypovolemia
Bayberry	-	-	Hypovolemia
Broom	-	-	-
Buckthorn	Albuminuria	-	Hypovolemia
Capsicum	-	-	Hypovolemia
Cascara	Albuminuria	-	Hypovolemia
Dandelion	-	-	Hypovolemia

Herb	Nephrotoxic	Aggravates CKD risk factor	Risky in CKD
Ginger	-	-	Hypoglycemia
Ginseng	-	-	Hypoglycemia
Horsetail	-	-	Hypoglycemia
Licorice	-	High BP	-
Ma huang	-	Hyperglycemia, high BP, kidney stones	Hypovolemia
Nettle	Acute or progressive kidney injury	Hyperglycemia	-
Noni	-	-	Hyperkalemia
Poke Root	-	-	Hypovolemia
Rhubarb	-	-	Hypovolemia
Senna	Acute or progressive kidney injury	-	Hypovolemia
Wormwood	Acute or progressive kidney injury, rhabdomyolysis	-	Hypovolemia
Yohimbe	Acute or progressive kidney injury, triggers lupus	-	-

Note: hypovolemia due to diarrhea and/or vomiting.

BP, blood pressure; NKF, National Kidney Foundation; CKD, chronic kidney disease

Herbs are not the only supplements we should be cautious about.

Study 29.4　Effect of B-Vitamin Therapy on Progression of Diabetic Nephropathy A Randomized Controlled Trial[6]

CONCLUSION:

Among patients with diabetic nephropathy, <u>high doses of B vitamins compared with placebo resulted in a greater decrease in GFR and an increase in vascular events.</u>

High doses of vitamins may also increase the rate of GFR decline. Be careful taking large doses of any vitamin. Remember, your kidneys can't process a normal amount of anything at this stage. Hitting them with 100% to 300% of your recommended daily allowance (RDA) is rolling the dice, in my eyes. You are going to get some vitamins and minerals through your diet. No need to go crazy with vitamins. A time-release vitamin for kidney patients with, say, 50% of the

RDA would be a good idea. This is not enough to cause us problems, but enough to ensure that we are not deficient when diet is taken into account.

As you can see, we need to be careful of what we read, watch or hear. We also need to apply a little common sense. If something sounds too good to be true, then it probably is.

You can feel safe when it comes to drugs or medical food products due to FDA regulation, inspection, testing, and audits. However, the unregulated supplement market is, well, just that: unregulated. We are trying to slow our disease, not take extra or unnecessary risks.

I will devote another chapter to supplements requested, but will have to release this as an update of the book. It is simply too much research to do at this point and still hit our publishing deadlines. If you are on the list at **www.stoppingkidneydisease.com**, you will get the chapter for free.

Bottom line:

Less is more when it comes to your kidneys. If you take any supplements at all, it should be with your doctor's approval, lots of good research, and be safe for your kidneys. Your blood and urine tests should also improve if the supplement is working. If not, you are likely wasting money and may be taking risks you are not aware of.

Putting extra workload on your kidneys or taking extra risks, either knowingly or unknowingly, has very little, if any, upside and could actually increase the rate of GFR decline in some cases.

Remember, less is more for kidney disease patients.

References

1. Underwood BD. A.G. Schneiderman Asks Major Retailers to Halt Sales of Certain Herbal Supplements as DNA Tests Fail to Detect Plant Materials Listed on Majority of Products Tested. 2015; https://ag.ny.gov/press-release/ag-schneiderman-asks-major-retailers-halt-sales-certain-herbal-supplements-dna-tests. Accessed 28 June, 2018.

2. USFDA. Tainted Products Marketed as Dietary Supplements_CDER. 2018; https://www.accessdata.fda.gov/scripts/sda/sdNavigation.cfm?sd=tainted_supplements_cder. Accessed 1 July, 2018.

3. Vamenta-Morris H, Dreisbach A, Shoemaker-Moyle M, Abdel-Rahman EM. Internet claims on dietary and herbal supplements in advanced nephropathy: truth or myth. *American journal of nephrology.* 2014;40(5):393-398.

4. Castillo-Rodriguez E, Fernandez-Prado R, Esteras R, et al. Impact of Altered Intestinal Microbiota on Chronic Kidney Disease Progression. *Toxins.* 2018;10(7):300.

5. Kirk J. A TO Z HEALTH GUIDE: Herbal Supplements and Kidney Disease. 2015; https://www.kidney.org/atoz/content/herbalsupp. Accessed 5 July, 2018.

6. House AA, Eliasziw M, Cattran DC, et al. Effect of B-vitamin therapy on progression of diabetic nephropathy: a randomized controlled trial. *Jama.* 2010;303(16):1603-1609.

"Factors" that Put the Brakes on Kidney Disease Progression

There are four strategies or things we can do to significantly affect the life of our kidneys that are different from controlling or treating the bad "Factors." These factors also slow heart disease progression. We need to get all of these "Factors" working for us to offset the bad "Factors" that increase the speed of kidney disease progression.

If you can get the bad "Factors" or comorbid conditions down to two and have all four of the good "Factors" working for you, your disease progression may slow dramatically. This takes time, and in my case, this process ended with remission.

As of 2019, science and research has given us a very good blueprint of what it takes to live a long time with a high quality of life.

Every kidney patient should implement the good "Factors." The research is so strong, it's not up for debate anymore.

CHAPTER 30

Magnesium: Getting a Survival Advantage

Magnesium is a catch-22 for people with kidney disease. As our disease progresses, our kidneys lose the ability to properly regulate magnesium. For this reason, magnesium consumption may be restricted, especially in stage 5. However, this is at odds with research showing that high magnesium levels decrease mortality rates and increase survival rates. Let's dig a little deeper and see how something that gives us a survival advantage is supposed to be bad for us.

We need to understand magnesium because it has the potential to lower mortality rates and slow the progression of heart disease. The first thing we must understand is the issue is not magnesium but magnesium clearance rates. Your kidneys are tasked with managing magnesium. As your kidney function declines, so does your ability to manage magnesium. For most people in stages 1, 2, 3, and even 4, the kidneys are still able to manage magnesium successfully. Your blood tests will be the final judge and jury, but research indicates that not until stage 5 does magnesium regulation become a real problem.

You may hear that you shouldn't take antacids that contain magnesium. Here is why: Milk of magnesia, an over-the counter laxative, has 1,100 to 2,200 mg of magnesium in the recommended dosage. The recommended daily amount (RDA) is 400 mg. In this case, you are dumping 1,100 mg of magnesium or more on your kidneys at one time. This is a problem and can lead to high magnesium levels. The same problem exists for magnesium-based laxatives like magnesium citrate. The recommended dosage of magnesium citrate for an adult is 7 to 10 ounces. Each ounce contains 290 mg of magnesium. The resulting dose of magnesium is 2,000 to 2,900 mg. This is four to five times the RDA delivered in one dose.

Our kidneys will suddenly have to deal with four to five times the normal daily amount in a few hours. Therefore, magnesium-based antacids or laxatives can be dangerous for people with kidney disease. Magnesium doses of more than 1,000 mg delivered to our bodies at one time may be too much for our kidneys to handle.

The good news is that this problem is easily handled. Taking a smaller dose of magnesium with each meal, or a time-release supplement, avoids much of this problem. For example, taking the RDA of 400 mg over three meals yields 133 mg at a time, but 400 mg over ten hours or so. 133 mg is very different than 1,000+ mg at one time.

Studies have shown that 360 mg to 720 mg a day of time release magnesium was well-tolerated and reduced the risk factors for vascular calcification in stage 3 and stage 4 patients.

It might take ten or more years to progress from stage 2 or 3 to stage 5, so why would we restrict magnesium during this ten-year period if we get a survival advantage? In addition, magnesium has other beneficial effects on our bodies.

Magnesium slows vascular calcification, lowers blood pressure, and is inversely correlated with inflammation.

In view of the benefits of magnesium, we want our magnesium levels to be at the highest end of the normal range. Let's see what we can find. First, let's look at vascular calcification. Hypermagnesemia is high magnesium and hypomagnesemia is low magnesium.

Study 30.1 — Oral Magnesium Supplementation in Chronic Kidney Disease Stages 3 and 4: Efficacy, Safety and Effect on Serum Calcification Propensity—A Prospective Randomized Double-Blinded Placebo-Controlled Clinical Trial[1]

RESULTS:

Thirty-four subjects completed the trial. Intracellular Mg remained stable throughout the trial despite significant increases in both serum and urine Mg. T_{50} increased significantly by 40 min from 256 ± 60 (mean $\pm$ SD) to 296 ± 64 minutes (95% confidence interval, 11–70, $P < 0.05$) in the Mg 30 mmol/d group after 8 weeks. No serious adverse events related to the study medication were reported during the study.

DISCUSSION:

Oral Mg supplementation was safe and well-tolerated in CKD stages 3 and 4 and improved T_{50}, but did not increase intracellular Mg. Further studies are needed to investigate the long-term effects of Mg supplementation in CKD stage 3 and 4 and whether improvement in calcification propensity is related to clinical endpoints.

Note: T_{50} is the term for serum calcification propensity. T_{50} is a mortality indicator. Higher T_{50} scores should reduce calcification of arteries. See next study.

Study 30.2 — Relationship between magnesium and clinical biomarkers on inhibition of vascular calcification.[18]

RESULTS:

Incubation of aortic segments in the presence of β-glycerophosphate and $NaH(2)PO(4)$ caused an increased tissue $Ca(2+)$ deposition compared to control conditions. This increased amount of $Ca(2+)$ in the aortic rings was significantly decreased in the presence of $Mg(2+)$. In CKD patients, but not in controls, magnesium serum concentration was associated with the IMT of the carotid arteries. In addition, CKD patients with higher magnesium serum concentration had a significantly lower PWV.

DISCUSSION AND CONCLUSION:

Elevated phosphate concentrations in the culture media induce ex vivo/in vitro medial calcification in intact rat aortic rings in the presence of alkaline phosphatase. Mg(2+) ions reduced ex vivo/in vitro vascular calcification despite increased phosphate concentration. This hypothesis is additionally based on the fact that CKD patients with high Mg(2) serum levels had significantly lower IMT and PWV values, which may result in a lower risk for cardiovascular events and mortality in these patients. Therefore, Mg(2+) supplementation may be an option for treatment and prevention of vascular calcification resulting in a reduction of cardiovascular events in CKD patients.

| Study 30.3 | Serum Calcification Propensity Predicts All-Cause Mortality in Predialysis CKD[2] |

ABSTRACT:

Medial arterial calcification is accelerated in patients with CKD and strongly associated with increased arterial rigidity and cardiovascular mortality. Recently, a novel *in vitro* blood test that provides an overall measure of calcification propensity by monitoring the maturation time (T_{50}) of calciprotein particles in serum was described. We used this test to measure serum T_{50} in a prospective cohort of 184 patients with stages 3 and 4 CKD, with a median of 5.3 years of follow-up. At baseline, the major determinants of serum calcification propensity included higher serum phosphate, ionized calcium, increased bone osteoclastic activity, and lower free fetuin-A, plasma pyrophosphate and albumin concentrations, which accounted for 49% of the variation in this parameter. Increased serum calcification propensity at baseline independently associated with aortic pulse wave velocity in the complete cohort and progressive aortic stiffening over 30 months in a subgroup of 93 patients. After adjustment for demographic, renal, cardiovascular and biochemical covariates, including serum phosphate, risk of death among patients in the lowest T_{50} tertile was more than two times the risk among patients in the highest T_{50} tertile (adjusted hazard ratio, 2.2; 95% confidence interval, 1.1 to 5.4; $P=0.04$). This effect was lost, however, after additional adjustment for aortic stiffness, suggesting a shared causal pathway. Longitudinally, serum calcification propensity measurements remained temporally stable (intraclass correlation=0.81). These results suggest that serum T_{50} may be helpful as a biomarker in designing methods to improve defenses against vascular calcification.

| Study 30.4 | Lower serum magnesium is associated with vascular calcification in peritoneal dialysis patients: a cross sectional study.[3] |

CONCLUSIONS:

Our findings suggest that Mg may inhibit vascular calcification. If this association is replicated across larger studies with serial Mg and vascular calcification measurements, interventions that increase serum Mg and their effect on vascular calcification warrant further investigation in the PD population.

Study 30.5 — Magnesium retards the progress of the arterial calcifications in hemodialysis patients: a pilot study.[4]

RESULTS:

Thirty-two patients of the Mg group and 27 of the Ca group completed the study. The mean time average values of the biochemical laboratories did not differ between the two groups, except serum Mg: 2.83 + 0.38 in the Mg group versus 2.52 + 0.27 mg/dl in the Ca group, $p = 0.001$. In 9/32 (28.12%) patients of the Mg group and in 12/27 (44.44%) patients of the Ca group, the arterial calcifications were worsened, $p = 0.276$. Moreover, in 4/32 (15.6%) patients of the Mg group and in 0/27 (0%) patients of the Ca group, they were improved, $p = 0.040$. The multivariate logistic regression analysis revealed that serum magnesium was an independent predictor for no progression of the arterial calcifications, $p = 0.047$.

CONCLUSIONS:

Magnesium probably retards the arterial calcifications in hemodialysis patients. Further clinical studies are needed to clarify whether magnesium provides cardiovascular protection to this group of patients.

Study 30.6 — Serum magnesium level and arterial calcification in end-stage renal disease.[5]

ABSTRACT:

In this paper, we examine the relationship of serum levels of Ca, P, Ca X P, P/Mg, Ca X P/Mg, alkaline phosphatase and iPTH to the development or regression of peripheral arterial calcifications (AC) in 44 patients with end-stage renal disease being treated by continuous ambulatory peritoneal dialysis (CAPD). The average follow-up time of this longitudinal study was 27 months (range 6-67 months). The patients were divided into two groups: Group A, those showing one or more increases of AC; and Group B, patients in whom AC either did not develop or decreased during the follow-up. There was no significant difference in serum Ca, P, Ca X P, alkaline phosphatase of iPTH between the two groups. However, serum Mg was significantly lower in Group A than in Group B (2.69 +/- 0.52 and 3.02 +/- 0.51 mg/dl, respectively, P less than 0.001), while the ratios P/Mg and Ca X P/Mg were significantly higher. Our observations suggest that in end-stage renal disease, hypermagnesemia may retard the development of arterial calcifications.

Study 30.7 — Hypomagnesemia is a significant predictor of cardiovascular and non-cardiovascular mortality in patients undergoing hemodialysis.[6]

ABSTRACT:

Although previous studies in the general population showed that hypomagnesemia is a risk for cardiovascular diseases (CVD), the impact of magnesium on the prognosis of patients on hemodialysis has been poorly investigated. To gain information on this, we conducted a nationwide registry-based cohort study of 142,555 hemodialysis patients to determine whether hypomagnesemia is an independent risk for increased mortality in this population. Study outcomes were 1-year all-cause and cause-specific mortality with baseline serum magnesium levels categorized into sextiles. During follow-up, a total of 11,454 deaths occurred, of which 4,774 had a CVD cause. In a fully adjusted model, there was a J-shaped association between serum magnesium and the odds ratio of all-cause mortality from the lowest to highest sextile, with significantly higher mortality in sextiles 1-3 and 6. Similar associations were found between magnesium and both CVD and non-CVD mortality. The proportion of patients with a baseline intact parathyroid hormone level under 50 pg/ml was significantly higher in the highest sextile; however, after excluding these patients, the CVD mortality risk in the highest sextile was attenuated. <u>Thus, hypomagnesemia was significantly associated with an increased risk of mortality in hemodialysis patients.</u>

Interventional studies are needed to clarify whether magnesium supplementation is beneficial for improving patient prognosis.

Now, Let's Look at Mortality Rates

Study 30.8 Serum Magnesium and Mortality in Hemodialysis Patients in the United States: A Cohort Study.[7]

CONCLUSION:

<u>Elevated serum magnesium levels > 2.10 mEq/L were associated with better survival than low serum magnesium levels < 1.30 mEq/L in HD patients.</u> Prospective studies may determine whether manipulation of low serum magnesium levels affects survival.

Study 30.9 Magnesium and Mortality in Patients with Diabetes and Early Chronic Kidney Disease[8]

RESULTS:

Patients' survival at 54 months in group 1, 2 and 3 was 27.8%, 73.8% and 80.2%, respectively (p<0.001). <u>Magnesium was found to be an independent predictor of both mortality and hospitalizations, with a statistically significant decrease in mortality and hospitalizations observed at higher levels of magnesium. Magnesium levels were also negatively correlated with known cardiovascular risk factors and with serum creatinine. Patients with lower magnesium level were more likely to start a renal replacement therapy.</u>

CONCLUSIONS:

<u>Lower magnesium levels result in a greater risk of cardiovascular mortality and hospitalization as well as an accelerated progression of renal disease to renal replacement therapy.</u>

Note: Magnesium was associated with better creatinine levels.

FIGURE 30.1: **Kaplan-Meier Survival Curve by Group Mg.**

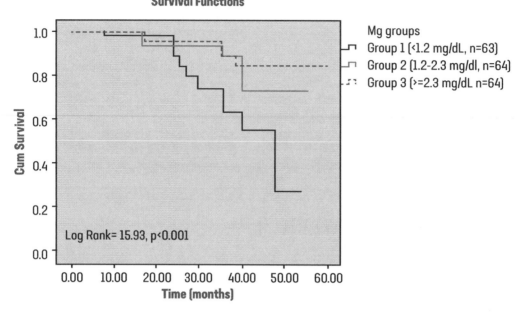

The chart shown above is from the same study. The group with magnesium greater than 2.3 mg/dl had much better survival rates. The normal magnesium range is 1.5 to 2.5 mg/dl.

Study 30.10 Association of serum magnesium (SMg) with all-cause mortality in patients with and without chronic kidney disease in the Dallas Heart Study.[9]

RESULTS:

Among 3,551 participants, 306 (8.6%) had prevalent CKD. Mean SMg was 2.08 ± 0.19 mg/dL (0.85 ± 0.08 mM, mean ± SD) in the CKD and 2.07 ± 0.18 mg/dL (0.85 ± 0.07 mM) in the nonCKD subgroups. During the follow-up period, 329 all-cause deaths and 306 CV deaths or events occurred. In a fully adjusted model, every 0.2 mg/ dL decrease in SMg was associated with ~20-40% increased hazard for all-cause death in both CKD and non-CKD subgroups. In CKD participants, the lowest SMg tertile was also independently associated with all-cause death (adjusted hazard ratio 2.31; 95% confidence interval 1.23-4.36 versus 1.15; 0.55-2.41; for low versus high tertile, respectively).

CONCLUSIONS:

Low SMg levels (1.4-1.9 mg/dL; 0.58-0.78 mM) were independently associated with all-cause death in patients with prevalent CKD in the DHS cohort. Randomized clinical trials are important to determine whether Mg supplementation affects survival in CKD patients.

Study 30.11 Magnesium level and mortality in chronic kidney disease and dialysis patients: a systematic review and meta analysis[10]

Cardiovascular disease (CVD) is a leading cause of death in chronic kidney disease (CKD) and end-stage renal disease patients. Although there have been studies establishing a link between high serum calcium and phosphate concentrations and mortality in this population, existing studies focusing on magnesium concentration and mortality still have inconclusive evidence. We, therefore, performed a systematic review and meta-analysis to evaluate the risk of mortality in dysmagnesemia in CKD and dialysis patients and to assess factors that predict this association. We comprehensively searched the databases of PubMed/MEDLINE and EMBASE from date of inception to September 2015. The inclusion criteria were published studies evaluating association of magnesium, hypomagnesemia, or hypermagnesemia and mortality in CKD or dialysis patients. A meta-analysis using a random-effects model comparing mortality between dysmagnesemia and normal serum magnesium groups was performed. We calculated pooled risk ratio (RR) of mortality. From 15 full-text articles, seven prospective observational studies involving 17,520 participants met our inclusion criteria and were included in the meta-analysis.

There was a significant association of hypomagnesemia and mortality with pooled RR = 1.42 (95% CI: 1.16- 1.79). However, hypermagnesemia is not associated with increase mortality with RR = 1.82 (95% CI: 0.66-1.03). Hypomagnesemia significantly increases the risk of mortality in the CKD or dialysis population. Physicians should be aware of this association. More prospective studies evaluating benefits of magnesium correction in CKD and dialysis patients should be performed.

Study 30.12 Magnesium and outcomes in patients with chronic kidney disease: focus on vascular calcification, atherosclerosis and survival[11]

ABSTRACT:

Patients with chronic kidney disease (CKD) have a high prevalence of vascular calcification, and cardiovascular disease is the leading cause of death in this population. However, the molecular mechanisms of vascular calcification, which are multifactorial, cell-mediated and dynamic, are not yet fully understood. We need to address ways to improve outcomes in CKD patients, both in terms of vascular calcification and cardiovascular morbidity and mortality—and to these ends, we investigate the role of magnesium. Magnesium's role in the pathogenesis of vascular calcification has not been extensively studied. Nonetheless, several *in vitro* and animal studies point towards a protective role of magnesium through multiple molecular mechanisms. Magnesium is a natural calcium antagonist, and both human and animal studies have shown that low circulating magnesium levels are associated with vascular calcification. Clinical evidence from observational studies of dialysis patients has shown that low magnesium levels occur concurrently with mitral annular calcification, peripheral arterial calcification and increased carotid intima-media thickness. Few interventional studies have been performed. Two interventional studies suggest that there may be benefits, such as retardation of arterial calcification and/or reductions in carotid intima–media thickness in response to magnesium supplementation in CKD patients, though both studies have limitations. Finally, observational studies have shown that low serum magnesium may be an independent risk factor for <u>premature death in CKD patients, and patients with mildly elevated serum magnesium levels could have a survival advantage over those with lower magnesium levels.</u>

Note: Patients with mildly elevated magnesium levels may have a survival advantage, yet we are told not to take magnesium. This is why understanding is so important for us.

Study 30.13 **Magnesium supplementation helps to improve carotid intima media thickness in patients on hemodialysis.**[12]

RESULTS:

At the end of two months, mean serum calcium, phosphorus and calcium x phosphorus product were not changed in both groups. <u>As expected, mean serum Mg level significantly increased in the Mg group at the end</u> of two months. In addition, serum parathyroid hormone (PTH) level <u>significantly decreased in the Mg group at the end of two months (P = 0.003). Baseline carotid IMT was similar between the groups. Bilateral carotid IMT was significantly improved in patients treated with magnesium citrate compared to initial values.</u>

CONCLUSION:

<u>Based on the present data, magnesium may play an important protective role in the progression of atherosclerosis in patients on dialysis.</u> Further studies are needed to assess more accurately the role of magnesium in atherosclerotic regression in dialysis patients.

Study 30.14 **Magnesium modifies the cardiovascular mortality risk associated with hyper-phosphatemia in patients undergoing hemodialysis: a cohort study.**[13]

RESULTS:

During follow-up, 11,401 deaths occurred, out of which 4,751 (41.7%) were ascribed to cardiovascular disease. <u>In multivariable analyses, an increase in serum phosphate levels elevated the risk of cardiovascular mortality in the lower- and intermediate-Mg groups, whereas no significant risk increment was observed in the higher-Mg group. Moreover, among patients with serum phosphate levels of ≥ 6.0 mg/dL, the cardiovascular mortality risk significantly decreased with increasing serum Mg levels</u> (adjusted odds ratios [95% confidence intervals] of the lower-, intermediate- and higher-Mg groups were 1.00 (reference), 0.81 [0.66-0.99] and 0.74 [0.56-0.97], respectively.). <u>An interaction between Mg and phosphate on the risk of cardiovascular mortality was statistically significant (P=0.03).</u>

CONCLUSION:

<u>Serum Mg levels significantly modified the mortality risk associated with hyperphosphatemia in patients undergoing hemodialysis.</u>

Study 30.15 Effects of Magnesium on the Phosphate Toxicity in Chronic Kidney Disease: Time for Intervention Studies[14]

ABSTRACT:

Magnesium, an essential mineral for human health, plays a pivotal role in the cardiovascular system. Epidemiological studies in the general population have found an association between lower dietary magnesium intake and an elevated risk of cardiovascular events. In addition, magnesium supplementation was shown to improve blood pressure control, insulin sensitivity and endothelial function. The relationship between magnesium and cardiovascular prognosis among patients with chronic kidney disease (CKD) has been increasingly investigated, as it is becoming evident that magnesium can inhibit vascular calcification, a prominent risk of cardiovascular events, which commonly occurs in CKD patients. Cohort studies in patients receiving dialysis have shown a lower serum magnesium level as a significant risk for cardiovascular mortality. Interestingly, the cardiovascular mortality risk associated with hyperphosphatemia is alleviated among those with high serum magnesium levels, consistent with in vitro evidence that magnesium inhibits high-phosphate-induced calcification of vascular smooth muscle cells. Furthermore, a harmful effect of high phosphate on the progression of CKD is also attenuated among those with high serum magnesium levels. The potential usefulness of magnesium as a remedy for phosphate toxicity should be further explored by future intervention studies.

Study 30.16 Magnesium Replacement Improves the Metabolic Profile in Obese and Pre-Diabetic Patients with Mild-to-Moderate Chronic Kidney Disease: A 3-Month, Randomized, Double-Blind, Placebo-Controlled Study.[15]

RESULTS:

At the end of follow-up, insulin resistance (-24.5 vs. -8.2%, P = 0.007), HOMA-IR index (-31.9 vs. -3.3%, P < 0.001), hemoglobin A1c (-6.6 vs. -0.16%, P < 0.001), insulin (-29.6 vs. -2.66%, P < 0.001), waist circumference (-4.8 vs. 0.55%, P < 0.001) and uric acid (-0.8 vs. 2.2%, P = 0.004) were significantly decreased in terms of mean changes; albumin (0.91 vs. -2.91%, P = 0.007) and magnesium (0.21 ± 0.18 vs. -0.04 ± 0.05 mg/dl, P < 0.001) were significantly increased in those taking magne-sium compared with a placebo. The decrease in metabolic syndrome (-10.5 vs. -4.9%, P = 0.183), obesity (-15.7 vs. -8.2%, P = 0.131), prediabetes (-17.5 vs. -9.8%, P = 0.140), and systolic (-5.0 ± 14.8 vs. 0.22 ± 14.9 mm Hg, P = 0.053) and diastolic (-3.07 ± 9.7 vs. 0.07 ± 9.6 mm Hg, P = 0.071) blood pressure did not achieve to a significant level after study.

CONCLUSION:

Our data support the argument that magnesium supplementation improves the metabolic status in hypomagnesemic CKD patients with pre-diabetes and obesity.

Study 30.17 The Role of Magnesium in Hypertension and Cardiovascular Disease[16]

Magnesium intake of 500 mg/d to 1,000 mg/d may reduce blood pressure (BP) as much as 5.6/2.8 mm Hg. However, clinical studies have a wide range of BP reduction, with some showing no change in BP. <u>The combination of increased intake of magnesium and potassium coupled with reduced sodium intake is more effective in reducing BP than single-mineral intake and is often as effective as one antihypertensive drug in treating hypertension</u>. Reducing intracellular sodium and calcium while increasing intracellular magnesium and potassium improves BP response. Magnesium also increases the effectiveness of all antihypertensive drug classes. It remains to be conclusively proven that cardiovascular disease, such as coronary heart disease, ischemic stroke and cardiac arrhythmias can be prevented or treated with magnesium intake. <u>Preliminary evidence suggests that insulin sensitivity, hyperglycemia, diabetes mellitus, left ventricular hypertrophy and dyslipidemia may be improved with increased magnesium intake</u>. Various genetic defects in magnesium transport are associated with hypertension, and possibly with cardiovascular disease. <u>Oral magnesium acts as a natural calcium channel blocker, increases nitric oxide, improves endothelial dysfunction, and induces direct and indirect vasodilation.</u>

Study 30.18 — Magnesium intake is inversely associated with coronary artery calcification: the Framingham Heart Study.[17]

CONCLUSIONS:

In community-dwelling participants free of cardiovascular disease, <u>self-reported magnesium intake was inversely associated with arterial calcification, which may play a contributing role in magnesium's protective associations in stroke and fatal coronary heart disease.</u>

Supplemental magnesium is also as effective as a phosphorus binder, which are used to lower phosphorus levels. Although calcium is normally used, again, magnesium may be a better option if we can tolerate the extra magnesium.

Study 30.19 — Magnesium carbonate is an effective phosphate binder for chronic hemodialysis patients: a pilot study.[19]

RESULTS:

Magnesium carbonate provided equal control of serum phosphorus (70.6% of the magnebind group and 62.5% of the calcium acetate group had their average serum phosphorus within the K-DOQI target during the efficacy phase), while significantly reducing daily elemental calcium ingestion from phosphate binders (908 +/- 24 vs. 1743 +/- 37 mg/day, P < .0001).

CONCLUSION:

<u>Magnesium carbonate was generally well-tolerated in this selected patient population, and was effective in controlling serum phosphorus while reducing elemental calcium ingestion.</u>

Study 30.20 — Use of magnesium as a drug in chronic kidney disease[20]

ABSTRACT:

From chronic kidney disease (CKD) Stage 4 onwards, phosphate binders are needed in many patients to prevent the development of hyperphosphataemia, which can result in disturbed bone and mineral metabolism, cardiovascular disease and secondary hyperparathyroidism. In this review, we re-examine the use of magnesium-containing phosphate binders for patients with CKD, particularly as their use circumvents problems such as calcium loading, aluminum toxicity and the high costs associated with other agents of this class. The use of magnesium hydroxide in the 1980s has been superseded by magnesium carbonate, as the hydroxide salt was associated with poor gastrointestinal tolerability, whereas studies with magnesium carbonate show much better gastrointestinal profiles. The use of combined magnesium- and calcium-based phosphate binder regi-mens allows a reduction in the calcium load, and magnesium and calcium regimen comparisons show that magnesium may be as effective a phosphate binder as calcium. A large, well-designed trial has recently shown that a drug combining calcium acetate and magnesium carbonate was non-inferior in terms of lowering serum phosphate to sevelamer-HCl and had an equally good tolerability profile. Because of the high cost of sevelamer and lanthanum carbonate, the use of magnesium carbonate could be advantageous, and drug acquisition cost savings would compensate for the cost of introducing routine magnesium monitoring, if this is thought to be necessary and not performed anyway. Moreover, given the potential cost savings, it may be time to re-investigate magnesium-containing phosphate binders for CKD patients with further well-designed clinical research using vascular end points.

As I keep saying, everything in kidney disease is related. There is a relationship between albumin levels and magnesium. 20% to 25% of magnesium is bound to albumin in our bodies. Low serum albumin can lead to low magnesium levels. High levels of albumin are correlated with higher levels of magnesium.

Study 30.21 Relationships between magnesium and protein concentrations in serum.[21]

ABSTRACT:

We determined concentrations of magnesium, total protein, albumin and globulin in more than 74,000 serum specimens from patients and noted a direct linear relationship between the concentration of magnesium in serum and the concentrations of total protein, albumin and globulin in serum. Albumin and magnesium concentrations are linearly related at high and low albumin concentrations; within the reference interval, however, the magnesium concentration is independent of the albumin concentration. Linear regression analysis suggests that 25% of the total serum magnesium is bound to albumin and 8% to globulins.

Study 30.22 Cardiovascular disease, mortality and magnesium in chronic kidney disease: growing interest in magnesium-related interventions[22]

EXCERPTS:

Serum Mg levels may be used as nutritional markers in dialysis patients because they correlate with serum albumin levels[23-28] body mass index[23,24,] normalized protein catabolic rate[24,26,28,] muscle mass[24] and strength[29], and subjective global assessment scores[24]. Of interest, the use of a low Mg PD dialysate induced a decrease in serum albumin levels[30].

At the end of this study, insulin resistance, glycemic control and uric acid levels were better in the former than in the latter patient group. <u>These improvements in metabolic indices were accompanied by an increase in not only serum Mg, but also albumin levels.</u>

Not surprisingly, magnesium is correlated with muscle quality, likely due to the relationship with albumin and protein.

Study 30.23 Significant positive relationship between serum magnesium and muscle quality in mainte-nance hemodialysis patients.[31]

RESULTS:

Serum Mg was 1.15 ± 0.16 mmol/L (2.8 ± 0.4 mg/dL), being higher than the reference range of normal subjects. There was a significant negative correlation between muscle quality and age ($r = -0.326$, $p<0.0001$) and duration of hemodialysis ($r = -0.253$, $p<0.0001$). The muscle quality of the diabetics was significantly lower than that of the non-diabetics ($p<0.001$). <u>There was a significant, positive correlation between muscle quality and serum Mg ($r = 0.118$, $p<0.05$), but not serum calcium or phosphate.</u> In multiple regression analysis, age, gender, hemodialysis duration, diabetes and serum Mg ($\beta = 0.129$, $p<0.05$) were significantly and independently associated with muscle quality ($R(2) = 0.298$, $p<0.0001$).

CONCLUSION:

<u>These results demonstrated that a lower serum Mg concentration was significantly associated with poor muscle quality in hemodialysis patients.</u> Further studies are needed to explore the mechanism by which lower serum Mg affects muscle quality.

Without a doubt, magnesium is good for us. However, before you go out and buy magnesium supplements, let's do some thinking. Magnesium consumption or supplementation depends on our current kidney function. Kidneys with GFR of 30 and above appear to have few issues with hypermagnesemia. Kidneys with GFR under 10 may not be able to control magnesium successfully. At this stage, dialysis is the best way to manage magnesium.

GFR between 10 and 20 may be a gray area and case-dependent.

Magnesium dosage from 360 mg to 720 mg a day appear to be safe if your GFR is high enough. This is true whether the dosage is time-released or smaller doses are taken several times a day. The recommended daily allowance is 320 mg for women and 420 mg for men.

It clear that we should always take magnesium instead of calcium if we have a choice. While it's tempting to take large doses to try to get a benefit, it's probably wise not to exceed the recommended daily amount. Another option is to use an equal amount of magnesium and calcium together if you cannot tolerate a dose of 400 or so mg.

The evidence is very strong that we need to keep magnesium levels as high as safely possible to slow vascular calcification, lower blood pressure, reduce phosphorus levels, and reduce inflammation. "Safely" means that you can handle magnesium supplementation without your magnesium levels going too high. This will be a little different for everyone depending on your current kidney function and diet. This is something you have to monitor with your doctor.

Magnesium reduces vascular calcification and phosphorus levels, which happens to be the exact combination that leads to heart disease killing us.

However, magnesium has to be used with some planning. Hypermagnesemia and hypomagnesemia are both risks, depending on your current health and kidney function.

Key Point of This Chapter

Early in your disease, you should be taking or consuming enough magnesium to keep your levels high, and as your disease progresses, you may have to reduce your magnesium intake. Your magnesium may stay high even as you reduce intake as your disease progresses. It may also be that as your disease gets better, you will need to increase magnesium intake to keep levels at the high end of the normal range.

Key Takeaway From This Chapter

Supplemental calcium intake should always be reduced to the lowest levels possible and supplemental magnesium intake should always be at the highest safe levels for your current stage of kidney disease.

Let Me Say This Again for Effect

Supplemental calcium intake should always be reduced to the lowest levels possible and supplemental magnesium intake should always be at the highest safe levels for your current stage of kidney disease.

Magnesium is one of the few things that seems to improve everything for us, if our levels don't get too high. A survival advantage appears to exist for those with magnesium levels on the high end or slightly exceeding the normal range. This is something we should all want to know about.

The common advice to stay away from single high doses of magnesium from antacids and laxatives is correct. However, it is not correct to say we don't need magnesium at the high end of the normal range. I can't advocate going outside the normal ranges, but keeping your magnesium levels at the top end of the normal range is a good strategy. Time-release or smaller doses with each meal is the right way to use magnesium.

Checking and actively managing magnesium levels should be required for every patient. The benefits are too big to ignore.

References

1. Bressendorff I, Hansen D, Schou M, et al. Oral magnesium supplementation in chronic kidney disease stages 3 and 4: efficacy, safety and effect on serum calcification propensity—a prospective randomized double-blinded placebo-controlled clinical trial. *Kidney International Reports.* 2017;2(3):380-389.

2. Smith ER, Ford ML, Tomlinson LA, et al. Serum calcification propensity predicts all-cause mortality in predialysis CKD. *Journal of the American Society of Nephrology.* 2014;25(2):339348.

3. Molnar AO, Biyani M, Hammond I, et al. Lower serum magnesium is associated with vascular calcification in peritoneal dialysis patients: a cross-sectional study. *BMC Nephrology.* 2017;18(1):129.

4. Tzanakis IP, Stamataki EE, Papadaki AN, Giannakis N, Damianakis NE, Oreopoulos DG. Magnesium retards the progress of the arterial calcifications in hemodialysis patients: a pilot study. *International Urology and Nephrology.* 2014;46(11):2199-2205.

5. Meema HE, Oreopoulos DG, Rapoport A. Serum magnesium level and arterial calcification in end-stage renal disease. *Kidney International.* 1987;32(3):388-394.

6. Sakaguchi Y, Fujii N, Shoji T, Hayashi T, Rakugi H, Isaka Y. Hypomagnesemia is a significant predictor of cardiovascular and non-cardiovascular mortality in patients undergoing hemodialysis. *Kidney International.* 2014;85(1):174-181.

7. Lacson E, Wang W, Ma L, Passlick-Deetjen J. Serum magnesium and mortality in hemodialysis patients in the United States: a cohort study. *American Journal of Kidney Diseases.* 2015;66(6):1056-1066.

8. Silva AP, Fragoso A, Silva C, et al. Magnesium and mortality in patients with diabetes and early chronic kidney disease. *J Diabetes Metab.* 2014;5(347):2.

9. Ferrè S, Li X, Adams-Huet B, et al. Association of serum magnesium with all-cause mortality in patients with and without chronic kidney disease in the Dallas Heart Study. *Nephrology Dialysis Transplantation.* 2017(gfx275).

10. Sanguankeo A, Upala S. Magnesium level and mortality in chronic kidney disease and dialysis patients a systematic review and meta analysis. *American Journal of Kidney Diseases.* 2016;67(5):A93.

11. Massy ZA, Drüeke TB. Magnesium and outcomes in patients with chronic kidney disease: focus on vascular calcification, atherosclerosis and survival. *Clinical Kidney Journal.* 2012;5(Suppl 1):i52-i61.

12. Turgut F, Kanbay M, Metin MR, Uz E, Akcay A, Covic A. Magnesium supplementation helps to improve carotid intima media thickness in patients on hemodialysis. *International Urology and Nephrology.* 2008;40(4):1075.

13. Sakaguchi Y, Fujii N, Shoji T, et al. Magnesium modifies the cardiovascular mortality risk associated with hyperphosphatemia in patients undergoing hemodialysis: a cohort study. *PLoS One.* 2014;9(12):e116273.

14. Sakaguchi Y, Hamano T, Isaka Y. Effects of magnesium on the phosphate toxicity in chronic kidney disease: time for intervention studies. *Nutrients.* 2017;9(2):112.

15. Toprak O, Kurt H, Sarı Y, Şarkış C, Us H, Kırık A. Magnesium replacement improves the metabolic profile in obese and prediabetic patients with mild-to-moderate chronic kidney disease: a 3-month, randomised, double-blind, placebo-controlled study. *Kidney and Blood Pressure Research.* 2017;42(1):33-42.

16. Houston M. The role of magnesium in hypertension and cardiovascular disease. *The Journal of Clinical Hypertension.* 2011;13(11):843-847.

17. Hruby A, O'Donnell CJ, Jacques PF, Meigs JB, Hoffmann U, McKeown NM. Magnesium intake is inversely associated with coronary artery calcification: the Framingham Heart Study. *JACC: Cardiovascular Imaging.* 2014;7(1):59-69.

18. Salem S, Bruck H, Bahlmann FH, et al. Relationship between magnesium and clinical biomarkers on inhibition of vascular calcification. *American Journal of Nephrology.* 2012;35(1):31-39.

19. Spiegel DM, Farmer B, Smits G, Chonchol M. Magnesium carbonate is an effective phosphate binder for chronic hemodialysis patients: a pilot study. *Journal of Renal Nutrition.* 2007;17(6):416-422.

20. Hutchison AJ, Wilkie M. Use of magnesium as a drug in chronic kidney disease. *Clinical Kidney Journal.* 2012;5(Suppl_1):i62-i70.

21. Kroll M, Elin R. Relationships between magnesium and protein concentrations in serum. *Clinical Chemistry.* 1985;31(2):244-246.

22. Ikee R. Cardiovascular disease, mortality and magnesium in chronic kidney disease: growing interest in magnesium-related interventions. *Renal Replacement Therapy.* 2018;4(1):1.

23. Ye H, Zhang X, Guo Q, et al. Prevalence and factors associated with hypomagnesemia in Southern Chinese continuous ambulatory peritoneal dialysis patients. *Peritoneal Dialysis International.* 2013;33(4):450-454.

24. Liu F, Zhang X, Qi H, et al. Correlation of serum magnesium with cardiovascular risk factors in maintenance hemodialysis patients–a cross-sectional study. *Magnesium Research.* 2013;26(3):100-108.

25. Lacson E, Wang W, Ma L, Passlick-Deetjen J. Serum magnesium and mortality in hemodialysis patients in the United States: a cohort study. *American Journal of Kidney Diseases.* 2015;66(6):1056-1066.

26. Li L, Streja E, Rhee CM, et al. Hypomagnesemia and mortality in incident hemodialysis patients. *American Journal of Kidney Diseases.* 2015;66(6):1047-1055.

27. Cai K, Luo Q, Dai Z, et al. Hypomagnesemia is associated with increased mortality among peritoneal dialysis patients. *PLoS One.* 2016;11(3):e0152488.

28. Ikee R, Toyoyama T, Endo T, Tsunoda M, Hashimoto N. Impact of sevelamer hydrochloride on serum magnesium concentrations in hemodialysis patients. *Magnesium Research.* 2016;29(4):184-190.

29. Okazaki H, Ishimura E, Okuno S, et al. Significant positive relationship between serum magnesium and muscle quality in maintenance hemodialysis patients. *Magnesium Research.* 2013;26(4):182-187.

30. Ejaz A, McShane A, Gandhi V, Leehey D, Ing T. Hypomagnesemia in continuous ambulatory peritoneal dialysis patients dialyzed with a low-magnesium peritoneal dialysis solution. *Peritoneal Dialysis International.* 1995;15(1):61-64.

31. Okazaki H, Ishimura E, Okuno S, et al. Significant positive relationship between serum magnesium and muscle quality in maintenance hemodialysis patients. *Magnesium Research.* 2013;26(4):182-187.

CHAPTER 31

Slowing the Progression of Kidney Disease by 50% or More

Keto Acid and Low-Protein Diets

Lowering dietary protein intake can slow kidney disease progression between 35% and 50% or more in many cases. Some people may go into remission using a combination of low- or very low-protein diets and the right protein supplement.

The catch is we have to know what we are doing in order to get the benefits or we could get no benefits at all. This means we can spend thousands of dollars and waste hundreds of hours with little or no benefit, not to mention the emotional toll it takes getting one bad blood test after another, thinking you are doing the right thing. Let my wasted years and money keep you from doing the same.

Keep in mind that slowing the progression by 50% or 60% is effectively a cure for many of us, depending on age. This is no small thing. If you would proceed to kidney failure in eight to ten years normally, then increasing that number to fifteen to twenty years or more is a huge benefit. Any number of things can happen, but it's not hard to imagine this delay could be life-saving for some.

There is a science to mastering these diets and protein supplements. The devil is in the details, so pay attention.

This is a big chapter that is broken into three parts:

> Protein supplements
>
> Low-protein or very low-protein diets
>
> Research and studies supporting keto acids

A low- (LPD) or very low-protein (VLPD) diet can slow the progression of your disease, but you can't be on a low-protein diet without compensating for the lack of protein. Some form of protein supplement is required to make a low-protein diet nutritionally safe. Low-protein diets and a protein supplement/food are tied together and cannot be separated. You cannot talk about one without the other.

Over one hundred studies are summarized at the end of the chapter. You can review them after reading the first two sections. I wanted to list every relevant study in the past ten years on keto acids and/or low protein. I went a little overboard, but this was needed, in my opinion. In the U.S. and many other countries, keto acids and low-protein diets are not used, for various reasons. One of those reasons is that there is not enough proof of their effectiveness. No one can say that ever again after this expanded chapter. Over eighty positive studies are shown, and I also list the studies that were inconclusive or had a negative outcome, in order to be fair. It would be wrong to cherry-pick or show only the positive studies.

Having more than eighty human studies showing the benefits of any drug, food, or supplement is fantastic when you think about it. The studies include different countries and different methodologies, spread across tens of thousands of patients. When someone (even your doctor, dietician, or nutritionist) tells you this is not proven, you can hit them over the head with over eighty studies from around the world.

A key part of making this type of dietary therapy effective is understanding how these diets and supplements affect your kidneys and overall health. Again, with understanding and education comes the power to make the best decisions possible for your health and slow the progression of your disease. I know it's a lot of reading, but I believe it's important to share all of the details.

Protein Supplements, Amino Acids, and Keto Acids

Protein is something we must have to survive and thrive. Our bodies can produce all but eight of the amino acids we need to survive.

The eight amino acids that our bodies cannot produce are called the essential amino acids. These amino acids must be provided by diet or supplementation. One other exception to this rule is tyrosine. Tyrosine can be produced by the body, but the hormone that tells our bodies to make tyrosine is produced by the kidneys. As kidney function declines, tyrosine production is reduced. For this reason, people with kidney disease often take tyrosine supplements along with the eight essential amino acids. However, all past keto acid supplements have been made for stage 5 patients with GFR below fifteen for end stage renal disease. Tyrosine is neither needed nor recommended for stage 2, 3 and most stage 4 patients. Those with earlier stages of kidney disease should not supplement tyrosine due to tyrosine's production of uremic toxins. You will learn to read the labels later in this chapter.

Protein Metabolism 101

Let's learn how our bodies digest protein. Amino acids have a nitrogen component. When you consume dietary protein, your body takes the amino acid and removes the nitrogen component. This is done in the liver in many cases, but other parts of the body contribute as well. This process produces urea (aka nitrogen waste) and ammonia. Both urea and ammonia are removed by healthy kidneys. However, in our case, we have a reduced ability to remove these waste products. This is important because both uremia and excess ammonia increase the speed of kidney disease progression.

As you have learned, urinary acid and ammonia excretion decrease as GFR decreases. Patients with the lowest rates of acid excretion have an 84% increased risk of fast decline in GFR. If we are unable to get rid of the urea and ammonia, we are driving 100 mph to kidney failure.

This is important because, to a large extent, you choose how much waste product and ammonia your body produces. If your kidneys can't do the work, you need to do it for them using your diet and supplement choices.

What Are Keto Acids

Again, amino acids contain nitrogen, but nitrogen is not used, present, or needed in the pathways that produce energy or nutrition from most of the essential amino acids.

Let's say this again: Dietary or supplemental amino acids (like those in the store) cannot be used by your body until the nitrogen component is removed for many (but not all) amino acids.

When the nitrogen is removed, the new amino acid form is called an "alpha ketoanalogue," usually referred to as "keto acids" for short. These new forms of the original amino acid are used by the body from a nutrition standpoint. The new "keto acid" is the same amino acid as before, with the nitrogen removed.

Let's keep repeating important information: Keto acids, or keto alpha analogues, are the same amino acids with the nitrogen component removed. Keto acids are ready to be used by our bodies for nutrition. You might say they are the nutritional form of amino acids. Keto acids are naturally occurring in the body.

An analogy might be removing the husk from corn. The outside husk has to be removed before we can eat the corn. After you remove them, you have a big pile of corn husks to dispose of. The parts of amino acids that we can't use have to be removed before our bodies can use them. In our case, these extra parts have to be disposed of by our kidneys. Keto acids are like buying corn that has had the husk removed. The corn is now ready to use if the husk is removed. As long as the nitrogen component is still present, your body can't use the amino acid for nutrition.

This process of removing the nitrogen component is one of the things driving us 100 mph toward kidney failure. The buildup of ammonia, urea, and uremic toxins speeds the progression of our disease and eventually kills us without dialysis.

The benefit of keto acids is they are ready for our bodies to use. Keto acids don't produce nitrogen or ammonia waste products that have to be filtered by our kidneys. Keto acids are in a form that is ready for our bodies to use without producing large amounts of urea or ammonia. Keto acids go right into our bloodstreams without putting a workload on our liver or kidneys.

All manner of protein supplements exist. There are hundreds of different options for healthy people, but for us, only two or three exist. Understanding how amino acid supplements stack up against both old and new keto acid supplements is mandatory.

It's all about the nitrogen

Let's start with the nitrogen amounts in each protein supplement for people with kidney disease. Reminder: Nitrogen intake is directly proportional to the amount of uremia and uremic toxins, and your blood urea nitrogen and creatinine levels. Lower your nitrogen intake and your blood tests will improve.

Type	Daily Nitrogen mgs
100% amino acids	1,200 to 1,500 mg
Generic 1980s calcium-based blend of amino/keto acids*	500 to 900 mg
Modern 2018 magnesium-based blend of amino/keto acids	150 to 250 mg

A pure amino acid supplement may have nine to ten times the nitrogen of a modern keto amino acid supplement, depending on dosage and exact formulation.

1980s generic formulations were an improvement over amino acids, but have a much higher nitrogen content than modern blends. The 1980s blends had very large amounts of calcium— over 1,100 mg at suggested doses. Remember the dangers of supplemental calcium and heart disease. If you take 1,000 mg of supplemental calcium or more, you've assumed that you're not getting any calcium from your diet, which is impossible. Even veggies have calcium. Many greens contain 180 to 220 mg per 3 ounces, or 100 grams. Many cheeses have 1,000 mg or more per serving. The idea that most of us are calcium-deficient has to be questioned for heart and kidney health. Vascular calcification is the number one killer of people with kidney disease, and supplemental calcium speeds vascular calcification. These should be avoided, when possible.

This is one of the reasons why I think innovation must come from us, the patients. The basic keto acid supplement formula hasn't changed in thirty years, despite an overwhelming amount of evidence regarding supplemental calcium intake and vascular calcification.

A modern up-to-date approach is needed. Modern keto/amino acid formulations benefit from nitrogen levels that are three to four times lower than older formulations, and have other big advantages, such as lower calcium, increased magnesium, lower renal acid load, lower uremic toxins, and more.

Toxin Convertible Nitrogen (TCN)

Toxin convertible nitrogen, or TCN, is a term used to describe how much nitrogen could be converted to uremic toxins. Approximately 70% of nitrogen can be converted to uremic toxins.

Now, let's look at the same nitrogen numbers again, considering the amount of uremic toxins we might be generating:

Type	Toxin Convertible Nitrogen
100% amino acids	1050 mg
Generic 1980s calcium blend of amino/keto acids*	630 mg
Modern 2018 blend of amino/keto acids	175 mg

Now we start to really see the difference. Amino acid supplements may create six times more uremic toxins than modern keto amino acid blends. Modern blends are several times lower than 1980s calcium and amino acid based supplements.

How Do We Know This Matters

We know this matters because multiple studies (as you will see later) show that keto acids work better than amino acids when it comes to slowing the progression of kidney disease. Nutritionally, they are the same. The difference is in the nitrogen and renal acid load.

Here are some of the aforementioned studies:

Study 31.1   **A crossover comparison of progression of chronic renal failure: Keto acids (KA) versus amino acids (AA)[21]**

We conclude that KA slow progression, relative to AA, independently of protein or phosphorus intake, in patients on this regimen.

Study 31.2   **Effect of a keto acid-amino acid-supplemented very low-protein diet on the progression of advanced renal disease: a reanalysis of the MDRD feasibility study.**

CONCLUSION:

The study suggests that supplementation of a very low-protein diet with the keto acid-amino acid mixture used in this feasibility study slowed the progression of advanced renal disease more than supplementation with an amino acid mixture.

Study 31.3   **Progression of chronic renal failure on substituting a keto acid supplement for an amino acid supplement[23]**

Viewed in light of previous evidence that progression seldom slows when treatment remains constant, the results suggest that this keto acid supplement slows progression by approximately half, compared with an essential amino acid supplement, with no change in diet.

Slowing progression of your disease by 50% is nothing to joke about. Keep reading.

Again, the big difference between amino acid supplements and keto acid supplements is the amount of nitrogen and the renal acid load. Nutrition is the same. Keto acids have other positive effects on the body, but protein nutrition is the same as amino acids.

Small amounts of nitrogen and ammonia waste really matter! Your kidneys are functioning at a greatly reduced capacity. A few hundred milligrams are important.

Dietary Nitrogen

Now, let's consider how much nitrogen is present in our daily diet. This has to be taken into account.

The standard recommendation is 0.8 grams per kilogram per day. A 75 kg person needs 60 grams of dietary protein per day.

For comparison, a 100- gram or 3.5-ounce small chicken breast contains 3,700 mg, or 3.7 grams, of nitrogen. The equivalent dosage of one of the Albutrix products contains approximately 187 mg, or .187 grams, of nitrogen.

For the same thirty grams of equivalent protein, one has 3,700 mg vs 187 mg in nitrogen. Doing the math, one has almost twenty times the nitrogen for the same amount of protein nutrition. This is a dramatic workload reduction. Assume three meals of 3.5 oz of protein plus assorted side dishes, you can easily be consuming 12,000 to 20,000 mg of nitrogen a day. High nitrogen foods are also high acid foods, a double whammy.

Healthy kidneys can dispose of this amount of nitrogen per day, whether it is 12,000 or 20,000 mg of nitrogen. However, our damaged kidneys cannot dispose of these waste products with the same efficiency. The excess urea and ammonia running through our veins and tissues shortens our lives. Don't forget, the entire reason dialysis was invented was to get rid of uremia/uremic toxins. Assume your kidneys completely failed. Without dialysis, your expected lifespan would be two to three weeks. Getting rid of waste products is a matter of life and death.

Another GFR analogy: Let's assume a healthy person with the highest GFR, 120, can process 12,000 mg of nitrogen a day. Therefore, a GFR of 100 can process 10,000 mg of nitrogen a day, and so on.

With each drop in GFR, our ability to handle nitrogen waste drops. Now let's assume that a patient with a GFR of 50 can handle 5,000 mg of nitrogen waste. A GFR of 20: 2,000 mg a day.

The lower the GFR, the lower the ability to process waste products.

If your kidneys can process 4,000 mg of nitrogen waste per day and you are eating 9,000 mg a day, we know what happens: uremia, acidosis, high phosphorus levels, accelerated heart disease, and so on. 100 mph toward kidney failure, if you don't make a change.

Now, let's assume you are consuming 3,000 mg of nitrogen per day, but your kidneys can process 4,000 mg per day. Over days or weeks, your blood work will start to move back into the normal ranges. Maybe not completely, but over time your body will think things are pretty normal again. On your next blood test, your eGFR will improve.

Your kidneys will be able to clean your blood of these waste products on a daily basis more like healthy kidneys. This is the basis of the kidney factor approach. When you clean up your blood, you can't help but start slowing the progression of your disease. One of the primary drivers of disease progression has now been stopped, slowed, or reduced.

You must eat below your capacity to clean your blood of nitrogen waste and acid load and to be able to do this, you need be able to calculate how much nitrogen you are consuming each day. Now that you know this, you can start improving your numbers through a combination of diet and regular blood tests. If your numbers are rising, you are eating too much protein. If your numbers are falling, you are eating less protein and getting closer to your kidneys' ability to handle the waste products you are throwing at them.

One more example, before we move on.

Let's consider the following numbers, assuming we can process 4,000 mg of nitrogen per day.

Dietary protein	Grams of protein	Nitrogen mg	Excess
Normal diet	100 grams a day	15,000	+ 9,000
Daily requirement	60 grams	9,000	+5,000
Break-even	27 grams	4,000	0
Eating below	22 grams	3,300	-700

In order to get below our daily workload of 4,000 mg a day, we have to limit protein consumption to less than 27 grams per day. This is an example to illustrate the idea, not an actual medical calculation.

If we are eating more than 27 grams a day, we are still contributing to all of the bad things that accelerate kidney disease. We might be contributing at a lower rate, but we are still likely contributing. We will get no or very little relief in symptoms or comorbid conditions if we are eating more than 27 grams a day in this example. In order to get real relief or an improvement in our system, we have to eat less than 27 grams for many weeks or months. Your blood urea nitrogen and creatinine clearance number will improve dramatically when your protein intake drops below your capacity to process the waste over several weeks and months.

Low-Protein (LPD) and Very Low-Protein diets (VLPD)

LPDs are usually 0.6 grams per kilogram and VLPDs use 0.3 grams per kilogram, as general guidelines. Going back to our example of 0.8 grams per day for a 75-kilogram person, here is what we get:

Diet	Recommendation per kg	Daily Protein in grams
Average diet	1.2 grams	90
Recommended	0.8 grams	60
LPD	0.6 grams	45
VLPD	0.3 grams	22.5

In order to get a real reduction in uremic toxins and waste, you have to get down in the 20s, using this example. A VLPD is a dramatic reduction compared to how most of us eat.

To cut to the chase, LPDs don't work as well as VLPDs for this reason. We aren't getting much of a break in terms of workload when we go from 60 grams to 45 grams of protein. An LPD equals a 25% reduction in workload, but a VLPD equals a 62% reduction in workload.

One key point: No standardized definition exists for LPD and VLPD, but 0.3 and 0.6 have been used in the past. However, 0.4 or 0.5 are fine. There is no magic number. It's more about your kidney function than about a static number or definition.

We already know that protein restriction slows kidney disease progression. However, the optimal dietary protein intake could not be confirmed. Why not?

Why can't a standard be developed for lower dietary protein to slow disease progression and the death rate by more than 50%? There are too many variables in these types of studies. Different diets, different stages of kidney disease, different levels of dietary compliance, different comorbid conditions, different study design and reporting, etc. Optimal amounts are not known, but we can figure it out very easily without a hundred medical studies. Maybe we can't know as a group, but individually we can figure out optimal intakes that work for ourselves using diet, blood work, and protein supplements.

Let's now look at what happens on a low-protein diet combined with different supplements.

No protein supplement, just diet restriction

LPD at 0.6 grams per day per kg	6,800 mg of nitrogen

Now let's add the recommendation from different protein supplements combined with the 0.6-kilogram LPD.

LPD + protein supplement	Nitrogen in mg
100% amino acids	8,300
Old keto/amino acids	7,700
Modern keto/amino acids	7,000

A LPD diet (0.6 grams per kilogram) combined with the recommended dosage of amino acids only reduces nitrogen load by 700 mg. 8,300 mg is pretty close to the 9,000 mg of nitrogen that we get with the RDA of 60 grams of protein a day. Let's think about this for a second: If our kidneys are operating at 35% capacity, or a GFR of around 35, does anyone think reducing nitrogen by 8% is going to help us? Our kidneys are working 65% less efficiently than healthy kidneys. How is an 8% reduction in workload going to help?

This is why LPD diets combined with amino acids have a poor record. We haven't reduced our kidney workload by a meaningful amount. A 7 to 8% reduction in workload when our kidneys are operating 60% to 70% less effectively is meaningless. This is most likely the reason these diets have such a poor record.

The reason VLPD diets combined with keto acids work better to reduce the load is we get a kidney workload reduction of 60%, which is more in line with a kidney that is operating at 30% of normal capacity. VLPDs with keto acids are the only combination that gives us a meaningful reduction in workload to match our reduced kidney function.

Now, let's do this again with a VLPD.

0.3 grams per kg	3,400 mg

Now with different protein supplements

100% amino acids	4,900 mg
Old keto/amino supplements	4,300 mg
Modern keto/amino	3,600 mg

Now we are getting somewhere in terms of real reductions in workload. The details matter here. The same diet with keto acids has a better outcome than with amino acids. In this case, 600 to 1,300 mg reduction in nitrogen helps make the difference. This is very telling and we need to pay attention. If your kidneys can only process 4,000 mg of nitrogen a day, an additional 1,300 mg reduction is a 32.5% reduction in nitrogen waste. This is what I mean when I say your choices can do the work for your kidneys. One choice is 30%+ reduction in workload than another choice with similar nutrition. These details matter when the capacity of your kidneys is 70% or 80% lower than normal. Keto acids have other benefits, but this also tells us that small amounts of nitrogen may make a difference in our success or failure. A number that looks small on paper may equal a 30% to 50% increase or decrease in workload on your kidneys. Don't forget this!

By reducing nitrogen by 5,000 or 6,000 mg a day, you effectively get a jump in GFR. As you reduce your nitrogen intake, your GFR will rise in most cases. The rise is because your kidneys can handle the workload better. Your kidneys are still functioning like before, but they can handle the lower workload better.

Now, let's compare combinations of diets and supplements.

Normal diet	9,000 mg+
100% amino acids + LPD	8,300 mg
Modern keto/amino + VPLD	3,600 mg

The normal diet has 2.5 times the amount of nitrogen and ammonia waste products compared to a VLPD diet and a modern keto/amino acid supplement.

Which diet and supplement combination do you think will have the best chances of lowering your uremia or uremic symptoms? As a patient, I had never this seen this math before. I had to beg and research to figure these things out.

Taking Diet Into Account

If these variables are not enough, the recommendations for dosage don't take into account dietary protein or the type of diet you are on. Again, a few examples make it easier to explain. High-quality proteins (meat) are around 15% to 18% amino acids.

It is recommended that a 75-kilogram person eat 60 grams of protein daily, which equals about 10 to 13 grams of amino acids.

Using the same 10 gram example, let's look at the current supplement recommendation to consume ten to eleven grams a day of essential amino acids. This advice is wrong, in my opinion. Let me show you why:

Supplement	Diet and amino acids in grams
100% amino acids + LPD diet at max recommended	18.5
1980s keto/amino + LPD at max recommended	20.75

Remember, you need only about 10 to 13 grams of essential amino acids per day in this example. Why are we being told to take more than we need? We are putting extra loads on our kidneys without any benefit. We are adding to the amount of uremic toxins or uremia by taking the recommended dosage, not to mention acidosis, hypercalcemia, hyperfiltration, and so on. This is one of the problems with diets and amino or keto acid supplements. It is assumed that you will get no amino acids from your diet, which is impossible. The goal is to take the workload off our kidneys—not increase it.

This is the second reason low-protein diets have a mixed record. In the real world where our kidneys live, we need to adjust for dietary protein to effectively minimize the workload on our kidneys. One issue that is real is the reduced ability to metabolize amino acids as we age. It is also true that acidosis, inflammation, and oxidative stress can reduce our ability to digest and effectively use amino acids. Some additional supplementation may be warranted, but let's let our blood test be our guide and not guess.

Using the same 75 kilogram example and 10 to 13 grams of essential amino acids per day. We will use 12 grams of amino acids for this example.

<u>Now let's go back to our diets and supplements to see what happens.</u>

Diet	Grams of amino acids	Shortfall in grams
Normal	12	0
LPD diet	7	5
VLPD diet	3.5	8.5

As you can see, you may never need to take 10+ grams of amino acid supplements a day. This is especially true if you are on a LPD diet or a very light protein restriction. Remember, our bodies are very good at getting rid of what we don't need. Eating more than we need causes extra workload on already damaged kidneys. This seems insane for someone with kidney disease.

We have to adjust our protein supplement dosages to reflect our current diets. In truth, someone on an LPD diet of 45 grams per day need only take 3 grams of amino or keto acids, not 10 grams. Meeting your nutritional needs while putting the lowest workload possible on your kidneys is the secret to these diets. This is especially true when you are starting out on a treatment plan.

You get the idea. You must lower supplemental protein intake when you increase dietary protein intake, and vice versa. Why this is not standard practice is a mystery to me. It seems so basic.

Once we calculate the protein we get from our diet, then we can calculate how much we need to compensate. One word of caution is warranted here. You need to increase the dosage only if your albumin is not rising after the first 90-day blood test or checkup. I personally did have to increase my dosage dramatically in order to get my albumin up, but this was before I was treating inflammation and oxidative stress. I was able to decrease my doses back to much lower than the recommended dosage when I got my inflammation and oxidative stress under control. The treatment plan takes this into account. If your albumin is not rising, then you can increase the amount of supplemental protein. The key is to do this later, when you have evidence that an increase is needed from your blood tests.

Most patients need only 5 to 9 grams of supplemental amino/ keto acids—not 11 or 14 grams. This lowers the workload on your kidneys and also saves you money. The same amount of protein supplement will last longer this way. This may seem trivial to some, but trust me—it matters to your kidneys and your pocketbook, as you will see.

We are trying to give our kidneys a sabbatical or an extended vacation—not work them overtime.

Fighting Incurable Diseases Should Not Be a High-Priced Crime

Price and access to keto acids has been a problem.

The average price of existing keto acid supplements, foods, and drugs is as follows for a one-month supply in U.S. dollars at the recommended dosage:

Brazil	$718
France	$380
Germany	$556
Hong Kong	$410
India	$291
Italy	$397
Mexico	$ 378
Average	$447
Plus shipping	$15
Plus taxes/tariffs	**variable**
Estimated cost	$462

It's expensive. I know because I paid many thousands of dollars for all kinds of products over the years when I was experimenting with different supplements and treatment plans. In countries with socialized medicine, cost may not be an issue. It is an issue in the U.S.

If cost wasn't bad enough, access is another issue. Keto acids were not and still are not available in many countries. This means patients had to break the law to try to stop an incurable disease.

One of the reasons I started this project was the idea that I had to pay through the nose and break the law while trying not to die young. I felt angry, frustrated, pissed off, helpless, and any other word you want to use. I had an incurable disease, would be out $6,000+ each year, and might have a criminal record if I got caught. No one should ever be in this position, and I mean ever.

I am bringing to market a keto acid supplement with the lowest amount of nitrogen ever made. I am also bringing a different formulation for each stage of kidney disease to reduce nitrogen at each stage. The retail price will be at least 60% lower than the average price in the rest of world. And if you take into account your dietary protein, you'll need less supplemental protein, so the effective cost is even lower.

I have very strong feelings on this issue as a fellow patient. One thing I can promise: We will be shipping our product, Albutrix, anywhere in the world it is legal to ship it. We won't break laws, but we will work with each and every one of you to find a way to ship to you if you want to try to slow the progression of your disease. Having worked with regulatory bodies in several countries already, I've found these people to be honest, compassionate people who want to help. It may not happen overnight in some cases, but it can happen. These diet and treatment plans are not for everyone, but I can't imagine saying no to a fellow patient after my experience. To this day, I am still angry about the situation we are put in trying to stop a deadly disease.

This means the effective price will be 50% to 80% lower than past keto acid supplements for people with kidney disease. This effort shows what one patient can do when other patients support the effort.

Unintended Consequences of Well-Meaning Advice of Taking Amino Acid Supplements or Kidney Related Supplements

One of my biggest frustrations is the lack of innovation for kidney patients. We are still clinging to information that is thirty to fifty years old for treatment or diet advice. A few examples for you to consider:

Someone I know socially, so I won't name them, lectured me for an hour one night on how I should be taking the amino acid ornithine. Ornithine is a non-essential amino acid involved in the urea and ammonia cycle. This person was very qualified with lots of letters behind their name and adamant that I should take supplemental ornithine.

However, after an hour of two or research I find that ornithine levels actually increased with kidney disease progression. I could find no study that said patients were deficient in ornithine. Turns out we are swimming in ornithine by the time we get to stage 5. We lose the ability to get rid of ornithine as kidney disease progresses. The following study shows ornithine levels increase in stages 4 and 5 by about 20% without supplementation. The reason is we can no longer get rid of ornithine. Excretion of ornithine drops by over 80% in stages 4 and 5.

Ornithine levels for different stages of kidney disease

Amino acid	Stage 2/3	Stage 4/5	Urinary excretion	Stage 2/3	a stage 4/5
Ornithine	53.9±22.6	66.9±21.8		15.4±57.1	1.8±5.1

In the 1970s and early 1980s Dr. Walser worked with ornithine and found ornithine supplementation wasn't helpful. When I told this person about my findings he replied "Oh well, in theory it made sense to me." This person dismissed my finding and never gave it another thought. We have to be careful about who is making recommendations to us and if they really know the implications of their advice.

My point here is not really about ornithine, it is that no one will ever care as much as a patient cares. This person may have meant well," but they really had no idea what they were recommending. Ornithine was tried in the 1970s and 1980s with no success when it comes to kidney patients. However, in 2017, 2018, and 2019, research on ornithine is pointing to something we didn't know about in the 1970s.

Study 31.4   Ornithine and its role in metabolic diseases: An appraisal.

ABSTRACT:

Ornithine is a nonessential amino acid produced as an intermediate molecule in urea cycle. It is a key substrate for the synthesis of proline, polyamines and citrulline. Ornithine also plays an important role in the regulation of several metabolic processes leading to diseases like hyperorithinemia, hyperammonemia, gyrate atrophy and cancer in humans. However, the mechanism of action behind the multi-faceted roles of ornithine is yet to be unraveled completely. Several types of cancers are also characterized by excessive polyamine synthesis from ornithine by different rate limiting enzymes. Hence, in this review we aim to provide extensive insights on poten-tial roles of ornithine in many of the disease related cellular processes and also on the structural features of ornithine interacting proteins, enabling development of therapeutic modalities.

Note: Polyamines are produced from ornithine.

Study 31.5 A Trans-omics Mathematical Analysis Reveals Novel Functions of the Ornithine Metabolic Pathway in Cancer Stem Cells.

ABSTRACT:

Bioinformatics and computational modelling are expected to offer innovative approaches in human medical science. In the present study, we performed computational analyses and made predictions using transcriptome and metabolome datasets obtained from fluorescence-based visualisations of chemotherapy-resistant cancer stem cells (CSCs) in the human oesophagus. This approach revealed an uncharacterized role for the ornithine metabolic pathway in the survival of chemotherapy-resistant CSCs. The present study fastens this rationale for further characterization that may lead to the discovery of innovative drugs against robust CSCs.

Note: This means ornithine and its related compounds may increase the survival rate of cancer cells that cannot be killed by current technology. This is the exact opposite of what we want.

Study 31.6 Dietary polyamine intake and risk of colorectal adenomatous polyps.

RESULTS:

A dietary intake of polyamines above the median amount in the study population was associated with 39% increased risk of colorectal adenoma at follow-up (adjusted OR: 1.39; 95% CI: 1.06, 1.83) in the pooled sample. In addition, younger participants (OR: 1.94; 95% CI: 1.23, 3.08), women (OR: 2.43; 95% CI: 1.48, 4.00), and ODC GG genotype carriers (OR: 1.59; 95% CI: 1.00, 2.53) had significantly increased odds of colorectal adenoma if they consumed above-median polyamine amounts.

CONCLUSIONS:

This study showed a role for dietary polyamines in colorectal adenoma risk. Corroboration of these findings would confirm a previously unrecognized, modifiable dietary risk factor for colorectal adenoma.

Note: ODC stands for ornithine decarboxylase. Polyamine are produced from ornithine and/or ornithine related byproducts. Adenoma is a form of tumor.

This can lead to a situation in which both ammonia and ornithine are too high, but guess what the treatment is for this condition? You guessed it, a low-protein diet. We can undo the benefits of certain treatments if we are not careful.

If we are already swimming in ornithine and ornithine intake even has a small chance of contributing to tumor growth and treatment-resistant cancer, why would we take a non-essential amino acid that we don't need? I am not saying ornithine will cause cancer. What I am saying is what was considered good advice and/or good medicine in the 1970s may be very different in 2019. We get all the risks with no proven benefit.

Here is what is looks like from a pro and con standpoint:

Pros

None proven

Cons

1. Increased renal acid load.

2. Increased nitrogen load.

3. Increased non-essential amino acid that we are not deficient in.

4. The latest science is linking ornithine byproducts to treatment-resistant cancer or tumor growth.

5. 1950s to 1980s research was not able to prove a benefit to kidney patients.

6. Works against the benefits of a low-protein diet.

This is what I mean by unintended consequences and well-meaning advice. What was a well-meaning and strong argument from one perspective turned out to be something very different in real life.

Another example is over-the-counter amino acid or protein supplements. You can buy essential amino acids in most health food stores or online. Nothing wrong with this, unless you are a kidney patient with reduced kidney function. The problem with this logic is the formulas are optimized for healthy patients, not those with kidney disease. Tyrosine is not present, as it is not an essential amino acid. This will work for earlier stages, but not for stage 5 patients. Again, the renal acid load and nitrogen load is much higher, with no nutritional benefit from the extra workload.

Yet another example is that past amino or keto acid formula are all based on stage 5 patients. No one seems to have ever cared about the rest of us in stage 3 or stage 4. We have different nutritional needs than stage five patients. If we want to optimize nutrition and reduce the workload on our kidneys, we need products specially designed for our health.

Taking a stage 5 supplement with lots of tyrosine is bad advice for stage 3 or stage 4 patients.

We need custom nutrition for each stage to give us the best odds.

Ornithine, essential amino acids, or stage 5 formulas are examples of unintended consequences that may affect our odds. As patients, we need more and better options..

Final Thought

I will leave you with one more analogy: The motorcycle I rode as a teen had a hard life. It was crashed who knows how many times, run until its tank was empty in 100-degree temperatures almost daily in the summer, and sat in the rain and cold. Maintenance was something I had never heard of. After a while, it became hard to start and ran rough.

It took an exacting combination for it to start and run halfway decently after years of abuse. Just the right amount of choke would get it started. Too little or too much left me out of breath and with a tired leg from kick starting. You couldn't ask too much of it, or it would cough and rattle. You couldn't take off too fast or cut the engine suddenly. I had to learn to keep everything just right to make it run anywhere close to a normal motorcycle. Our kidneys are much like my old but beloved motorcycle. We are looking for the right combination to keep our damaged or crashed kidneys working as close to normal kidneys as possible.

It's going to take some effort and some trial and error to keep them running, but it can be done in many cases. It will be frustrating and you will be cursing some part of the plan, and not every blood test will come back like you expect or want. However, if you keep trying, you will find a combination that allows your kidneys to keep running as long as possible.

Our kidneys need the lowest amount of nitrogen possible and we need the maximum amount of nutrition possible, given our restrictions. The lowest nitrogen combinations of diet and protein supplements give us the best chances of slowing our disease. The evidence is overwhelming, as you are about to see.

102 Keto Acid Studies

I almost made this section a separate book called something like *The Big Book of Keto Acid Research*. I pared it down and used summaries instead. 102 studies are included this report and, to my knowledge, it is the most comprehensive ever published. Everything is cited as usual, so you can dig deeper if you want to.

Negative studies and inconclusive studies are also included, to be fair. You need all of the information to make an informed decision on your treatment plan, not just a few cherry-picked reports.

When I was floundering around, looking for a better treatment, I started researching keto acids based on Dr. Walser's advice. I was angry, bitter, and frustrated at this point. I wanted to trust everything while, at the same time, I trusted no cure or treatment. Every treatment and every doctor failed me at this point (for the record, it was not any doctor's fault; it's just how I felt at the time). I needed research to restore my faith in a new treatment plan. Here is an updated version. Summary of the research in the following pages:

Positive animal studies:

CKD: 9

Exercise: 1

TOTAL: 10

Negative animal studies:

0

Inconclusive:

0

Positive human studies:

CKD: 74

ESRD: 4

Exercise: 6

TOTAL: 84

Negative Human studies:

0

Inconclusive Human studies:

CKD: 7

ESRD: 1

TOTAL: 8

What you will find is 84 positive studies spread across hundreds of patients and several countries. You will find no toxicity issues, as keto acids are naturally occurring in the body.

My perspective was: I have an incurable kidney disease, keto acids have a strong record of slowing disease progression, and they won't hurt me. What could I lose?

I have underlined a few sentences in each study to streamline things for you. Please reread the chapter on keto acids and then browse or read these studies again. Pay special attention to the studies that apply to your disease or situation. I know it's a lot of data and technical info, but hey, it's your life we're talking about. Study up and become an expert.

I am not aware of any other treatment option for us once drugs have failed or if drugs are not an option. Diet, exercise, nutrition, and understanding how your kidneys work is the only treatment plan you have left in 2019.

This is what we have to work with, and now it will be available to everyone. You may choose not to pursue a low- or very low-protein diet supplemented with keto acids. It's your choice, and no one should judge you for it. However, as someone who fought the battle and watched people I cared about in a slow decline robbing them of years of life, I think this is about as low risk as it gets for treatment plans for a deadly disease. No surgery or strong drugs with equally strong side effects. It's a form of amino acid your body makes normally, combined with a heart- and kidney-healthy, nutrient-dense diet.

As you browse (or hopefully read) these studies, keep in mind the difference between LPD and VLPD diets. You will even see that keto acids have a beneficial effect on exercise by reducing ammonia production. This is an extra benefit for us and exercise is a little harder for us.

Please read, reread, highlight, mark it up, and whatever it takes to get a handle on this chapter and the studies. It's really important for every one of us and our doctors, dietitians, and nutritionists to be familiar with this information.

Animal and Human Studies

PART 1: Positive Animal Studies

1.1. Chronic Kidney Disease

Low-protein diet + keto-acids and/or amino acids

Study 1

Title: Effect of a low-protein diet supplemented with keto-acids on autophagy and inflammation in 5/6 nephrectomized rats[1]

Main outcomes: Effects on skeletal muscle

SUMMARY:

In summary, the present study demonstrated that autophagy/mitophagy was increased and inflammation was aggravated in skeletal muscle in CKD rats. In addition, a LPD supplemented with KA improved the loss in muscle mass and blocked the activation of autophagy/mitophagy and inflammation in the skeletal muscle of CKD rats. Thus, these findings may provide relevant preclinical data for the use of a LPD supplemented with KA in patients with CKD.

Study 2

Title: Supplementation of ketoacids contributes to the up-regulation of the Wnt7a/Akt/p70S6K path way and the down-regulation of apoptotic and ubiquitin– proteasome systems in the muscle of 5/6 nephrectomised rats[2]

Main outcomes: Effects on skeletal muscle

CONCLUSION:

In summary, the present study provides a novel molecular explanation of KA in improving muscle atrophy in CKD-LPD. The results obtained lend strong support to the view that KA supplementation enhances muscle mass by preventing the activation of the UPS and caspase-3-dependent apoptosis and upregulating the Wnt7a/Akt/p70S6K signalling pathway in the muscle of CKD-LPD rats. The present findings about the beneficial effects of KA illuminate that KA might be a better therapeutic strategy for muscle atrophy in CKD-LPD. More studies are still needed to deter mine the precise mechanism in which KA improves muscle atrophy in CKD.

Study 3

Title: Autophagy-lysosome pathway in skeletal muscle of diabetic nephropathy rats and the effect of low-protein diet plus $_a$-keto acids on it[3]

Main outcomes: Effects on skeletal muscle

CONCLUSION:

ALP (autophagy-lysosome pathway) is activated in skeletal muscle of diabetic nephropathy rats. And low protein plus $_\alpha$-keto acid decrease the activation of ALP and improve muscle wasting.

Study 4

Title: Effect of a Low-Protein Diet Supplemented with Ketoacids on Skeletal Muscle Atrophy and Autophagy in Rats with Type 2 Diabetic Nephropathy[4]

Main outcomes: Effects on skeletal muscle and proteinuria

ABSTRACT:

A low-protein diet supplemented with ketoacids maintains nutritional status in patients with diabetic nephropathy. The activation of autophagy has been shown in the skeletal muscle of diabetic and uremic rats. This study aimed to determine whether a low-protein diet supplemented with keto acids improves muscle atrophy and decreases the increased autophagy observed in rats with type 2 diabetic nephropathy. In this study, 24-week-old Goto-Kakizaki male rats were randomly divided into groups that received either a normal protein diet (NPD group), a low-protein diet (LPD group) or a low-protein diet supplemented with ketoacids (LPD +KA group) for 24 weeks. Age- and weight-matched Wistar rats served as control animals and received a normal protein diet (control group). We found that protein restriction attenuated proteinuria and decreased blood urea nitrogen and serum creatinine levels. Compared with the NPD and LPD groups, the LPD +KA group showed a delay in body weight loss, an attenuation in soleus muscle mass loss and a decrease of the mean cross-sectional area of soleus muscle fibers. The mRNA and protein expression of autophagy-related genes, such as Beclin-1, LC3B, Bnip3, p62 and Cathepsin L, were increased in the soleus muscle of GK rats fed with NPD compared to Wistar rats. Impor-tantly, LPD resulted in a slight reduction in the expression of autophagy-related genes; however, these differences were not statistically significant. In addition, LPD+ KA abolished the upregulation of autophagy-related gene expression. Furthermore, the activation of autophagy in the NPD and LPD groups was confirmed by the appearance of autophagosomes or autolysosomes using electron microscopy, when compared with the Control and LPD +KA groups. Our results showed that LPD +KA abolished the activation of autophagy in skeletal muscle and decreased muscle loss in rats with type 2 diabetic nephropathy.

Study 5

Title: Low-protein diet supplemented with ketoacids reduces the severity of renal disease in 5/6 nephrectomized rats: a role for KLF15[5]

Main outcomes: Effects on proteinuria

ABSTRACT:

Dietary protein restriction is an important treatment for chronic kidney disease. Herein, we tested the effect of low-protein or low-protein plus ketoacids (KA) diet in a remnant kidney model. Rats with a remnant kidney were randomized to receive normal protein diet (22%), low-protein (6%) diet (LPD), or low-protein (5%) plus KA (1%) diet for 6 months. Protein restriction prevented proteinuria, decreased blood urea nitrogen levels, and renal lesions; however, the LPD retarded growth and decreased serum albumin levels. Supplementation with KA corrected these abnormalities and provided superior renal protection compared with protein restriction alone. The levels of Kruppel-like factor-15 (KLF15), a transcription factor shown to reduce cardiac fibrosis, were decreased in remnant kidneys. Protein restriction, which increased KLF15 levels in the normal kidney, partially recovered the levels of KLF15 in remnant kidney. The expression of KLF15 in mesangial cells was repressed by oxidative stress, transforming growth factor-β, and tumor necrosis factor (TNF)-α. The suppressive effect of TNF-α on KLF15 expression was mediated by TNF receptor-1 and nuclear factor-$\kappa\beta$. Over-expression of KLF15 in mesangial and HEK293 cells significantly decreased fibronectin and type IV collagen mRNA levels. Furthermore, KLF15 knockout mice developed glomerulosclerosis following uninephrectomy. Thus, KLF15 may be an antifibrotic factor in the kidney, and its decreased expression may contribute to the progression of kidney disease.

Study 6

Title: A low-protein diet supplemented with ketoacids plays a more protective role against oxidative stress of rat kidney tissue with 5/6 nephrectomy than a low-protein diet alone[6]

Main outcomes: Effects on proteinuria

ABSTRACT:

Dietary protein restriction is one major therapy in chronic kidney disease (CKD), and ketoacids have been evaluated in CKD patients during restricted-protein diets. The objective of the present study was to compare the efficacy of a low-protein diet supplemented with ketoacids (LPD+KA) and a low-protein diet alone (LPD) in halting the development of renal lesions in CKD. 5/6 Nephrectomy Sprague– Dawley rats were randomly divided into three groups, and fed with either 22 % protein (normal-protein diet; NPD), 6 % protein (LPD) or 5 % protein plus 1 %ketoacids (LPD+KA) for 24 weeks. Sham-operated rats were used as controls. Each 5/6 nephrectomy group included fifteen rats and the control group included twelve rats. Proteinuria, decreased renal func-tion, glomerular sclerosis and tubulointerstitial fibrosis were found in the remnant kidneys of the NPD group. Protein restriction ameliorated these changes, and the effect was more obvious in the LPD+KA group after 5/6 nephrectomy. Lower body weight and serum albumin levels were found in the LPD group, indicating protein malnutrition. Lipid and protein oxidative prod-ucts were significantly increased in the LPD group compared with the LPD+KA group. These findings indicate that a LPD supplemented with ketoacids is more effective than a LPD alone in protecting the function of remnant kidneys from progressive injury, which may be medi-ated by ketoacids ameliorating protein malnutrition and oxidative stress injury in remnant kidney tissue.

Study 7

Title: Effects of Low-Protein Diets Supplemented with Ketoacid on Expression of TGF-β and Its Receptors in Diabetic Rats[7]

Main outcomes: Effects on proteinuria and kidney functions

SUMMARY:

In summary, our study has demonstrated that the levels of TGF-β1, TβRI, and TβRII were increased in the renal tissue in DN rats. In addition, a low-protein diet supplemented with ketoacids decreased the expression of TGF-β1, TβRI, and TβRII in the renal tissue of DN rats. Low-protein diets supplemented with ketoacid have been demonstrated to provide a protective effect on the renal function as represented by reduced SCr, BUN, and urinary protein excretion, probably through down-regulating the gene expression of TGF-β1 and its receptors in LPD + KA group.

Study 8

Title: Low-protein diet supplemented with ketoacids ameliorates proteinuria in ¾ nephrectomised rats by directly inhibiting the intrarenal renin–angiotensin system[8]

Main outcomes: Effects on oxidative stress and proteinuria

ABSTRACT:

Low-protein diet plus ketoacids (LPD + KA) has been reported to decrease proteinuria in patients with chronic kidney diseases (CKD). However, the mechanisms have not been clarified. As over-activation of intrarenal renin–angiotensin system (RAS) has been shown to play a key role in the progression of CKD, the current study was performed to investigate the direct effects of LPD + KA on intrarenal RAS, independently of renal haemodynamics. In this study, 3/4 subtotal renal ablated rats were fed 18 % normal-protein diet (Nx-NPD), 6 % low-protein diet (Nx-LPD) or 5 % low-protein diet plus 1 % ketoacids (Nx-LPD + KA) for 12 weeks. Sham-operated rats fed NPD served as controls. The level of proteinuria and expression of renin, angiotensin II (AngII) and its type 1 receptors (AT1R) in the renal cortex were markedly higher in Nx-NPD group than in the sham group. LPD + KA significantly decreased the proteinuria and inhibited intrarenal RAS activation. To exclude renal haemodynamic impact on intrarenal RAS, the serum samples derived from the different groups were added to the culture medium of mesangial cells. It showed that the serum from NxNPD directly induced higher expression of AngII, AT1R, fibronectin and transforming growth factor-β 1 in the mesangial cells than in the control group. Nx-LPD + KA serum significantly inhibited these abnormalities. Then, proteomics and biochemical detection suggested that the mechanisms underlying these beneficial effects of LPD + KA might be amelioration of the nutritional metabolic disorders and oxidative stress. In conclusion, LPD + KA could directly inhibit the intrarenal RAS activation, independently of renal haemodynamics, thus attenuating the proteinuria in CKD rats.

Study 9

Title: Keto acid metabolites of branched-chain amino acids inhibit oxidative stress-induced necrosis and attenuate myocardial ischemia–reperfusion injury[9]

Main outcomes: Effects on oxidative stress.

ABSTRACT:

Branched chain $_\alpha$-keto acids (BCKAs) are endogenous metabolites of branched-chain amino acids (BCAAs). BCAA and BCKA are significantly elevated in pathologically stressed heart and contribute to chronic pathological re-modeling and dysfunction. However, their direct impact on acute cardiac injury is unknown. Here, we demonstrated that elevated BCKAs significantly attenuated ischemia–reperfusion (I/R) injury and preserved post I/R function in isolated mouse hearts. BCKAs protected cardiomyocytes from oxidative stress-induced cell death in vitro. Mechanistically, BCKA protected oxidative stress induced cell death by inhibiting necrosis without affecting apoptosis or autophagy. Furthermore, BCKAs, but not BCAAs, protected mitochondria and energy production from oxidative injury. Finally, administration of BCKAs during reperfusion was sufficient to significantly attenuate cardiac I/R injury. These findings uncover an unexpected role of BCAA metabolites in cardioprotection against acute ischemia/reperfusion injury, and demonstrate the potential use of BCKA treatment to preserve ischemic tissue during reperfusion.

1.2. Exercise

Study 1

Title: Acute supplementation with keto analogues and amino acids in rats during resistance exercise[10]

Main outcomes: Effects on biomarkers of muscle damage during exercise

ABSTRACT:

During exercise, ammonia levels are related to the appearance of both central and peripheral fatigue. Therefore, controlling the increase in ammonia levels is an important strategy in ameliorating the metabolic response to exercise and in improving athletic performance. Free amino acids can be used as substrates for ATP synthesis that produces ammonia as a side product. Keto analogues act in an opposite way, being used to synthesize amino acids whilst decreasing free ammonia in the blood. Adult male rats were divided into four groups based on receiving either keto analogues associated with amino acids (KAAA) or a placebo and resistance exercise or no exercise. There was an approximately 40 % increase in ammonaemia due to KAAA supplementation in resting animals. Exercise increased ammonia levels twofold with respect to the control, with a smaller increase (about 20 %) in ammonia levels due to exercise. Exercise itself causes a significant increase in blood urea levels (17 %). However, KAAA reduced blood urea levels to 75

% of the pre-exercise values. Blood urate levels increased 28 % in the KAAA group, independent of exercise. Supplementation increased glucose levels by 10 % compared with control animals. Exercise did not change glucose levels in either the control or supplemented groups. Exercise promoted a 57 % increase in lactate levels in the control group.

Supplementation promoted a twofold exercise-induced increase in blood lactate levels. The present results suggest that an acute supplementation of KAAA can decrease hyperammonaemia induced by exercise.

PART 2: Negative Animal Studies

> No negative animal studies related to kidney disease were found.

> However, two negative studies were found which were related to maple syrup disease.

PART 3: Inconclusive Animal Studies

> No studies were found.

PART 4: Positive Human Studies

4.1. Chronic kidney disease

Low Protein Diet + Keto Acids and/or Amino Acids

Study 1

Title: Do Ketoanalogues Still Have a Role in Delaying Dialysis Initiation in CKD Predialysis Patients?[11]

Main outcomes: Effects on progression of the disease

ABSTRACT:

Early versus later start of dialysis is still a matter of debate. Low-protein diets have been used for many decades to delay dialysis initiation. Protein-restricted diets (0.3–0.6 g protein/kg/day) supplemented with essential amino acids and ketoanalogues (sVLPD) can be offered, in association with pharmacological treatment, to motivated stage 4–5 chronic kidney disease (CKD) patients not having severe comorbid conditions; they probably represent 30–40% of the concerned population. A satisfactory adherence to such dietary prescription is observed in approximately 50% of the patients. While the results of the studies on the effects of this diet on the rate of progression of renal failure remain inconclusive, they are highly significant when initiation of dialysis is the primary outcome. The correction of uremic symptoms allows for initiation of dialysis treatment at a level of residual renal function lower than that usually recommended. Most of the CKD-associated complications of cardiovascular and metabolic origin, which hamper both lifespan and quality of life, are positively influenced by the diet. Lastly, with regular monitoring jointly assumed by physicians and dietitians, nutritional status is well preserved as confirmed by a very low mortality rate and by the absence of detrimental effect on the long-term outcome of patients on cerenal replacement therapy is initiated. On account of its feasibility, efficacy and safety, sVLPD deserves a place in the management of selected patients to safely delay the time needed for dialysis.

Study 2

Title: Effect of Low-Protein Diet Supplemented with Keto Acids on Progression of Chronic Kidney Disease[12]

Main outcomes: Effects on progression of the disease

ABSTRACT:

Hypoproteic diets are most often discussed for patients with chronic kidney disease (CKD) who do not receive dialysis. A very low-protein diet supplemented with ketoanalogues of essential amino acids (keto-diet) proved effective in ameliorating metabolic disturbances of advanced CKD and delaying the initiation of dialysis without deleterious effects on nutritional status. Several recent studies report that the keto-diet could also slow down the rate of decline in renal function, with better outcomes after the initiation of dialysis. Results of a single-center randomized controlled trial addressing the rate of CKD progression revealed a 57% slower decline in renal function with the keto-diet compared with a conventional low-protein diet (LPD). The keto-diet allowed the safe management of selected patients with stage 4-5 CKD, delaying dialysis for almost 1 year, with a major impact on patient quality of life and health expenditures. Therefore, the keto-diet could be a link in the integrated care model. Careful selection of patients, nutritional monitoring, and dietary counseling are required.

Study 3

Title: Management of protein-energy wasting in nondialysis-dependent chronic kidney disease: reconciling low protein intake with nutritional therapy[13]

Main outcomes: Effects on progression of the disease

SUMMARY:

A strategy used to enhance the potential beneficial effects of a protein-restricted diet is to reduce protein intake to 0.3 g/kg/day of mixed biological protein [very-low-protein diet (VLPD)] and provide a daily supplement of 0.28 g/kg of a combination of some EAAs and keto acids or hydroxy acid analogues of the other EAAs. These supplements of the VLPD are necessary to provide adequate total protein/amino acids and EAAs to meet a patient's nutritional needs; they may also possibly provide an anabolic stimulus and are free of phosphorus compounds, which may have additional advantages given the association of hyperphosphatemia with CKD progression.

Furthermore, the keto acid and hydroxy acid analogues provide EAA precursors without the nitrogen load from EAAs. Hence, these SVLPDs appear to generate less toxic metabolic products than similar amounts of protein from LPDs. These VLPDs, and LPDs in general, also appear to reduce proteinuria.

Study 4

Title: Efficacy of the Essential Amino Acids and KetoAnalogues on the CKD progression rate in real practice in Russia-city nephrology registry data for outpatient clinic[14]

Main outcomes: Effects on progression of the disease

CONCLUSION:

LPD combined with EAA/KA supplementation lead to the decrease of the CKD progression both in well-designed clinical study and in real nephrology practice in wide variety diseases and settings.

Study 5

Title: Vegetarian low-protein diets supplemented with ketoanalogues: a niche for the few or an option for many?[15]

Main outcomes: Effects on progression of the disease

CONCLUSION:

The data obtained in this feasibility study may support a wider offer of LPD-KA to patients with severe and progressive CKD, as 'success' of at least 6 months on the diet can be obtained in elderly patients with high co-morbidities and low educational level, further underlining the importance of individual choices and empowerment in CKD patients. Such a dietary programme is feasible, safe and adaptable to a routine clinical setting, and it can provide promising results in terms of slowing the progression of CKD, even though these results must be confirmed by studies using control groups and exploring its implementation in different clinical settings.

Study 6

Title: Better preservation of residual renal function in peritoneal dialysis patients treated with a low-protein diet supplemented with keto acids: a prospective, randomized trial[16]

Main outcomes: Effects on progression of the disease

CONCLUSION:

A diet containing 0.6–0.8 g of protein/kg IBW/day is safe and, when combined with keto acids, is associated with an improved preservation of RRF (Residual Renal Function) in relatively new PD (peritoneal dialysis) patients without significant malnutrition or inflammation.

Study 7

Title: Analysis of the Effectiveness of Renoprotection of Low-Protein Diet and Ketoanalogues of Amino Acids In Patients With Chronic Kidney Disease[17]

Main outcomes: Effects on progression of the disease

CONCLUSION:

Renoprotection based on the use KA/AA in patients with CKD stages 3-4 proved to be more effective than without it in slowing the rate of decline in GFR, hypertension correction, proteinuria reduction, maintaining the level of Hb, prevention of disorders of protein and calcium-phosphate metabolism, as well as correction of the lipid metabolism.

Study 8

Title: The role of balanced low-protein diet in inhibition of predialysis chronic kidney disease progression in patients with systemic diseases[18]

Main outcomes: Effects on progression of the disease

CONCLUSION:

Early (predialysis) restriction of diet protein (0.6 g/ kg/day) with addition of highly energetic mixture and essential keto/amino acids improves a nutritive status of CDK patients and inhibits GFR decline.

Study 9

Title: The effect of low-protein diet supplemented with ketoacids in patients with chronic renal failure[19]

Main outcomes: Effects on progression of the disease

ABSTRACT:

It is known that dietary protein restriction slows the progression of chronic renal disease. If daily protein intake is less than 0.5-0.6 g/kg bw, the diet has to be supplemented with essential amino acids/ketoacids. In this study the authors evaluate the long-term effect of low-protein diet supplemented with ketoacids on the progression of chronic renal failure, calcium and phosphorus metabolism, nutritional status, the compliance of patients and the permanent dietary education for the compliance. 51 predialysis patients have been treated with ketoacids supplemented low-protein diet during 12-57 months (mean treatment period: 26 months). Serum creatinine raised from 349.72+/-78.04 micromol/l to 460.66+/-206.66 micromol/l (27 micromol/l/year or 2.3micromol/l/ month), glomerular filtration rate (GFR) decreased from 21.52+/-7.84 ml/ min to18.22+/-7.76 ml/min (0.83 ml/min/year or 0.07 ml/min/month). The slope of 1/ serum creatinine versus time was 0.0018 by linear regression analysis. Serum parathormone decreased significantly, but serum calcium and phosphorus did not change. Nutritional status of patients did not change significantly during the follow-up period. Protein intake decreased significantly and remained at this lower level during the treatment period. According to results: low-protein diet supplemented with ketoacids was effective in slowing progression of chronic renal fail-ure, decreased PTH, did not change nutritional status. With permanent and good education it was possible to keep patients on low-protein diet for a long period.

Study 10

Title: Adaptive responses to very low protein diets: The first comparison of ketoacids to essential amino acids[20]

Main outcomes: Effects on progression of the disease

CONCLUSION:

In summary, this study indicates that a VLPD (very low protein diet) supplemented with either KA (ketoacid) or EAA (essential amino acids) should produce neutral nitrogen balance in most patients with CRF (chronic renal failure). Successful adaptation to the VLPD regimen involved a marked reduction in amino acid oxidation and a postprandial inhibition of protein degradation, resulting in more efficient utilization of amino acids. Thus, the adaptive responses to dietary protein restriction remain intact in CRF patients consuming the VLPD regimen. Finally, evidence indicating that a VLPD supplemented with KA slows progression compared to an identical diet plus EAA.

Study 11

Title: A crossover comparison of progression of chronic renal failure: Ketoacids versus amino acids[21]

Main outcomes: Effects on progression of the disease

CONCLUSION:

In summary, we found that when 16 patients were alternately provided with KA or AA supplements for three or four treatment periods, 13 of them exhibited slower progression on KA supplements and three exhibited slower progression on AA supplements. This difference is statistically significant. One further patient had observations during two treatment periods, but he failed to complete the three period protocol. Even if this patient is included, so that 13 out of 17 progress more slowly on KA, this result remains significant (P <0.05) by the sign test.

Study 12

Title: Randomized, Double-Blind, Placebo-Controlled Trial to Evaluate Efficacy of Keto diet in Predialytic Chronic Renal Failure[22]

Main outcomes: Effects on progression of the disease

CONCLUSION:

This study was designed to assess whether a keto diet, a combination of ketoanalogs of essential amino acids (KAs) and a very low–protein diet, retards progression of chronic renal failure and maintains nutritional status. Over a 9-month period, very low–protein diet supplemented with ketoanalogs helped CRF patients to preserve GFR and maintain BMI. KAs were safe and efficacious in retarding the progression of renal failure and preserving the nutritional status of CRF patients.

Study 13

Title: Progression of Chronic Renal Failure on Substituting a Ketoacid Supplement for an Amino Acid Supplement[23]

Main outcomes: Effects on progression of the disease

CONCLUSION:

The results suggest that this ketoacid supplement slows progression by approximately half, compared with an essential amino acid supplement, with no change in diet.

Study 14

Title: Progression of chronic renal failure in patients given ketoacids following amino acids[24]

Main outcomes: Effects on progression of the disease

ABSTRACT:

Twelve patients with chronic renal failure who exhibited a progressive decline in 24-hour creatinine clearance, despite being given for 2 to 10 months a diet containing 0.3 g per kg ideal weight of protein and 7 to 9 g mg per kg ideal weight of phosphorus, supplemented with vitamins, CaCO3, and 10 g per day of essential amino acids, were changed to a supplement containing predominantly ketoacids. In six patients whose serum creatinine was 7.5 mg/dl or greater at change over, progression continued unabated. In six patients with serum creatinine levels at changeover of 6.6 to 7.4 mg/ dl, one was non-compliant with the diet and progressed to dialysis. In the other five, progression, measured as the rate of change of a bimonthly radioisotope clearance, has been undetectable during the ensuing one to two years. There has been no change in urea appearance, blood pressure, phosphaturia or proteinuria. Nutri-tion has been maintained. Thus this ketoacid supplemented regimen apparently halted the progression of moderately—severe chronic renal failure for at least a year in a small group of patients in whom restriction of protein and phosphate intake without ketoacids failed to halt progression. In more severe renal failure, no effect on progression was seen.

Study 15

Title: Progression of chronic renal failure is related to glucocorticoid production[25]

Main outcomes: Effects on progression of the disease

CONCLUSION:

Changing from essential amino acids to ketoacids (or vice versa) without change in diet was associated with lower 17-hydroxycorticosteroid excretion on ketoacids (but not when factored by GFR). Therefore, progression of chronic renal failure is related to glucocorticoid production (and to triglyceridemia, which is correlated with it). Ketoacids appear to slow progression in part by suppressing production of glucocorticoids.

Study 16

Title: Branched-Chain Amino-Acid Metabolism in Renal Failure[26]

Main outcomes: Effects on progression of the disease

CONCLUSION:

In conclusion, abnormal branched-chain amino acid metabolism is a well-known phenomenon in CKD patients, and is always associated with disturbed muscle and hepatosplanchnic amino acid metabolism. In predialysis care, branched-chain keto acid/amino acid supplements are integrated into a therapeutic strategy that includes protein restriction and supplementation with other essential amino acids, to improve uremic toxicity, delay the progression of renal disease, and correct the metabolic complications associated with CKD. In dialysis patients, it was reported that the normalization of plasma BCAAs and the overall improvement of protein metabolism by BCAA supplementation were associated with improvements in appetite and nutritional status.

Study 17

Title: Effect of Low-Protein Diet Supplemented with Keto Acids on Progression of Disease in Patients with Chronic Renal Failure[27]

Main outcomes: Effects on progression of the disease

CONCLUSION:

Together, these findings suggest that a low-protein diet supplemented with ketoacids is well tolerated by the patients, and seems to be a good alternative in the treatment of CRF patients. It seems to be crucial that the patient must follow strictly the rules of the diet program to achieve success of the therapy.

Study 18

Title: Low protein diets are mainstay for management of chronic kidney disease[28]

Main outcomes: Effects on progression of the disease

CONCLUSION:

Low protein diets, made either of natural foods or of L-essential amino acids and/or their nitrogen-free ketoanalogues, are feasible, safe, and efficient means to reduce disease progression in patients with chronic kidney disease and do not prejudice patient outcomes once they get into Renal Replacement Therapy. They ameliorate symptomatology, grant a posi-tive nitrogen balance, reduce proteinuria, improve osteodystrophy and lipid profile, reduce serum concentra-tions of uric acid, phosphate, and maintain plasma bicarbonate within nor-mal limits thus pre-venting metabolic acidosis. They also reduce the number of hypotensive drugs and the quantity of erythropoietin to be administered to achieve target hemoglobin concentrations, and do not deteriorate quality of life. On the contrary, they retard progression of chronic kidney disease. There is a need to motivate patients to increase adherence to.

Study 19

Title: Effect of a ketoacid-aminoacid-supplemented very low protein diet on the progression of advanced renal disease: a reanalysis of the MDRD feasibility study[29]

Main outcomes: Effects on progression of the disease

CONCLUSION:

The study suggests that supplementation of a very low protein diet with the ketoacid-aminoacid mixture used in this feasibility study slowed the progression of advanced renal disease more than supplementation with an amino acid mixture.

Study 20

Title: Low protein diet and ketosteril in predialysis patients with renal failure[30]

Main outcomes: Effects on progression of the disease

ABSTRACT:

A low protein diet with increased content of essential amino acids and their keto-analogues does not deteriorate the nitrogen balance of patients with chronic renal failure. By adding essential amino acids and keto-analogues a normal protein metabolism is maintained in spite of the reduce intake of protein substances with the diet. Supplementation of the diet of chronic renal failure patients with essential amino acids and keto-analogues allows a considerable reduction of the protein intake to be achieved which brings about reduction of glomerular hyperfiltration which actually retards the progression of renal failure and improves its short-term prognosis.

Study 21

Title: The effect of dietary protein restriction on the progression of diabetic and nondiabetic renal diseases: a meta-analysis[31]

Main outcomes: Effects on progression of the disease

BACKGROUND:

Dietary protein has long been thought to play a role in the progression of chronic renal disease, but clinical trials to date have not consistently shown that dietary protein restriction is beneficial.

DATA SYNTHESIS:

The relative risk for progression of renal disease in patients receiving a low-protein diet compared with patients receiving a usual-protein diet was calculated by using a random-effects model. In five studies of nondiabetic renal disease, a low-protein diet significantly reduced the risk for renal failure or death (relative risk, 0.67 [95% Cl, 0.50 to 0.89]). In five studies of insulin-dependent diabetes mellitus, a low-protein diet significantly slowed the increase in urinary albumin level or the decline in glomerular filtration rate or creatinine clearance (relative risk, 0.56 [Cl, 0.40 to 0.77]). Tests for heterogeneity showed no significant differences in relative risk among studies of either diabetic or nondiabetic renal disease. No significant differences were seen between diet groups in pooled mean arterial blood pressure (diabetic and nondiabetic patients) or glycosylated hemoglobin level (diabetic patients only).

CONCLUSION:

Dietary protein restriction effectively slows the progression of both diabetic and nondiabetic renal diseases.

Study 22

Title: Effect of restricted protein diet supplemented with keto analogues in chronic kidney disease: a systematic review and meta-analysis[32]

Main outcomes: Effects on progression of the disease

ABSTRACT:

Restricted protein diet supplemented with keto analogues (s(v)LPD) could delay the progression of CKD effectively without causing malnutrition.

Study 23

Title: Low protein diets for chronic renal failure in non-diabetic adults[33]

Main outcomes: Effects on progression of the disease

BACKGROUND:

For more than fifty years, low protein diets have been proposed to patients with kidney failure. However, the effects of these diets in preventing severe renal failure and the need for maintenance dialysis have not been resolved.

OBJECTIVES:

To determine the efficacy of low protein diets in delaying the need to start maintenance dialysis.

MAIN RESULTS:

Eight trials were identified from over 40 studies. A total of 1524 patients were analysed, 763 had received reduced protein intake and 761 a higher protein intake. Two hundred and fifty one renal deaths were recorded, 103 in the low protein diet and 148 in the higher protein diet group (RR 0.69, 95% CI 0.56 to 0.86, P = 0.0007). To avoid one renal death, 2 to 56 patients need to be treated with a low protein diet during one year.

AUTHORS' CONCLUSIONS:

<u>Reducing protein intake in patients with chronic kidney disease reduces the occurrence of renal death by 31% as compared with higher or unrestricted protein intake.</u> The optimal level of protein intake cannot be confirmed from these studies.

Study 24

Title: Reduction of morbidity related to emergency access to dialysis with very low protein diet supplemented with ketoacids (VLPD+KA)[34]

Main outcomes: Effects on nutritional status

CONCLUSION:

<u>The VLPD+KA is safe to maintain the nutritional status</u> of patients of CKD until the AV fistula is made or the <u>PD (peritoneal dialysis) training is given.</u>

Study 25

Title: Keto acid-supplemented low-protein diet for treatment of adult patients with hepatitis B virus infection and chronic glomerulonephritis[35]

Main outcomes: Effects on nutritional status

CONCLUSION:

To our knowledge, the current study is the first prospective, randomized trial of low-protein diets in patients with stage I–II CKD, and suggests that a low-protein diet supplemented with keto acids can be useful in patients with chronic glomerulonephritis and HBV infection. <u>A keto acid-supplemented low-protein diet was both nutritionally safe and associated with improvements in malnutrition, in the present study. Keto acid supplementation also resulted in significant improvements in serum albumin and prealbumin compared with a non-supplemented diet</u> in the present study, but there were no between-group differences in serum creatinine concentrations or the eGFR. This may be due to the limited duration of the study. <u>Keto acid supplementation resulted in a significant reduction</u> in urinary protein excretion and microalbuminuria in <u>the present study, possibly mediated by decreased levels of fibrotic factors such as transforming growth factor-β.</u>

Study 26

Title: Influence of ketoanalogs supplementation on the progression in chronic kidney disease patients who had training on low-protein diet[36]

Main outcomes: Effects on nutritional status

CONCLUSION:

In conclusion, KA supplementation on over LPD (Low protein diet) delayed the progression of CKD without deteriorating nutritional status, and patients with diabetes or those with a better nutritional status showed a greater likelihood of benefiting from the diet.

Study 27

Title: Keto-analogues and essential amino acids and other supplements in the conservative management of chronic kidney disease[37]

Main outcomes: Effects on nutritional status

ABSTRACT:

The manipulation of dietary protein intake is the mainstay of nutritional treatment of patients affected by chronic renal insufficiency, with the aim to reduce the burden of uremic toxins in order to decrease uremic toxicity and delay the need for dialysis. Consensus exists regarding the benefit of progressive protein restriction towards delaying the progression of renal failure and the need for dialysis, provided adequate energy supply. Although pivotal, protein restriction is only one aspect of the dietary management of chronic kidney disease (CKD) patients. Additional features, though strictly related to proteins, include modifications in sodium, phosphorus and energy intake, as well as in the source (animal or plant derived) of protein and lipids. In addition, supplements play an important role as a means to obtain both beneficial effects and nutritional safety in the renal patient. Essential amino acid and ketoacid mixtures are the most utilized types of supplementation in CKD patients on restricted protein regimens. The essential amino acids plus ketoacid supplementation is mandatory in conjunction with a very low-protein diet in order to assure an adequate essential amino acid supply. It is needed to safely implement a very low protein (and phosphorus) intake, so as to obtain the beneficial effect of a severe protein restriction while preventing malnutrition. Protein-free products and energy supplements are also crucial for the prevention of protein-energy wasting in CKD patients. Calcium, iron, native vitamin D and omega-3 PUFAs are other types of supplementation of potential benefits in the CKD patients on conservative management.

Study 28

Title: Effects of keto/amino acids and a low-protein diet on the nutritional status of patients with Stages 3B-4 chronic kidney disease[38]

Main outcomes: Effects on nutritional status

CONCLUSION:

The keto/amino acids ketosteril or ketoaminol are an important component of LPD, which prevents malnutrition and an additional source of calcium that inhibits hyperphosphatemia and slows the development of uremic hyperparathyroidism. Incorporation of keto/ amino acids into LPD leads to a less pronounced reduction in s-Klotho protein in relation to the degree of renal failure than does LPD without keto/amino acids.

Study 29

Title: Nephroprotective role of early correction of impaired nutritional status in patients with chronic disease of the kidneys at a predialysis stage[39]

Main outcomes: Effects on nutritional status

CONCLUSION:

Early (predialysis) use of low-protein diet balanced by addition of amino- and keto-acids and high-energy nutritional mixes has a positive influence on nutritional status of patients with chronic renal insufficiency and can inhibit GFR lowering.

Study 30

Title: Long-term adaptive responses to dietary protein restriction in chronic renal failure[40]

Main outcomes: Effects on nutritional status

CONCLUSION:

In summary, our results can indicate that VLPD/KA regimen can maintain nutritional status during long-term therapy. The leucine turnover results identified the compensatory response(s) leading to neutral BN with this restrictive regimen and provide the first direct evidence that the adaptive responses to dietary protein restriction are maintained during long-term therapy.

Study 31

Title: Long-term effects of a new ketoacid—amino acid supplement in patients with chronic renal failure[41]

Main outcomes: Effects on nutritional status

ABSTRACT:

Nine patients with severe chronic renal failure (mean glomerular filtration rate 4.8 ml/mm; mean serum creatinine 11.3 mg/dl) who were previously on a protein-restricted diet were treated with a diet containing an average of 33 kcal/kg and 22.5 g/day of mixed quality protein, supplemented by a combination of amino acids and mixed salts formed between basic amino acids and keto-analogues of essential amino acids. The supplement was designed to minimize or reverse the amino acid abnormalities of chronic renal failure rather than to meet the normal requirements for the essential amino acids; it contained tyrosine, ornithine, and a high proportion of branched-chain ketoacids, but no phenylalanine or tryptophan and very little methionine. Within one month, serum urea nitrogen fell and serum albumin and transferrin rose significantly; serum creatinine fell slightly. Hyper-phosphatemia (present in three patients) was corrected. Nitrogen balance, measured in seven of the nine patients, on the average was neutral, as it was in a preceding control period on a 40 to 50 g/day protein diet. Plasma tyrosine and threonine, which were subnormal before therapy, rose to normal or high normal levels.

Branched-chain amino acids did not change. During a total of 63 patient-months of therapy, no side effects or toxicity were observed, and serum albumin and transferrin did not change further. It is concluded that this specially designed supplement added to a 20 to 25 g/d protein diet is an acceptable regimen which can improve or maintain protein nutrition in patients with severe chronic renal failure who would otherwise require dialysis.

Study 32

Title: Oral essential amino acid and keto acid supplements in children with chronic renal failure[42]

Main outcomes: Effects on nutritional status

ABSTRACT:

The effects on growth, body composition, and metabolism of a protein-restricted diet supplemented with essential amino acids, the calcium-ketoacids of valine, leucine, isoleucine, and phenylalanine, and the calcium-hydroxy acid of methionine, were investigated in seven growth-retarded children with chronic renal failure. During 0.4 to 1.0 years of treatment there were significant increases in growth velocity and upper arm circumference so scores, body cell mass (intracellular water calculated as tritium space minus corrected sodium bromide space) and serum transferrin. Blood urea and urea: creatinine ratio fell in all children. Renal function assessed from plasma creatinine and 51Cr EDTA clearance did not change significantly. During treatment there was an increase in plasma calcium, high levels necessitating brief interruption of therapy in two children, and a decrease in plasma phosphate. Levels of serum parathormone fell in all children, and were correlated inversely with plasma calcium and positively with plasma phosphate. Abnormalities compared to control children in blood amino-acid and branched-chain ketoacid levels were unaffected by treatment. These results suggest that a protein-restricted diet supplemented with essential amino acids and calcium-keto and hydroxy acids may be useful to improve linear growth and nutritional status in children with chronic renal failure, and that a reduction in hyperparathyroidism may be partly responsible for some of the beneficial effects observed.

Study 33

Title: Protein-restricted diets plus keto/amino acids—a valid therapeutic approach for chronic kidney disease patients [43]

Main outcomes: Effects on nutritional status

ABSTRACT:

Chronic kidney disease (CKD) is increasingly common, and there is an increasing awareness that every strategy should be used to avoid complications of CKD. Restriction of dietary protein intake has been a relevant part of the management of CKD for more than 100 years, but even today, the principal goal of protein-restricted regimens is to decrease the accumulation of nitrogen waste products, hydrogen ions, phosphates, and inorganic ions while maintaining an adequate nutritional status to avoid secondary problems such as metabolic acidosis, bone disease, and insulin resistance, as well as proteinuria and deterioration of renal function. This supplement focuses on recent experimental and clinical findings related to an optimized dietary management of predialysis, dialysis, and transplanted patients as an important aspect of patient care. Nutritional treatment strategies are linked toward ameliorating metabolic and endocrine disturbances, improving/maintaining nutritional status, as well as delaying the renal replacement initiation and improving outcomes in CKD patients. A final consensus states that dietary manipulations should be considered as one of the main approaches in the management program of CKD patients and that a reasonable number of patients with moderate or severe CKD benefit from dietary protein/phosphorus restriction.

Study 34

Title: Short-term effects of a very-low-protein diet (VLPD) supplemented with ketoacids (KA) in non-dialyzed chronic kidney disease (CKD) patients[44]

Main outcomes: Effects on nutritional status

CONCLUSION:

This study indicates that a VLPD+KA can maintain the nutritional status of the patients similarly to a conventional LPD. Besides, an improvement in calcium and phosphorus metabolism and a reduction in serum urea nitrogen were attained only with the VLPD+KA. Thus, VLPD+KA can constitute another efficient therapeutic alternative in the treatment of CKD patients.

Study 35

Title: The role of keto acids in the supportive treatment of children with chronic renal failure[45]

Main outcomes: Effects on nutritional status

CONCLUSION:

In conclusion, in our study, the nutritional status of patients with chronic renal failure improved with the administration of a keto-acid diet, and consequently, the growth rate increased and progression to end stage renal failure was delayed.

Study 36

Title: The effect of a keto acid supplement on the course of chronic renal failure and nutritional parameters in predialysis patients and patients on regular hemodialysis therapy: the Hungarian Ketosteril Cohort Study[46]

Main outcomes: Effects on nutritional status

CONCLUSION:

In a large group of PRE (predialysis) patients prescription of a low protein diet supplemented with KA is feasible and leads to a diminution of 1/sCr equation slopes independent from the degree of renal dysfunction, suggesting a retardation in the rate of CRF (chronic renal failure) progression. There was an improvement in nutritional parameters both in PRE and DIA (dialysis patients) patients, the latter being characterized by improved SGA (subjective global assessment) scores.

Study 37

Title: Controlled trial of two keto acid supplements on renal function, nutritional status, and bone metabolism in uremic patients[47]

Main outcomes: Effects on nutritional status

ABSTRACT:

In this matched, controlled study, two different types of EAA/KA supplements were compared in uremic patients fed a 30 g protein restricted diet. The patients were paired for age, sex, and underlying renal disease. The supplement with the higher BCKA content resulted in an improvement of renal function, bone metabolism, and a normalization of plasma BCAA concentrations. With both supplements, adequate nutritional status of the patients was maintained. We conclude that the BCKA content of the supplement is of considerable importance for uremic patients on low protein diets.

Study 38

Title: Nutrition and outcome on renal replacement therapy of patients with chronic renal failure treated by a supplemented very low protein diet[48]

Main outcomes: Effects on nutritional status

ABSTRACT:

Protein-restricted diets are prescribed in patients with chronic renal failure (CRF) to alleviate uremic symptoms and to slow the progression of CRF. The potential deleterious effects of protein restriction on nutritional status and clinical outcome of patients with CRF have raised concern. In this study, data were collected from 1985 to 1998 on 239 consecutive patients (age 50.2 +/- 15.6 yr) with advanced CRF (GFR 13.1 +/- 4.8 ml/min) to whom a supplemented very low protein diet (SVLPD) providing 0.3 g protein, 35 kcal, and 5 to 7 mg of inorganic phosphorus per kg per day was administered for a mean duration of 29.6 +/- 25.1 mo. The diet was supplemented with essential amino acids and ketoanalogs, calcium carbonate, iron, and multivitamins. During SVLPD, protein intake decreased from 0.85 +/- 0.23 to 0.43 +/- 0.11 g/kg per d, and body mass index and serum albumin concentration remained unchanged overall. Fourteen patients died during SVLPD; death was unrelated to nutritional parameters. Hemodialysis was initiated after SVLPD in 165 patients at a mean GFR of 5.8 +/-1.5 ml/min. During an average of 54 mo on hemodialysis, mortality was low (2.4% after 1 yr) and correlated to age only, not to nutritional parameters observed at the end of SVLPD. Similar results were obtained in 66 transplanted patients (12 were not dialyzed before transplantation). SVLPD can be safely used in patients with CRF without adverse effects on the clinical and nutritional status of the patients. Due to the preservation of nutritional status and the correction of uremic symptoms, the initiation of dialysis was deferred in these patients. The outcome of patients on renal replacement therapy is not affected by prior treatment with SVLPD during the predialysis phase of CRF.

Study 39

Title: Nutritional Therapy in Patients with Chronic Kidney Disease: Protein-Restricted Diets Supplemented with Keto/Amino Acids[49]

Main outcomes: Effects on nutritional status

> Should We Still Prescribe a Reduction in Protein Intake for CKD Patients?[50]

In summary, there is strong evidence that low protein diets are effective in reducing 'renal death' and it has been proven repeatedly that these diets are nutritionally safe. Although there remains uncertainty about the influence of a low protein diet on protection from loss of kidney function, many experimental data are consistent with a benefit of this type of treatment for CKD patients. Other considerations include a patient's quality of life (especially with respect to the aspect of not starting dialysis) and the reduction of health care costs. The latter reflects the expected growth in the number of CKD patients. Evidence about an additive benefit from a well designed low protein diet should be added to other renal preservation strategies. The aim for an optimal management of CKD should be the inclusion of nutritional care in a more general CKD patient follow-up

> Cardiovascular Risk Factors in Severe Chronic Kidney Disease: The Role of Protein-Restricted Diets Supplemented with Keto/Amino Acids[51]

In summary, a well constructed dietary treatment strategy for CKD patients consisting of protein-restricted diets supplemented with keto/amino acids can exert favorable effects on several cardiovascular risk factors. Reduction in the intake of protein, phosphorus and sodium while preserving an adequate energy intake will benefit the patient. The benefits seem to be augmented by the mainly or totally vegetarian nature of the diet and the effects of keto/amino acids supplementation. The improvements to be expected include better control of arterial blood pressure and anemia, an improved lipoprotein profile, prevention or correction of hyperphosphatemia and secondary hyperparathyroidism, amelioration of insulin sensitivity and improved metabolic control for diabetic patients. Finally, the diet may reduce the degree of inflammation and oxidative stress.

> Low Protein Diets and Proteinuria: Renal and Cardiac Outcomes[52]

In summary, an effective reduction of urinary albuminuria/proteinuria can reduce the risk of doubling serum creatinine, ESRD or death or/and reducing the risk of having a stroke, heart attack and congestive heart failure. Furthermore, dietary interventions such as protein-restricted diets supplemented with ketoacids can be considered as a safe therapy to contribute to the reduction of proteinuria.

> Influence of SVLPD on the Evolution of Proteinuria and the Potential Correlation with the Outcome of Blood Pressure and Renal Function[53]

In conclusion, very low protein diets supplemented with keto/amino acids have an early antiproteinuric effect in most CKD patients. However, this benefit is not long-lasting in all patients. On the other hand, the greater the degree of reduction in albuminuria/ proteinuria during the initial 3 months, the greater the degree of 'renal protection'. As occurring with ACE-inhibitor therapies, the predictive value of decreased proteinuria is particularly strong in patients with higher urinary protein excretion at baseline. In general, a reduction in proteinuria should be a specific target for renoprotective treatment, especially in nephrotic patients.

> Paradigm Shift of Ketoacid Treatment in Patients with Hypoalbuminemia?[54]

Based on these results plus the calculated protein equivalent of the daily Ketosteril intake it is speculated that the effect of this keto/amino acid supplement is not only of quantitative nature, but also based on modulation of metabolism. The modulation of metabolism includes changes induced by keto/amino acids, especially BCAA, on appetite regulation, on regulation of protein synthesis and degradation as well as on biomarkers of acute-phase inflammation (TNF-$_\alpha$, CRP) and oxidative stress, which is a well-known explanation for the observed findings.

> Outcome of Old Patients on Supplemented Very Low Protein Diets (VLPD) – Short Communication[55]

In conclusion, elderly patients can comply with a supplemented very low protein diet and it extends their status far below the GFR limits that are suggested by DOQI recommendations. At the same time, these patients maintain a satisfactory nutritional status and a good quality of life. Once they begin dialysis, these patients have a survival rate, which favorably can be compared with that of patients of similar age.

> How to Manage Older Patients with Keto/Amino Acids?[56]

Based on these results, it can be concluded that the metabolic actions of keto/amino acids occurring during long-term therapy do not significantly affect renal hemodynamics. There could be an associated change in the tubular transport mechanism that decreases the renal excretion of branched-chain amino acids. Compared to previous data obtained from the younger CKD patients, there were no significant changes in the outcome parameters. We conclude that low protein diets supplemented with keto/amino acids can be considered safe in older CKD patients.

> Long-Term Results under Ketoacid Substituted Low Protein Diet–German Experience[57]

In conclusion, these results not only confirm the beneficial effects of very low protein diets supplemented with keto/amino acids in terms of maintaining nutritional status, and delaying the onset of dialysis, but they also show improved control of calcium-phosphate metabolism and correction of dynamic histological features in bone. Finally, the outcome of patients who subsequently began dialysis was not negatively affected by the nutritional intervention during the predialysis period.

> Level of β2 Microglobulin in Urine of Patients with Diabetic Nephropathy and CKD Treated with a Low Protein Diet and Ketosteril[58]

In conclusion, our preliminary, short-term results show that keto/amino acid-supplemented proteinrestricted diets significantly reduce urinary β2 microglobulin levels. The results support the hypothesis that this type of dietary treatment based on supplementation of the diet with keto/ amino acids can improve tubular re-absorption mechanisms in CKD patients. Furthermore, the results indicate that in future the renal function evaluation must include specific tubular functions tests.

> Keto Acid Therapy and Residual Function in CAPD and HD Patients[59]

In conclusion, individualized keto/amino acid supplemented diet combined with adequate dialysis treatment significantly helps control the metabolic status of hemodialysis patients with malnutrition. The regimen can also stabilize residual renal function.

> Beneficial responses to modified diets in treating patients with chronic kidney disease[60]

Successful dietary manipulation can ameliorate many complications of CKD. Low-protein diets are nutritionally safe, they reduce the accumulation of metabolic products, and they can suppress progressive loss of kidney function. Dietary manipulation should be an integral part of the therapy for patients with progressive CKD.

Study 40

Title: Adherence to ketoacids/essential amino acids supplemented low protein diets and new indications for patients with chronic kidney disease[61]

Main outcomes: Effects on proteinuria

CONCLUSION:

Taken together, these new research data confirm an overall picture that a low protein diet providing 0.3–0.6 g/kg Body Weight/day with added KA (ketoanalogues) / EAA (essential amino acids) supplements may improve proteinuria and delays time until dialysis has to be started. The latter most likely occurs because uremic toxicity is reduced.

Study 41

Title: Protein-Restricted Diets Plus Keto/Amino Acids - A Valid Therapeutic Approach for Chronic Kidney Disease Patients[62]

Main outcomes: Effects on proteinuria and metabolic products

ABSTRACT:

Chronic kidney disease (CKD) is increasingly common, and there is an increasing awareness that every strategy should be used to avoid complications of CKD. Restriction of dietary protein intake has been a relevant part of the management of CKD for more than 100 years, but even today, the principal goal of protein restricted regimens is to decrease the accumulation of nitrogen waste products, hydrogen ions, phosphates, and inorganic ions while maintaining an adequate nutritional status to avoid secondary problems such as metabolic acidosis, bone disease, and insulin resistance, as well as proteinuria and deterioration of renal function. This supplement focuses on recent experimental and clinical findings related to an optimized dietary management of predialysis, dialysis, and transplanted patients as an important aspect of patient care. Nutritional treatment strategies are linked toward ameliorating metabolic and endocrine disturbances, improving/maintaining nutritional status, as well as delaying the renal replacement initiation and improving outcomes in CKD patients. A final consensus states that dietary manipulations should be considered as one of the main approaches in the management program of CKD patients and that a reasonable number of patients with moderate or severe CKD benefit from dietary protein/phosphorus restriction.

Study 42

Title: Metabolic effects of two low protein diets in chronic kidney disease stage 4-5—a randomized controlled trial[63]

Main outcomes: Effects on proteinuria and metabolic products

BACKGROUND:

International guidelines have not reached a complete agreement about the optimal amount of dietary proteins in chronic kidney disease (CKD). The aim of this study was to compare, with a randomized controlled design, the metabolic effects of two diets with different protein content (0.55 vs 0.80 g/kg/day) in patients with CKD stages 4-5.

RESULTS:

Mean age was 61+/-18 years, 44% were women, mean eGFR was 18+/-7 ml/min/month. Three months after the dietary assignment and throughout the study period the two groups had a significantly different protein intake (0.72 vs 0.92 g/kg/day). The intention to treat analysis did not show any difference between the two groups. Compliance to the two test diets was significantly different ($P < 0.05$): 27% in the 0.55-Group and 53% in the 0.8-Group, with male gender and protein content (0.8 g/kg/day) predicting adherence to the assigned diet. The per protocol analysis, conversely, showed that serum urea nitrogen, similar at the time of randomization, significantly increased in the 0.8-Group vs 0.55-Group by 15% ($P < 0.05$). Serum phosphate, PTH and bicarbonate resulted similar in the two groups throughout the study. The 24 h urinary urea nitrogen significantly decreased after the first 3 months in 0.55-Group ($P < 0.05$), as well as the excretion of creatinine, sodium and phosphate ($P < 0.05$ vs baseline) and were significantly lower than the 0.8-Group. The prescription of phosphate binders, allopurinol, bicarbonate supplements and diuretics resulted significantly less frequent in the 0.55-Group ($P < 0.05$).

CONCLUSIONS:

This study represents the first evidence that in CKD patients a protein intake of 0.55 g/kg/day, compared with a 0.8 g/kg/day, guarantees a better metabolic control and a reduced need of drugs, without a substantial risk of malnutrition.

Study 43

Title: Eleven reasons to control the protein intake of patients with chronic kidney disease[64]

Main outcomes: Effects on proteinuria and metabolic products

ABSTRACT:

For many years patients with chronic kidney disease have been advised to control the protein content of their diet. This advice has been given on the basis of a number of reported metabolic effects of lowering protein intake, such as lowering serum urea nitrogen levels, improving phosphocalcic metabolism and insulin resistance and, more recently, ameliorating proteinuria (independent of antiproteinuric medications). The effects on the progression of kidney disease, although spectacular in experimental studies, have been less convincing in humans. It is possible that flawed design of clinical trials is responsible for this discrepancy. In this Review, we comment on experimental findings that indicate that limiting protein intake protects the kidney and ameliorates uremic symptoms, outline how the body adapts to a reduction in protein intake, and describe the metabolic benefits to the patient. We then review the evidence from randomized controlled trials and meta-analyses that pertains to the effects of low-protein diets in adults with chronic kidney disease.

Study 44

Title: Effect of Keto Acids on Asymmetric Dimethylarginine, Muscle, and Fat Tissue in Chronic Kidney Disease and After Kidney Transplantation[65]

Main outcomes: Effects on proteinuria

CONCLUSION:

In conclusion, both studies clearly demonstrated that in obese non-transplant and transplanted CKD patients, a long-term low-protein diet supplemented with keto acids/amino acids can reduce BMI and body fat mass, decrease plasma concentrations of ADMA (Assymteric Dimethylarginine), and reduce proteinuria.

Study 45

Title: Comparison of the effects of alpha-keto/ amino acid supplemented low protein diet and diabetes diet in patients with diabetic nephropathy[66]

Main outcomes: Effects on proteinuria

CONCLUSION:

Alpha-keto/amino acid can reduce proteinuria more effectively, while improve renal function and nutritional status in diabetic nephropathy patients with well toleration.

Study 46

Title: Keto-Acid Therapy in Predialysis Chronic Kidney Disease Patients: Consensus Statements[67]

Main outcomes: Effects on proteinuria and metabolic products

CONCLUSION:

Keto acid/amino acid-supplemented protein-restricted diets:

> Decrease uremic toxins;

> Reduce proteinuria;

> Improve calcium-phosphate metabolism/hyper parathyroidism;

> Improve the lipid profile;

> May slow the progression of CKD;

> Will delay the time until dialysis is required to treat uremic symptoms;

> Do not induce malnutrition; and

> Improve quality of life.

Study 47

Title: Keto-supplemented Low Protein Diet: A Valid

Therapeutic Approach For Patients With Steroid-Resistant Proteinuria During Early-Stage Chronic Kidney Disease[68]

Main outcomes: Effects on proteinuria and renal protection

CONCLUSION:

sLPD (Supplemented low protein diet) is both nutritionally safe and beneficial, providing nephroprotective effects for early-stage CKD patients with steroid-resistant proteinuria.

Study 48

Title: Effects of low-protein diet supplemented with ketoacids and erythropoietin in chronic renal failure: a long-term metabolic study[69]

Main outcomes: Effects on proteinuria and kidney function

ABSTRACT:

Ketoacids (KA) and recombinant human erythropoietin (rHuEPO) may each, on their own, influence the metabolic status of patients with chronic renal failure (CRF). A long-term prospective randomized study was designed to monitor the metabolic and nutritional status and progression of CRF using three therapeutic protocols: (A) low-protein diet (LPD) with 0.6 g of protein and 35kcal/kg/day, with recombinant human erythropoietin (rHuEPO) at a dose of 40 U kg/week and ketoacids (KA) 100 mg/kg/day, (Group I), (B) LPD and rHuEPO (Group II), and (C) LPD only (Group III).A total of 105 patients (50M/55F), aged 26-78 years, CCr 22-36 ml/min, were monitored at the beginning, and at every 6 months for 3 years in the above three study groups. Group I comprised 35 patients, Group II 38 patients and Group III 32 patients. During follow-up, a significantly smaller decrease in GFR (CCr, Cin) and in I/SCr, and an increase in serum albumin, transferrin, leucine, body mass, index and HDL-cholesterol were found in Group I (all $p < 0.01$). In addition, significant decreases were also seen in proteinuria, renal fractional leucine excretion and serum triglycerides level ($p < 0.01$). Co-administration of LPD, rHuEPO and KA thus constitutes an effective alternative to conservative management of CRF, delaying in follow-up period progression of renal failure and correction of metabolic parameters.

Study 49

Title: Conservative treatment with ketoacid and amino acid supplemented low-protein diets in chronic renal failure[70]

Main outcomes: Effects on kidney function

ABSTRACT:

Twenty-six patients with advanced renal failure (glomerular filtration rate less than 6 ml/min) were treated with a mixed quality low protein diet and ketoacid analogues. An improvement in nitrogen balance, serum transferrin and phosphate, and base excess was observed after 2 weeks of treatment. In a longer term study, the result of 20 patients treated with ketoacids for up to 14 months were compared to a group 40 patients who received a low-protein diet with essential amino acids. Patients responded similarly to the two diets; however, the group receiving ketoacids had a significantly lower glomerular filtration rate.

There was improvement in calcium and phosphate metabolism with ketoacid treatment. The patients were able to tolerate treatment with both the ketoacids and vitamin D.

Study 50

Title: Effect of protein restriction diet on renal function and metabolic control in patients with type 2 diabetes: a randomized clinical trial[71]

Main outcomes: Effects on kidney function

ABSTRACT:

A randomized clinical trial was conducted on 60 patients with type 2 diabetes in primary care -19 with normoalbuminuria, 22 with microalbuminuria, and 19 with macroalbuminuria. All patients experienced a screening phase during the 3 months, and were designated according to percentages of daily caloric intake (e.g., carbohydrates 50%, fat 30%, and 20% of protein). After this period, they were randomly assigned to receive either LPD (0.6-0.8 g/kg per day) or normal protein diet (NPD) (1.0-1.2 g/kg per day) for a period of 4 months. Twenty nine patients received LPD and 31 received NPD. Primary endpoints included measures of renal function (UAER, serum creatinine and GFR) and glycemic control (fasting glucose and glycosylated hemoglobin A1c).

RESULTS:

Renal function improved among patients with macroalbuminuria who received LPD: UAER decreased (1,280.7 +/- 1,139.7 to 444.4 +/- 329.8 mg/24 h; $p < 0.05$) and GFR increased (56.3 +/- 29.0-74.2 +/- 40.4 ml/min; $p < 0.05$). In normoalbuminuric and microalbuminuric patients, there were no significant changes in UAER or GFR after either diet. HbA1c decreased significantly among microalbuminuric patients on both diets (LPD, 8.2 +/- 1.6-7.2 +/- 1.8%; $p < 0.05$; NPD, 8.8 +/- 1.9-7.1 +/- 0.8%; $p < 0.05$) and among macroalbuminuric patients who received NPD (8.1 +/- 1.8-6.9 +/- 1.6%; $p < 0.05$).

CONCLUSIONS:

A moderated protein restriction diet improved the renal function in patients with type diabetes 2 and macroalbuminuria.

Study 51

Title: Treatment of chronic kidney disease patients with ketoanalogue-supplemented low-protein diet and ketoanalogue-supplemented very-low-protein diet[72]

Main outcomes: Effects on renal functions

CONCLUSIONS:

The CKD patients on sLPD (supplemented low protein diet) and sVLPD (supplemented very low protein diet) showed improvement in renal function, metabolic status, and nutrition.

Study 52

Title: Is There a Role for Ketoacid Supplements in the Management of CKD?[73]

Main outcomes: Effects on production of toxic metabolic products

ABSTRACT:

Ketoacid (KA) analogues of essential amino acids (EAAs) provide several potential advantages for people with advanced chronic kidney disease (CKD). Because KAs lack the amino group bound to the $_\alpha$ carbon of an amino acid, they can be converted to their respective amino acids without providing additional nitrogen. It has been well established that a diet with 0.3 to 0.4 g of protein per kilogram per day that is supplemented with KAs and EAAs reduces the generation of potentially toxic metabolic products, as well as the burden of potassium, phosphorus, and possibly sodium, while still providing calcium. These KA/EAA-supplemented very-low-protein diets (VLPDs) can maintain good nutrition, but the appropriate dose of the KA/EAA supplement has not been established. Thus, a KA/ EAA dose-response study for good nutrition clearly is needed. Similarly, the composition of the KA/EAA supplement needs to be reexamined; for example, some KA/EAA preparations contain neither the EAA phenylalanine nor its analogue. Indications concerning when to inaugurate a KA/EAA-supplemented VLPD therapy also are unclear. Evidence strongly suggests that these diets can delay the need for maintenance dialysis therapy, but whether they slow the loss of glomerular filtration rate in patients with CKD is less clear, particularly in this era of more vigorous blood pressure control and use of angiotensin/ aldosterone blockade. Some clinicians prescribe KA/ EAA supplements for patients with CKD or treated with maintenance dialysis, but with diets that have much higher protein levels than the VLPDs in which these supplements have been studied. More research is needed to examine the effectiveness of KA/EAA supplements with higher protein intakes.

Study 53

Title: Pharmaco-Economic Evaluation of Keto Acid/ Amino Acid-Supplemented Protein-Restricted Diets[74]

Main outcomes: Effects on production of metabolic products

CONCLUSION:

In conclusion, the severely protein-restricted diet supplemented with keto analogues of essential amino acids seems to be effective and safe in ameliorating nitrogen waste-product retention and acid-base and calcium-phosphorus metabolism disturbances, and in delaying the initiation of RRT (Renal Replacement Therapy), with no deleterious effects on nutritional status in some patients with CKD.

Study 54

Title: Conservative long-term treatment of chronic renal failure with keto acid and amino acid supplementation[75]

Main outcomes: Effects on production of metabolic products

CONCLUSION:

It can be concluded that a low-protein diet supplemented with EAA or KA can improve the uremic metabolism, rehabilitation status and safely postpone the start of maintenance dialysis.

Study 55

Title: Ketoanalogue-Supplemented Vegetarian Very Low–Protein Diet and CKD Progression[76]

Main outcomes: Effects on metabolic products

ABSTRACT:

Dietary protein restriction may improve determinants of CKD progression. However, the extent of improvement and effect of ketoanalogue supplementation are unclear. We conducted a prospective, randomized, controlled trial of safety and efficacy of ketoanalogue– supplemented vegetarian very low–protein diet (KD) compared with conventional low–protein diet (LPD). Primary end point was RRT initiation or .50% reduction in initial eGFR. Non-diabetic adults with stable eGFR,30 ml/min per 1.73 m^2, proteinuria ,1 g/g urinary creatinine, good nutritional status, and good diet compliance entered a run-in phase on LPD. After 3 months, compliant patients were randomized to KD (0.3 g/kg vegetable proteins and 1 cps/5 kg ketoanalogues per day) or continue LPD (0.6 g/kg per day) for 15 months. Only 14% of screened patients were randomized, with no differences between groups. Adjusted numbers needed to treat (NNTs; 95% confidence interval) to avoid composite primary end point in intention to treat and per-protocol analyses in one patient were 4.4 (4.2 to 5.1) and 4.0 (3.9 to 4.4), respectively, for patients with eGFR, 30 ml/min per 1.73 m^2. Adjusted NNT (95% confidence interval) to avoid dialysis was 22.4 (21.5 to 25.1) for patients with eGFR, 30 ml/min per 1.73 m^2 but decreased to 2.7 (2.6 to 3.1) for patients with eGFR, 20 ml/min per 1.73 m^2 in intention to treat analysis. Correction of metabolic abnormalities occurred only with KD (Keto supplemented low protein diet). Compliance to diet was good, with no changes in nutritional parameters and no adverse reactions. Thus, this KD seems nutritionally safe and could defer dialysis initiation in some patients with CKD.

Study 56

Title: Metabolic effects of keto acid—amino acid supplementation in patients with chronic renal insufficiency receiving a low-protein diet and recombinant human erythropoietin—a randomized controlled trial[77]

Main outcomes: Effects on oxidative stress

ABSTRACT:

Supplement with keto acids/amino acids (KA) and erythropoietin can independently improve the metabolic sequels of chronic renal insufficiency. Our study was designed to establish whether a supplementation with keto acids/amino acids (KA) exerts additional beneficial metabolic effects in patients with chronic renal insufficiency (CRF) treated with a low-protein diet (LPD) and recombinant human erythropoietin (EPO). In a prospective randomized controlled trial over a period of 12 months, we evaluated a total of 38 patients (20 M/18 F) aged 32-68 years with a creatinine clearance (CCr) of 20-36 ml/min. All patients were receiving EPO (40 U/kg twice a week s.c.) and a low-protein diet (0.6 g protein/kg/day and 145 kJ/kg/day). The diet of 20 patients (Group I) was supplemented with KA at a dosage of 100 mg/kg/day while 18 patients (Group II) received no supplementation. During the study period, the glomerular filtration rate slightly decreased (CCr from28.2 +/- 3.4 to 26.4 +/- 4.1 ml/min and 29.6 +/- 4.8 to 23.4 +/- 4.4 ml/min in groups I and II, respectively and Cin); this however was more marked in Group II (Group I vs. Group II, $p < 0.01$). The serum levels of urea also declined ($p < 0.01$), more pronouncedly in Group I ($p < 0.025$). In Group I, there was a significant rise in the levels of leucine ($p < 0.01$), isoleucine ($p < 0.01$), valine ($p < 0.02$) and albumin ($p < 0.01$) and a decrease in proteinuria ($p < 0.01$). Analysis of the lipid spectrum revealed a mild yet significant decrease in total cholesterol and LDL cholesterol ($p < 0.02$), more pronounced in Group I. In Group I, there was a decrease in plasma triglycerides (from4.2 +/- 0.8 down to values a low as 2.2 +/- 0.6 mmol/L; $p < 0.01$) whereas HDL-cholesterol levels increased (from 0.9 +/- 0.1 to 1.2 +/- 0.1 mmol/L, $p < 0.01$). A further remarkable finding was a reduction in the serum concentration of free radicals ($p < 0.01$). We conclude that a KA supplementation in patients with CRF receiving LPD and EPO potentiates the beneficial effects on metabolism of proteins, amino acids and surprisingly, also lipids.

Study 57

Title: Cardiovascular risk factors in severe chronic renal failure: the role of dietary treatment[78]

Main outcomes: Effects on oxidative stress

CONCLUSION:

Aim of this study was to investigate the influence of vegan diet supplemented with essential amino acids (EAA) and ketoanalogues (VSD) on both traditional and nontraditional cardiovascular risk factors (CVRF). These results indicate a better lipoprotein profile in patients on vegan diet including nontraditional CVRF. In particular, these patients show a reduced oxidative stress with a reduced acute-phase response (CRP) as compared to patients on conventional diet. We hypothesize that urea, significantly lower in patients on VSD, may account, possibly together with the reduction of other protein break down products, for the decreased acute-phase response observed in these patients. Our findings suggest that low-protein diets, and vegan in particular, may exert a beneficial effect on the development of cardiovascular disease in patients with end-stage renal disease (ESRD).

Study 58

Title: Keto diet, physiological calcium intake and native vitamin D improve renal osteodystrophy[79]

Main outcomes: Effects on renal osteodystrophy

CONCLUSION:

In patients with advanced renal failure (GFR<20 ml/ min) a VLPD (very low protein diet) supplemented with calcium salts of keto analogues, 1 g of calcium carbonate, and 1,000 IU of vitamin D2 has a favorable effect on both components of renal osteodystrophy. The beneficial effect on osteitis fibrosa is mainly explained by the decrease of plasma PTH levels secondary to a decrease in plasma phosphate independently of permanent changes in plasma concentration of calcium and calcitriol, possibly in association with the correction of acidosis and the increase in plasma 25 OH vitamin D. The beneficial effect on osteomalacia also occurs without significant changes in plasma calcium and calcitriol, and is mainly explained by the correction of acidosis.

Study 59

Title: Role of keto acids in the prophylaxis and treatment of renal osteopathy[80]

Main outcomes: Effects on renal osteopathy

ABSTRACT:

KA administration given in addition to a low-protein diet leads to a reduction of PTH secretion followed by diminishing of osteofibrosis. Osteomalacia will also be reduced by a better control of the calcium-phosphate metabolism, an increase of 1,25-(OH)2-D levels, and a lower burden of aluminum. Therapeutic levels of 25-OH-D and calcitonin (caused by simultaneous administration of vitamin D) are probably necessary to achieve this effect. KA are not only the optimum form of substitution in the nutritional treatment of chronic renal failure, but they seem to be very effective in the treatment of renal osteodystrophy.

Study 60

Title: Long-term outcome on renal replacement therapy in patients who previously received a keto acid–supplemented very-low-protein diet[81]

Main outcomes: Effects on mortality

CONCLUSION:

The lack of correlation between death rate and duration of diet and the moderate mortality rate observed during the first 10 y of renal replacement therapy confirm that a supplemented very-low-protein diet has no detrimental effect on the outcome of patients with chronic kidney disease who receive renal replacement therapy.

Study 61

Title: Survival on Dialysis Among Chronic Renal Failure Patients Treated With a Supplemented Low-Protein Diet Before Dialysis[82]

Main outcomes: Effects on mortality

CONCLUSION:

The data presented suggest that a supplemented low-protein diet plus close follow-up of patients with CRF (Chronic renal failure) may substantially reduce the early mortality on dialysis.

Study 62

Title: Low-protein diet in chronic kidney disease: from questions of effectiveness to those of feasibility[83]

Main outcomes: Effects on quality of life and mortality

SUMMARY:

At present, as the safety of LPD and its beneficial effects on uraemic symptoms are obvious, its prescription to most CKD patients seems justified, even if its effect on CKD progression remains controversial. Indeed, by reducing uraemic symptoms, late dialysis may be safely considered, which is probably the most important point for the patient in terms of quality of life and midterm mortality.

Study 63

Title: Low protein diet supplemented with ketoanalogues makes hemodialysis withdrawal possible[84]

Main outcomes: Effects on long-term survival

CONCLUSION:

In conclusion, for selected, well-informed patients having residual kidney function and able to adhere to a supplemented low-protein diet and medication control, long-term survival after hemodialysis withdrawal can be successfully achieved.

Study 64

Title: Effects of a supplemented very low protein diet in predialysis patients on the serum albumin level, proteinuria, and subsequent survival on dialysis[85]

Main outcomes: Effects on survival

ABSTRACT:

A very low protein diet (0.3 g/kg ideal body weight) supplemented with essential amino acids (or ketoanalogues) is seldom employed at present in chronic renal failure for fear of inducing protein deficiency, especially in patients who also have the nephrotic syndrome. Nevertheless, we have used this dietary regimen in predialysis patients for a number of years. We have shown that when these patients reach the end stage, they rarely exhibit hypoalbuminemia, in contrast to the reported 25-50% hypoalbuminemia at the onset of dialysis nationwide. Furthermore, their survival for the first 2 years on dialysis is much improved, in comparison with the national experience, adjusted for age, sex, and cause of renal disease. When nephrotic patients are given this regimen, they exhibit some improvement in parameters of the nephrotic state, but nevertheless progress to dialysis, provided their initial glomerular filtration rate (GFR) is < 30 ml/min. However, if their initial GFR is > 30 ml/ min, they may show gradual but complete remission of the nephrotic syndrome, even when the underlying disease is diabetic nephropathy or focal segmental glomerulosclerosis. We conclude that this dietary regimen is not only safe in patients with renal failure, with or without the nephritic syndrome, but may be of substantial benefit. The mechanism remains to be explained.

Study 65

Title: The beneficial effect of ketoacids on serum phosphate and parathyroid hormone in patients with chronic uremia[86]

Main outcomes: Effects on phosphate level

ABSTRACT:

Hyperphosphatemia and secondary hyperparathyroidism are regular complications in patients suffering from advanced renal failure. As aluminum-containing drugs carry the well-known risk of aluminum intoxication, we were interested in testing in a prospective study a mixture of ketoanalogues and amino acids which have been shown to lower the serum phosphate and parathyroid hormone in uremic patients. For 3 months, in addition to their diet, 17 uremic patients and 12 hemodialysis patients received a daily supplement of this mixture. Although no additional phosphate binders were administered, serum phosphate decreased significantly in the former group and was slightly lower in the latter. The serum parathyroid hormone level was consistently lowered when the initial concentration was not higher than 20 times normal.

Study 66

Title: Very Low Protein Diet Reduces Indoxyl Sulfate

Levels in Chronic Kidney Disease[87]

Main outcomes: Effects on indoxyl sulfate levels

CONCLUSION:

High levels of indoxyl sulfate (IS) are associated with chronic kidney disease (CKD) progression and increased mortality in CKD patients. VLPD supplemented with ketoanalogues reduced IS serum levels in CKD patients not yet on dialysis.

Study 67

Title: Acute Effects of Very-Low-Protein Diet on FGF23 Levels: A Randomized Study[88]

Main outcomes: Effects on fibroblast growth factor 23 levels

CONCLUSION:

High levels of fibroblast growth factor 23 are associated with mortality, CKD progression, and calcification in CKD patients. A very-low -protein diet supplemented with ketoanalogues reduced fibroblast growth factor 23 levels in CKD patients not yet on dialysis.

Study 68

Title: Effects of dietary protein restriction on albumin and fibrinogen synthesis in macroalbuminuric type 2 diabetic patients[89]

Main outcomes: Effects on albumin and fibrinogen

CONCLUSION:

LPD in type 2 diabetic patients with diabetic nephropathy reduces low-grade inflammatory state, proteinuria, albuminuria, whole-body proteolysis and ASR of fibrinogen, while increasing albumin FSR, ASR and serum concentration.

Study 69

Title: Reduction of plasma asymmetric dimethylarginine in obese patients with chronic kidney disease after three years of a low-protein diet supplemented with keto-amino acids: a randomized controlled trial[90]

Main outcomes: Effects on plasma asymmetric dimethylarginine levels

CONCLUSION:

Compared with the placebo group, long term coadministration of a low-protein diet and keto-amino acids in CKD patients with obesity led to decreases of ADMA, visceral body fat and proteinuria. Concomitant decreases of glycated hemoglobin, LDL-cholesterol and pentosidine may also contribute to the delay in progression of renal failure.

Study 70

Title: Protein synthesis in skeletal muscle of uremic patients: effect of low-protein diet and supplementation with ketoacids[91]

Main outcomes: Effects on protein synthesis

ABSTRACT:

The purpose of this study was to investigate the modifications of muscle protein synthesis activity in uremic patients fed a low-protein diet and a low-protein diet supplemented with a keto acid-amino acid mixture. The protein synthesis activity was evaluated in vitro on isolated muscle ribosomes incubated in a cell-free medium with tritiated leucine. Simultaneously, nitrogen kinetics and amino acid patterns were examined. Protein synthesis activity is correlated with the protein content of the diet in uremic patients. The keto acid-amino acid supplementation enhances protein synthesis. Variations of protein synthesis can be correlated with the variations of nitrogen balance which implies a major role of protein synthesis activity in muscle protein metabolism. Variations in plasma levels of the essential amino acids, mainly leucine and valine, can be correlated with the variations of protein synthesis activity, and these amino acids seem therefore to be mediators of the dietary effects on protein synthesis in uremia.

Study 71

Title: Comparative evaluation of efficacy and safety profile of rhubarb and $_\alpha$-keto analogs of essential amino acids supplementation in patients with diabetic nephropathy[92]

Main outcomes: Effects on clinical and biochemical features

ABSTRACT:

To determine the efficacy and safety profile of rhubarb and $_\alpha$-keto analogs of essential amino acids supplementation in patients of diabetic nephropathy (DN), we studied 96 patients of DN attending a tertiary care center of the North India. The patients were randomly divided into three equal interventional groups. Group I (control) that received conservative management along with placebo, Group II (rhubarb) that received conservative management along with rhubarb capsule (350 mg, thrice daily), and Group III [keto amino acid (KAA)] that received conservative management along with $_\alpha$-keto analogs of essential amino acids (600 mg, thrice daily). The treatment was continued for 12 weeks. Clinical and biochemical parameters were assessed at 0, 4, 8, and 12 weeks of treatment. A progressive improvement in clinical features and biochemical parameters was seen in all three groups after 12 weeks of treatment. The KAA group showed more marked improvement in clinical features as well as biochemical parameters compared to the rhubarb group. There was a reduction in blood glucose, blood urea, serum creatinine, and 24h total urine protein. There was an increase in hemoglobin, 24h total urine volume, and glomerular filtration rate. There was no statistical difference between the rhubarb band KAA groups with respect to side effects ($P > 0.05$). Our study suggests that KAA is more effective than rhubarb as add-on therapy with conservative management in patients of DN.

Study 72

Title: Effects of a Supplemented Hypoproteic Diet in Chronic Kidney Disease[93]

Main outcomes: Effects on nitrogen waste products retention

CONCLUSION:

The SVLPD seems to be effective and safe in ameliorating nitrogen waste products retention and acid-base and calcium-phosphorus metabolism disturbances, and in delaying the RRT initiation, with no deleterious effect on the nutritional status of patients with CKD.

Study 73

Title: Effect of dietary protein restriction on prognosis in patients with diabetic nephropathy[94]

Main outcomes: Effects on prognosis of the disease

CONCLUSION:

Moderate dietary protein restriction improves prognosis in type 1 diabetic patients with progressive diabetic nephropathy in addition to the beneficial effect of antihypertensive treatment.

Study 74

Title: Economic effects of treatment of chronic kidney disease with low-protein diet[95]

Main outcomes: Effects on economic evaluation

CONCLUSION:

The results of these simulations indicate that the treatment of CKD patients with a very low-protein diet is cost-effective relative to a moderate low-protein diet in an Italian setting. Further studies should test this model in other countries with different dialysis costs and dietary support.

4.2. End Stage Renal Disease Studies

Study 1

Title: Very low-protein diet plus ketoacids in chronic kidney disease and risk of death during end-stage renal disease: a historical cohort controlled study[96]

Main outcomes: Effects on mortality

CONCLUSION:

s-VLPD during CKD does not increase mortality in the subsequent RRT (Renal Replacement Therapy) period.

Study 2

Title: Ketoanalogues supplementation decreases dialysis and mortality risk in patients with anemic advanced chronic kidney disease[97]

Main outcomes: Effects on mortality

CONCLUSION:

A total of 1113 events of initiating long-term dialysis and 1228 events of the composite out-come of long-term dialysis or death occurred in patients with advanced CKD after a mean follow-up of 1.57 years. Data analysis suggests KA supplementation is associated with a lower risk for long-term dialysis and the composite outcome when daily dosage is more than 5.5 tablets. The beneficial effect was consistent in subgroup analysis, independent of age, sex, and co-morbidities.

Study 3

Title: Very low protein diets supplemented with ketoanalogues in ESRD predialysis patients and its effect on vascular stiffness and AVF Maturation[98]

Main outcomes: Effects on vascular stiffness

CONCLUSION:

VLPD supplemented with KA/EAA appear to improve the native AVF (arteriovenous fistula) primary outcome, decreasing the initial vascular stiffness, possible by preserving vascular wall quality in CKD patients through a better serum phosphate levels control and the limitation of inflammatory response.

Study 4

Title: Effect of restricted protein diet supplemented with keto analogues in end-stage renal disease: a systematic review and meta-analysis[99]

Main outcomes: Effects on nutritional status

CONCLUSION:

Meta-analysis results indicated that, compared with normal protein diet, low-protein diet (LPD) supplemented with keto analogues (sLPD) could improve serum albumin (P < 0.00001), hyperparathyroidism (P < 0.00001) and hyperphosphatemia (P= 0.008). No differences in triglyceride, cholesterol, hemoglobin, Kt /v and CRP were observed between different protein intake groups. Our meta-analysis indicated that restricted protein diet supplemented with keto analogues may improve nutritional status and prevent hyperparathyroidism in ESRD (End-stage renal disease) patients.

4.3. Exercise

Study 1

Title: Keto analogues and amino acids supplementation induces a decrease of white blood cell counts and a reduction of muscle damage during intense exercise under thermoneutral conditions[100]

Main outcomes: Effects on biomarkers of muscle damage during exercise

ABSTRACT:

This study evaluated the acute effect of keto analogue and amino acid (AA-KAAA) supplementation on both white blood cell counts and the established biomarkers of muscle damage during exercise under thermoneutral conditions. Sixteen male cyclists received a ketogenic diet for two days and were divided into two equal groups: a group taking AA-KAAA (KA) or a control group (PL). The athletes performed a two hour cycling session followed by a maximum incremental test until voluntary exhaustion (VExh). Blood samples were obtained at rest and during exercise for further hematological and biochemical analyses. Exercise-induced ammonemia increased in the PL group at VExh (75%) but remained unchanged in the KA group. Both groups exhibited a significant increase in leukocyte and neutrophil counts of ~85% (~13 × 109L^{-1}), but the shape of the lymphocytes and the eosinophil counts suggest that AA-KAAA supplementation helps prevent lymphocytosis. AA-KAAA supplementation induced a decrease in creatine kinase and aspartate aminotransferase levels at VExh while showing a significant decrease in lactate dehydrogenase at 120 min. We found that AA-KAAA supplementation decreases both the lymphocyte count response in blood and the established biomarkers of muscle damage after intense exercise under a low heat stress environment.

Study 2

Title: Keto analogue and amino acid supplementation and its effects on ammonemia and performance under thermoneutral conditions[101]

Main outcomes: Effects on biomarkers of muscle damage during exercise

ABSTRACT:

Alterations of cerebral function, fatigue and disturbance in cognitive-motor performance can be caused by hyperammonemia and/or hot environmental conditions during exercise. Exercise-induced hyperammonemia can be reduced through supplementation with either amino acids or combined keto analogues and amino acids (KAAA) to improve exercise tolerance. In the present study, we evaluated KAAA supplementation on ammonia metabolism and cognitive-motor performance after high-intensity exercise under a low heat stress environment. Sixteen male cyclists received a ketogenic diet for 2 d and were divided into two groups, KAAA (KEx) or placebo (CEx) supplementation. The athletes performed a 2 h cycling session followed by a maximum test (MAX), and blood samples were obtained at rest and during exercise. Cognitive-motor tasks were performed before and after the protocol, and the exhaustion time was used to evaluate physical performance. The hydration status was also evaluated. The CEx group showed a significant increase (~70%) in ammonia concentration at MAX, which did not change in the KEx group. The non-supplemented group showed a significant increase in uremia. Both the groups has a significant increase in blood urate concentrations at 120 min, and an early significant increase from 120 min was observed in the CEx group. There was no change in the glucose concentrations of the two groups. A significant increase in lactate was observed at the MAX moment in both groups. There was no significant difference in the exhaustion times between the groups. No changes were observed in the cognitive-motor tasks after the protocol. We suggest that KAAA supplementation decreases ammonia concentration during high-intensity exercise but does not affect physical or cognitive-motor performances under a low heat stress environment.

Study 3

Title: The supportive effect of supplementation with α-keto acids on physical training in type 2 diabetes mellitus[102]

Main outcomes: Effects on biomarkers of muscle damage during exercise

ABSTRACT:

The maintenance of physical activity is crucial for the prevention and management of type 2 diabetes(T2D), and exercise induced changes including production of metabolites like ammonia can result in fatigue and exercise intolerance. Nutritional supplements may serve as an effective measure in supporting patients undergoing physical training by acting on their metabolism. This study investigates the effects of supplementation with $_\alpha$-keto acids (KAS) on exercise tolerance and glucose control in T2D patients. In a double-blind, placebo-controlled, randomized study 28 T2D patients underwent 6 weeks training on a cycle ergometer while they were supplemented with either a placebo or KAS (0.2 g kg^{-1} body weight each day). The weekly training volume, power output at maximum and lactic threshold, leg muscle torque, the plasma concentration and 8 h urinary discharge of glucose, ammonia and urea were determined before and after the training as well as after one week of recovery. With KAS the patients did significantly more voluntary exercise (213 vs. 62 min, P <0.01), reached a higher VO2max (27. 3 vs. 24.8 ml min^{-1} kg^{-1}), higher power output (224 vs. 193 watts, P < 0.05) and greater endurance capacity (108 vs. 96 watts at lactic threshold, P < 0.05). Although the patients without KAS improved their glucose control after the training (P < 0.05), this effect could not be maintained after recovery as it was in the KAS group, where there was a prolonged benefit in glucose control. KAS also affected the ammonia and urea metabolism. KAS delivered supportive effects on the physical training along with a prolonged benefit in glucose control in T2D patients.

Study 4

Title: Keto analogue and amino acid supplementation affects the ammonaemia response during exercise under ketogenic conditions[103]

Main outcomes: Effects on biomarkers of muscle damage during exercise

ABSTRACT:

Hyperammonaemia is related to both central and peripheral fatigue during exercise. Hyperammonaemia in response to exercise can be reduced through supplementation with either amino acids or combined keto analogues and amino acids (KAAA). In the present study, we determined the effect of short-term KAAA supplementation on ammonia production in subjects eating a low-carbohydrate diet who exercise. A total of thirteen male cyclists eating a ketogenic diet for 3 d were divided into two groups receiving either KAAA (KEx) or lactose (control group; LEx) supplements. Athletes cycled indoors for 2 h, and blood samples were obtained at rest, during exercise and over the course of 1 h during the recovery period. Exercise-induced ammonaemia increased to a maximum of 35 % in the control group, but no significant increase was observed in the supplemented group. Both groups had a significant increase (approximately 35 %) in uraemia in response to exercise. The resting urate levels of the two groups were equivalent and remained statistically unchanged in the KEx group after 90 min of exercise; an earlier increase was observed in the LEx group. Glucose levels did not change, either during the trial time or between the groups. An increase in lactate levels was observed during the first 30 min of exercise in both groups, but there was no difference between the groups. The present results suggest that the acute use of KAAA diminishes exercise-induced hyperammonaemia.

Study 5

Title: Improved training tolerance by supplementation with α -Keto acids in untrained young adults: a randomized, double blind, placebo-controlled trial[104]

Main outcomes: Effects on exercise tolerance

CONCLUSION:

Under KAS (α -keto acid supplementation), subjects could bear a higher training volume and reach a higher power output and peak muscle torque, accompanied by a better stress-recovery-state. Thus, KAS improves exercise tolerance and training effects along with a better stress-recovery state. Whether the improved training tolerance by KAS is associated with effects on ammonia homeostasis requires further observation.

Study 6

Title: Nitrogen Sparing Induced by a Mixture of Essential Amino Acids Given Chiefly as Their Keto-Analogues during Prolonged Starvation in Obese Subjects[105]

Main outcomes: Effects on starvation

CONCLUSION:

These experiments show that when physiologic mechanisms for conserving nitrogen during starvation reach a maximum, nitrogen losses can be further reduced by infusion of ketoacids. No toxicity or metabolic derangements were observed and no accumulation of ketoacids in plasma occurred.

PART 5: Negative Human Studies

> No studies were found

PART 6: Inconclusive Human Studies

6.1. Chronic Kidney Disease

Study 1

Title: Effect of dietary protein restriction on nutritional status in the Modification of Diet in Renal Disease Study[106]

Main outcomes: Effects on nutritional status

ABSTRACT:

The safety of dietary protein and phosphorous restriction was evaluated in the Modification of Diet in Renal Disease (MDRD) Study. In Study A, 585 patients with a glomerular filtration rate (GFR) of 25 to SS ml/min/l.73 m^2 were randomly assigned to a usual protein diet (1.3 g/kg/day) or a low-protein diet (0.58 g/kg/day). In Study B, 255 patients with a GFR of 13 to 24 ml/min/l.73 m^2 were randomly assigned to the low-protein diet or a very-low-protein diet (0.28g/kg/day), supplemented with a ketoacid-amino acid mixture (0.28 g/kg/day). The low-protein and very-low-protein diets were also low in phosphorus. Mean duration of follow-up was 2.2 years in both studies. Protein and energy intakes were lower in the low-protein and very-low-protein diet groups than in the usual-protein group. Two patients in Study B reached a "stop point" for malnutrition. There was no difference between randomized groups in the rates of death, first hospitalizations, or other "stop points" in either study. Mean values for various indices of nutritional status remained within the normal range during follow-up in each diet group. However, there were small but significant changes from baseline in some nutritional indices, and differences between the randomized groups in some of these changes. In the low-protein and very-low-protein diet groups, serum albumin rose, while serum transferrin, body wt, percent body fat, arm muscle area and urine creatinine excretion declined. Combining patients in both diet groups in each study, a lower achieved protein intake (from food and supplement) was not correlated with a higher rate of death, hospitalization or stop points, or with a progressive decline in any of the indices of nutritional status after controlling for baseline nutritional status and follow-up energy intake. These analyses suggest that the low-protein and very-low-protein diets used in the MDRD Study are safe for periods of two to three years. Nonetheless, both protein and energy intake declined and there were small but significant declines in various indices of nutritional status. These declines are of concern because of the adverse effect of protein calorie malnutrition in patients with end-stage renal disease. Physicians who prescribe low-protein diets must carefully monitor patients' protein and energy intake and nutritional status.

Study 2

Title: Nutritional Status and Dietary Manipulation in Predialysis Chronic Renal Failure Patients[107]

Main outcomes: Effects on nutritional status

CONCLUSION:

Our findings are also consistent with the concept that nutritional status can be maintained in patients eating a very-low-protein diet, supplemented with essential amino acids and ketoacids; there may even be some benefit to this diet in comparison to the standard LPD diet, at least in patients with advanced CRF. On the other hand, we have not identified a mechanism for any benefit of the KAD regimen, and it could be that patients adhering to this diet may simply be more highly motivated, resulting in a much better dietary compliance.

Study 3

Title: Can Renal Replacement Be Deferred by a Supplemented Very Low Protein Diet?[108]

Main outcomes: Effects on renal replacement therapy

ABSTRACT:

Patients with chronic renal failure are commonly started on renal replacement therapy (RRT) as soon as (or, in some centers, before) the usual criteria for severity are met, i.e., GFR,10 ml/min for nondiabetic patients and 15 ml/min for diabetic patients. To determine whether RRT can safely be deferred beyond this point, adults with all types of chronic renal failure who met these criteria on presentation (23 patients) or who reached these levels of severity during treatment (53 patients) were managed conservatively until RRT was judged necessary by their chosen dialysis or transplantation team, without input into this decision from the present authors. Patients were prescribed a very low protein diet (0.3g/kg) plus supplemental essential amino acids and/or ketoacids and followed closely. The intervals between the time at which GFR became less than 10 ml/min (15 ml/min in diabetic patients) and the date at which renal replacement therapy was started were used as estimates of renal survival on nutritional therapy. Kaplan–Meier analysis showed median renal survival of 353 d. Acidosis and hypercholesterolemia were both predictive of shorter renal survival. Signs of malnutrition did not develop. Final GFR averaged 5.6 6 1.9 ml/min. Two patients died; thus, annual mortality was only 2.5%. Hospitalizations totaled 19 in 93 patient-years of treatment, or 0.2 per year. Thus, these well motivated patients with GFR, 10 ml/min (15 ml/min in diabetic patients) were safely managed by diet and close follow-up for a median of nearly 1 yr without dialysis. It is concluded that further study of this approach is indicated.

Study 4

Title: Effect of a keto acid-amino acid supplement on the metabolism and renal elimination of branched-chain amino acids in patients with chronic renal insufficiency on a low protein diet[109]

Main outcomes: Effects on renal amino acid and protein excretion

ABSTRACT:

The aim of our study was to evaluate the effect of a low-protein diet supplemented with keto acids-amino acids on renal function and urinary excretion of branched-chain amino acids (BCAA) in patients with chronic renal insufficiency (CRI). In a prospective investigation 28 patients with CRI (16 male, 12 female, aged 28-66 yrs, CCr 18.6 +/- 10.2 ml/min) on a low-protein diet (0.6 g of protein /kg BW/day and energy intake 140 kJ/kg BW/day) for a period of one month were included. Subsequently, this low protein diet was supplemented with keto acids-amino acids at a dose of 0.1g/kg BW/day orally for a period of 3 months. Examinations performed at baseline and at the end of the follow-up period revealed significant increase in the serum levels of BCAA leucine ($p < 0.02$), isoleucine ($p < 0.03$), and valine ($p < 0.02$) while their renal fractional excretion declined ($p < 0.02$, $p< 0.01$ resp.). Keto acid-amino acid administration had no effect on renal function and on the clearance of inulin, paraamino hippuric acid. Endogenous creatinine and urea clearance remained unaltered. A significant correlation between fractional excretion of sodium and leucine ($p < 0.05$) and a hyperbolic relationship between inulin clearance and fractional excretion of BCAA ($p < 0.01$) were seen. Moreover, a significant decrease in proteinuria ($p < 0.02$), plasma urea concentration and renal urea excretion and a rise in albumin level ($p < 0.03$) were noted. We conclude that in patients with CRI on a low protein diet the supplementation of keto acids-amino acids does not affect renal hemodynamics, but is associated—despite increases in plasma concentrations—with a reduction of renal amino acid and protein excretion suggesting induction of alterations in the tubular transport mechanisms.

Study 5

Title: The effect of oral essential amino acids and their ketoanalogues on children receiving regular haemodialysis[110]

Main outcomes: Effects on renal amino acid and protein excretion

ABSTRACT:

The plasma aminogram in uremic children receiving conservative treatment or undergoing hemodialysis demonstrated a similar profile to that first described in adults and children. We were able to demonstrate that dialysis did not correct the abnormal plasma amino acid pattern and that free amino acid losses in the dialysate during hemodialysis could not be compensated for by children receiving an adequate protein intake. Oral supplementation with essential amino acids (EAA) or ketoanalogues (KAA) only partially corrected the amino acid abnormalities and biochemical improvement in protein metabolism was not observed, however, increasing the relative proportions of branch chain amino acids in the supplement might be associated with improvement in metabolism. These data are in contrast to previous studies on the use of EAA or KAA in adults and children in which patients received a reduced protein intake, whereas in the present study protein intake was not restricted. The raised plasma levels of methionine and 3-methyl-histidinewere not associated with side effects.

Study 6

Title: A meta-analysis of the effects of dietary protein restriction on the rate of decline in renal function[111]

Main outcomes: Effects on progression of the disease

ABSTRACT:

Dietary protein restriction has been reported to delay the need for renal replacement therapy in clinical trials and meta-analyses. However, less clear is what effect dietary protein has on the rate of decline in renal function. We pooled the results of 13 randomized controlled trials (n = 1,919 patients) and found that dietary protein restriction reduced the rate of decline in estimated glomerular filtration rate by only 0.53 mL/min/yr (95% confidence interval [CI], 0.08 to 0.98 mL/min/yr). We also used weighted regression analysis to determine the reasons for the differences in the results of these 13 randomized trials along with 11 other nonrandomized controlled trials (n = 2,248 patients). The effect of dietary protein restriction (glomerular filtration rate decline in treatment minus control) was substantially less in randomized versus nonrandomized trials (regression coefficient, -5.2 mL/ min/yr; 95% CI, -7.8 to -2.5 mL/min/yr; P < 0.05) and relatively greater among diabetic versus nondiabetic patients (5.4 mL/min/yr; 95% CI, 0.3 to 10.5 mL/ min/yr; P < 0.05), while there was a trend toward a greater effect with each additional year of follow-up (2.1 mL/min/yr; 95% CI, -0.05 to 4.2 mL/min/yr; P = NS). However, the number of diabetic patients studied was small and the duration of follow-up was short in most trials. No other patient or study characteristics altered the effect of dietary protein restriction on the rate of decline in renal function. Thus, although dietary protein restriction retards the rate of renal function decline, the relatively weak magnitude of this effect suggests that better therapies are needed to slow the rate of renal disease progression.

Study 7

Title: Effect of dietary protein restriction on the progression of kidney disease: long-term follow-up of the Modification of Diet in Renal Disease (MDRD) Study[112]

Main outcomes: Effects on progression of the disease

CONCLUSION:

The efficacy of a 2- to 3-year intervention of dietary protein restriction on progression of non-diabetic kidney disease remains inconclusive. Future studies should include a longer duration of intervention and follow-up.

6.2. End Stage Renal Disease

Study 1

Title: Effects of severe protein restriction with ketoanalogues in advanced renal failure[113]

Main outcomes: Effects on kidney functions and phosphocalcic plasma parameters

CONCLUSION:

Compared to a moderate protein restriction (0.65 g/ kg/day), a severe protein restriction (0.3 g/ kg/day) supplemented by ketoanologues does not limit GFR decrease when GFR is below 20 mL/ min/1.73m2, but improves phosphocalcic plasma parameters.

References

1. Zhang Y, Huang J, Yang M, Gu L, Ji J, Wang L, et al. Effect of a low-protein diet supplemented with keto-acids on autophagy and inflammation in 5 / 6 nephrectomized rats. 2015;1–13.

2. Wang D-T, Lu L, Shi Y, Geng Z-B, Yin Y, Wang M, et al. Supplementation of ketoacids contributes to the up-regulation of the Wnt7a/Akt/p70S6K pathway and the down-regulation of apoptotic and ubiquitin-proteasome systems in the muscle of 5/6 nephrectomised rats. *Br J Nutr*. 2014 May;111(9):1536–48.

3. Huang J, Yuan W, Wang J, Gu L, Yin J, Dong T, et al. Autophagylysosome pathway in skeletal muscle of diabetic nephropathy rats and the effect of low-protein diet plus $_a$-keto acids on it. *Zhonghua Yi Xue Za Zhi*. 2013 Nov 26;93(44):3551–5.

4. Huang J, Wang J, Gu L, Bao J, Yin J, Tang Z, et al. Effect of a Low-Protein Diet Supplemented with Ketoacids on Skeletal Muscle Atrophy and Autophagy in Rats with Type 2 Diabetic Nephropathy. 2013;8(11):1–12.

5. Gao X, Huang L, Grosjean F, Esposito V, Wu J, Fu L, et al. Lowprotein diet supplemented with ketoacids reduces the severity of renal disease in 5/6 nephrectomized rats: a role for KLF15. *Kidney Int*. 2011 May;79(9):987–96.

6. Gao X, Wu J, Dong Z, Hua C, Hu H, Mei C. A low-protein diet supplemented with ketoacids plays a more protective role against oxidative stress of rat kidney tissue with 5/6 nephrectomy than a low-protein diet alone. *Br J Nutr*. 2010 Feb 2;103(04):608.

7. Yang X, Yang M, Cheng M, Ma L-B, Xie X-C, Han S, et al. Effects of Low-Protein Diets Supplemented with Ketoacid on Expression of TGF-$_β$ and Its Receptors in Diabetic Rats. *Biomed Res Int*. 2015;2015:1–7.

8. Zhang J, Yin Y, Ni L, Long Q, You L, Zhang Q, et al. Low-protein diet supplemented with ketoacids ameliorates proteinuria in 3/4 nephrectomised rats by directly inhibiting the intrarenal renin– angiotensin system. *Br J Nutr*. 2016 Nov 18;116(09):1491–501.

9. Dong W, Zhou M, Dong M, Pan B, Liu Y, Shao J, et al. Keto acid metabolites of branched-chain amino acids inhibit oxidative stress-induced necrosis and attenuate myocardial ischemia– reperfusion injury. *J Mol Cell Cardiol*. 2016 Dec;101:90–8.

10. de Almeida RD, Seixas Prado E, Daniel Llosa C, Magalhães-Neto A, Cameron L-C. Acute supplementation with keto analogues and amino acids in rats during resistance exercise. *Br J Nutr*. 2010 Nov 2;104(10):1438–42.

11. Aparicio M, Bellizzi V, Chauveau P, Cupisti A, Ecder T, Fouque D, et al. Do Ketoanalogues Still Have a Role in Delaying Dialysis Initiation in CKD Predialysis Patients? *Semin Dial*. 2013 Nov;26(6):714–9.

12. Garneata L, Mircescu G. Effect of Low-Protein Diet Supplemented With Keto Acids on Progression of Chronic Kidney Disease. *J Ren Nutr*. 2013 May;23(3):210–3.

13. Kovesdy CP, Kopple JD, Kalantar-Zadeh K. Management of protein-energy wasting in non-dialysis-dependent chronic kidney disease: reconciling low protein intake with nutritional therapy. *Am J Clin Nutr.* 2013 Jun 1;97(6):1163–77.

14. Zemchenkov A, Konakova IN. Efficacy of the Essential Amino Acids and Keto-Analogues on the CKD progression rate in real practice in Russia - city nephrology registry data for outpatient clinic. *BMC Nephrol.* 2016 Dec 7;17(1):62.

15. Piccoli GB, Ferraresi M, Deagostini MC, Vigotti FN, Consiglio V, Scognamiglio S, et al. Vegetarian low-protein diets supplemented with keto analogues: a niche for the few or an option for many? *Nephrol Dial Transplant.* 2013 Sep 1;28(9):2295–305.

16. Jiang N, Qian J, Sun W, Lin A, Cao L, Wang Q, et al. Better preservation of residual renal function in peritoneal dialysis patients treated with a low-protein diet supplemented with keto acids: a prospective, randomized trial. *Nephrol Dial Transplant.* 2009 Aug 1;24(8):2551–8.

17. Sigitova ON, Arkhipov E V, Kim TY. Analysis of the Effectiveness of Renoprotection of Low-Protein Diet and Ketoanalogues of Amino Acids In Patients With Chronic Kidney Disease. *Kardiologiia.* 2015;55(9):43–9.

18. Milovanov IS, Lysenko L V, Milovanova LI, Dobrosmyslov IA. The role of balanced low-protein diet in inhibition of predialysis chronic kidney disease progression in patients with systemic diseases. *Ter Arkh.* 2009;81(8):52–7.

19. Molnár M, Szekeresné Izsák M, Nagy J, Figler M. The effect of low-protein diet supplemented with ketoacids in patients with chronic renal failure. *Orv Hetil.* 2009 Feb;150(5):217–24.

20. Masud T, Young VR, Chapman T, Maroni BJ. Adaptive responses to very low protein diets: the first comparison of ketoacids to essential amino acids. *Kidney Int.* 1994 Apr;45(4):1182–92.

21. Walser M, Hill SB, Ward L, Magder L. A crossover comparison of progression of chronic renal failure: ketoacids versus amino acids. *Kidney Int.* 1993 Apr;43(4):933–9.

22. Prakash S, Pande DP, Sharma S, Sharma D, Bal CS, Kulkarni H. Randomized, double-blind, placebo-controlled trial to evaluate efficacy of ketodiet in predialytic chronic renal failure. *J Ren Nutr.* 2004 Apr;14(2):89–96.

23. Walser M, Hill S, Ward L. Progression of chronic renal failure on substituting a ketoacid supplement for an amino acid supplement. *J Am Soc Nephrol.* 1992 Jan;2(7):1178–85.

24. Walser M, LaFrance ND, Ward L, VanDuyn MA. Progression of chronic renal failure in patients given ketoacids following amino acids. *Kidney Int.* 1987 Jul;32(1):123–8.

25. Walser M, Ward L. Progression of chronic renal failure is related to glucocorticoid production. *Kidney Int.* 1988 Dec;34(6):859–66.

26. Cano NJM. Branched-Chain Amino-Acid Metabolism in Renal Failure. *J Ren Nutr*. 2009 Sep;19(5):S22–4.

27. Deniz Ayli M, Ayli M, Ensari C, Mandiroglu F, Allioglu M. Effect of Low-Protein Diet Supplemented with Keto Acids on Progression of Disease in Patients with Chronic Renal Failure. *Nephron*. 2000;84(3):288–9.

28. De Santo NG, Perna A, Cirillo M. Low protein diets are mainstay for management of chronic kidney disease. *Front Biosci*. 2011 Jun 1;3:1432–42.

29. Teschan PE, Beck GJ, Dwyer JT, Greene T, Klahr S, Levy AS, et al. Effect of a ketoacid-aminoacid-supplemented very low protein diet on the progression of advanced renal disease: a reanalysis of the MDRD feasibility study. *Clin Nephrol*. 1998 Nov;50(5):273– 83.

30. Tzekov VD, Tilkian EE, Pandeva SM, Nikolov DG, Kumchev EP, Manev EI, et al. Low protein diet and ketosteril in predialysis patients with renal failure. *Folia Med*. 2000;42(2):34–7.

31. Pedrini MT, Levey AS, Lau J, Chalmers TC, Wang PH. The effect of dietary protein restriction on the progression of diabetic and nondiabetic renal diseases: a meta-analysis. *Ann Intern Med*. 1996 Apr 1;124(7):627–32.

32. Jiang Z, Zhang X, Yang L, Li Z, Qin W. Effect of restricted protein diet supplemented with keto analogues in chronic kidney disease: a systematic review and meta-analysis. *Int Urol Nephrol*. 2016 Mar;48(3):409–18.

33. Fouque D, Laville M, Boissel JP. Low protein diets for chronic kidney disease in non diabetic adults. *Cochrane database Syst Rev*. 2006 Apr 19;(2):CD001892.

34. Duenhas M, Gonçalves E, Dias M, Leme G, Laranja S. Reduction of morbidity related to emergency access to dialysis with very low protein diet supplemented with ketoacids (VLP-D+KA). *Clin Nephrol*. 2013 May 1;79(05):387–93.

35. Mou S, Li J, Yu Z, Wang Q, Ni Z. Keto acid-supplemented lowprotein diet for treatment of adult patients with hepatitis B virus infection and chronic glomerulonephritis. *J Int Med Res*. 2013 Feb 24;41(1):129–37.

36. CHANG JH, KIM DK, PARK JT, KANG EW, YOO TH, KIM BS, et al. Influence of ketoanalogs supplementation on the progression in chronic kidney disease patients who had training on low-protein diet. *Nephrology*. 2009 Dec;14(8):750–7.

37. Cupisti A, Bolasco P. Keto-analogues and essential aminoacids and other supplements in the conservative management of chronic kidney disease. *Panminerva Med*. 2017 Jun;59(2):149–56.

38. Milovanova SY, Milovanov YS, Taranova M V., Dobrosmyslov IA. Effects of keto/amino acids and a low-protein diet on the nutritional status of patients with Stages 3B-4 chronic kidney disease. *Ter Arkh*. 2017;89(6):30.

39. Milovanov IS, Kozlovskaia L V, Milovanova LI. Nephroprotective role of early correction of impaired nutritional status in patients with chronic disease of the kidneys at a predialysis stage. *Ter Arkh*. 2008;80(6):29–33.

40. Tom K, Young VR, Chapman T, Masud T, Akpele L, Maroni BJ. Long-term adaptive responses to dietary protein restriction in chronic renal failure. *Am J Physiol Metab*. 1995 Apr;268(4):E668–77.

41. Mitch WE, Abras E, Walser M. Long-term effects of a new ketoacid-amino acid supplement in patients with chronic renal failure. *Kidney Int*. 1982 Jul;22(1):48–53.

42. Jones R, Dalton N, Turner C, Start K, Haycock G, Chantler C. Oral essential amino-acid and ketoacid supplements in children with chronic renal failure. *Kidney Int*. 1983 Jul;24(1):95–103.

43. Aparicio M, Bellizzi V, Chauveau P, Cupisti A, Ecder T, Fouque D, et al. Protein-restricted diets plus keto/amino acids—a valid therapeutic approach for chronic kidney disease patients. *J Ren Nutr*. 2012 Mar;22(2 Suppl):S1-21.

44. Feiten SF, Draibe SA, Watanabe R, Duenhas MR, Baxmann AC, Nerbass FB, et al. Short-term effects of a very-low-protein diet supplemented with ketoacids in nondialyzed chronic kidney disease patients. *Eur J Clin Nutr*. 2005 Jan 8;59(1):129–36.

45. Mir S, Özkayin N, Akgun A. The role of keto acids in the supportive treatment of children with chronic renal failure. *Pediatr Nephrol*. 2005 Jul 26;20(7):950–5. 6

46. Zakar G, Hungarian Ketosteril Cohort Study. The effect of a keto acid supplement on the course of chronic renal failure and nutritional parameters in predialysis patients and patients on regular hemodialysis therapy: the Hungarian Ketosteril Cohort Study. *Wien Klin Wochenschr*. 2001 Sep 17;113(17–18):688–94.

47. Meisinger E, Strauch M. Controlled trial of two keto acid supplements on renal function, nutritional status, and bone metabolism in uremic patients. *Kidney Int Suppl*. 1987 Oct;22:S170-3.

48. Aparicio M, Chauveau P, De Précigout V, Bouchet JL, Lasseur C, Combe C. Nutrition and outcome on renal replacement therapy of patients with chronic renal failure treated by a supplemented very low protein diet. *J Am Soc Nephrol*. 2000 Apr;11(4):708–16.

49. Aparicio M, Aguirre RDB, Cupisti A et al. Nutritional therapy in patients with chronic kidney disease: protein-restricted diets supplemented with keto/amino acids. Abstracts from the International Advisory Board Meeting 2006. *Am J Nephrol* [Internet]. 2006;26(Suppl 1):1–28.

50. Fouque D. Should we still prescribe a reduction in protein intake for CKD patients? *Am J Nephrol*. 2006;26(Suppl 1):7–9.

51. Cupisti A. Cardiovascular risk factors in severe chronic kidney disease: The role of protein-restricted diets supplemented with keto/amino acids. *Am J Nephrol*. 2006;26(1):10–2.

52. Mitch WE. Low Protein Diets and Proteinuria: Renal and Cardiac Outcomes. *Am J Nephrol.* 2006;26(Suppl 1):9–10.

53. Aparicio M. Influence of SVLPD on the Evolution of Proteinuria and the Potential Correlation with the Outcome of Blood Pressure and Renal Function. *Am J Nephrol.* 2006;26(Suppl 1):12–3.

54. Zakar G. Paradigm Shift of Ketoacid Treatment in Patients with Hypoalbuminemia? *Am J Nephrol.* 2006;26(Suppl 1):13–4.

55. Aparicio M. Outcome of Old Patients on Supplemented Very Low Protein Diets (VLPD) – Short Communication. *Am J Nephrol.* 2006;26(Suppl 1):15–6.

56. Teplan V. How to Manage Older Patients with Keto/Amino Acids? *Am J Nephrol.* 2006;26(Suppl 1):16–8.

57. Frhling P. Long-Term Results under Ketoacid Substituted Low Protein Diet – German Experience. *Am J Nephrol.* 2006;26(Suppl 1):19.

58. Aguirre R. Level of $_\beta$2 Microglobulin in Urine of Patients with Diabetic Nephropathy and CKD Treated with a Low Protein Diet and Ketosteril. *Am J Nephrol.* 2006;26(Suppl 1):20–1.

59. Teplan V. Keto Acid Therapy and Residual Function in CAPD and HD Patients. *Am J Nephrol.* 2006;26(Suppl 1):23–4.

60. Mitch WE. Beneficial responses to modified diets in treating patients with chronic kidney disease. *Kidney Int.* 2005 Apr;67:S133–5.

61. Fouque D, Chen J, Chen W, Garneata L, Hwang S, KalantarZadeh K, et al. Adherence to ketoacids/essential amino acidssupplemented low protein diets and new indications for patients with chronic kidney disease. *BMC Nephrol.* 2016 Dec 7;17(1):63.

62. Aparicio M, Bellizzi V, Chauveau P, Cupisti A, Ecder T, Fouque D, et al. Protein-Restricted Diets Plus Keto/Amino Acids - A Valid Therapeutic Approach for Chronic Kidney Disease Patients. *J Ren Nutr.* 2012 Mar;22(2):S1–21.

63. Cianciaruso B, Pota A, Pisani A, Torraca S, Annecchini R, Lombardi P, et al. Metabolic effects of two low protein diets in chronic kidney disease stage 4-5—a randomized controlled trial. *Nephrol Dial Transplant.* 2008 Feb;23(2):636–44.

64. Fouque D, Aparicio M. Eleven reasons to control the protein intake of patients with chronic kidney disease. *Nat Clin Pract Nephrol.* 2007 Jul;3(7):383–92.

65. Teplan V. Effect of Keto Acids on Asymmetric Dimethylarginine, Muscle, and Fat Tissue in Chronic Kidney Disease and After Kidney Transplantation. *J Ren Nutr.* 2009 Sep;19(5):S27–9.

66. Qiu H, Liu F, Zhao L, Huang S, Zuo C, Zhong H, et al. Comparison of the effects of alpha-keto/ amino acid supplemented low protein diet and diabetes diet in patients with diabetic nephropathy. *Sichuan Da Xue Xue Bao Yi Xue Ban.* 2012 May;43(3):425–8.

67. Aparicio M, Cano NJM, Cupisti A, Ecder T, Fouque D, Garneata L, et al. Keto-Acid Therapy in Predialysis Chronic Kidney Disease Patients: Consensus Statements. *J Ren Nutr.* 2009 Sep;19(5):S33–5.

68. Zhang J, Xie H, Fang M, Wang K, Chen J, Sun W, et al. Ketosupplemented low protein diet: A valid therapeutic approach for patients with steroid-resistant proteinuria during earlystage chronic kidney disease. *J Nutr Health Aging.* 2016 Apr 23;20(4):420–7.

69. Teplan V, Schück O, Knotek A, Hajný J, Horácková M, Skibová J, et al. Effects of low-protein diet supplemented with ketoacids and erythropoietin in chronic renal failure: a long-term metabolic study. *Ann Transplant.* 2001;6(1):47–53.

70. Frohling PT, Schmicker R, Vetter K, Kaschube I, Gotz KH, Jacopian M, et al. Conservative treatment with ketoacid and amino acid supplemented low-protein diets in chronic renal failure. *Am J Clin Nutr.* 1980 Jul 1;33(7):1667–72.

71. Velázquez López L, Sil Acosta MJ, Goycochea Robles M V, Torres Tamayo M, Castañeda Limones R. Effect of protein restriction diet on renal function and metabolic control in patients with type 2 diabetes: a randomized clinical trial. *Nutr Hosp.* 23(2):141–7.

72. Subhramanyam SV, Lakshmi V, Nayak KS. Treatment of chronic kidney disease patients with ketoanalogue-supplemented lowprotein diet and ketoanalogue-supplemented very-low-protein diet. *Hong Kong J Nephrol.* 2014 Oct;16(2):34–41.

73. Shah AP, Kalantar-Zadeh K, Kopple JD. Is There a Role for Ketoacid Supplements in the Management of CKD? *Am J Kidney Dis.* 2015 May;65(5):659–73.

74. Garneata L. Pharmaco-Economic Evaluation of Keto Acid/Amino Acid-Supplemented Protein-Restricted Diets. *J Ren Nutr.* 2009 Sep;19(5):S19–21.

75. Schmicker R, Vetter K, Lindenau K, Fröhling PT, Kokot F. Conservative Long-Term Treatment of Chronic Renal Failure with Keto Acid and Amino Acid Supplementation. *Transfus Med Hemotherapy.* 1987;14(5):34–8.

76. Garneata L, Stancu A, Dragomir D, Stefan G, Mircescu G. Ketoanalogue-Supplemented Vegetarian Very Low-Protein Diet and CKD Progression. *J Am Soc Nephrol.* 2016 Jul 1;27(7):2164–76.

77. Teplan V, Schück O, Votruba M, Poledne R, Kazdová L, Skibová J, et al. Metabolic effects of keto acid—amino acid supplementation in patients with chronic renal insufficiency receiving a low-protein diet and recombinant human erythropoietin—a randomized controlled trial. *Wien Klin Wochenschr.* 2001 Sep 17;113(17–18):661–9.

78. Bergesio F, Monzani G, Guasparini A, Ciuti R, Gallucci M, Cristofano C, et al. Cardiovascular risk factors in severe chronic renal failure: the role of dietary treatment. *Clin Nephrol.* 2005 Aug;64(2):103–12.

79. Lafage MH, Combe C, Fournier A, Aparicio M. Ketodiet, physiological calcium intake and native vitamin D improve renal osteodystrophy. *Kidney Int.* 1992 Nov;42(5):1217–25.

80. Fröhling PT, Schmicker R, Lindenau K, Vetter K, Kokot F. Role of keto acids in the prophylaxis and treatment of renal osteopathy. *Contrib Nephrol.* 1988;65:123–9.

81. Chauveau P, Couzi L, Vendrely B, de Précigout V, Combe C, Fouque D, et al. Long-term outcome on renal replacement therapy in patients who previously received a keto acid– supplemented very-low-protein diet. *Am J Clin Nutr.* 2009 Oct 1;90(4):969–74.

82. Coresh J, Walser M, Hill S. Survival on dialysis among chronic renal failure patients treated with a supplemented low-protein diet before dialysis. *J Am Soc Nephrol.* 1995 Nov;6(5):1379–85.

83. Thilly N. Low-protein diet in chronic kidney disease: from questions of effectiveness to those of feasibility. *Nephrol Dial Transplant.* 2013 Sep 1;28(9):2203–5.

84. Kao T-W, Liao C-T, Shiao C-C, Kuo Y-H, Hung K-Y, Wu K-D. Low Protein Diet Supplemented With Ketoanalogues Makes Hemodialysis Withdrawal Possible. *Am J Kidney Dis.* 2008 Jan;51(1):160–1.

85. Walser M. Effects of a supplemented very low protein diet in predialysis patients on the serum albumin level, proteinuria, and subsequent survival on dialysis. *Miner Electrolyte Metab.* 1998;24(1):64–71.

86. Schaefer K, von Herrath D, Asmus G, Umlauf E. The beneficial effect of ketoacids on serum phosphate and parathyroid hormone in patients with chronic uremia. *Clin Nephrol.* 1988 Aug;30(2):93–6.

87. Marzocco S, Dal Piaz F, Di Micco L, Torraca S, Sirico ML, Tartaglia D, et al. Very Low Protein Diet Reduces Indoxyl Sulfate Levels in Chronic Kidney Disease. *Blood Purif.* 2013;35(1–3):196–201.

88. Di Iorio B, Di Micco L, Torraca S, Sirico ML, Russo L, Pota A, et al. Acute Effects of Very-Low-Protein Diet on FGF23 Levels: A Randomized Study. *Clin J Am Soc Nephrol.* 2012 Apr 1;7(4):581–7.

89. Giordano M, Lucidi P, Ciarambino T, Gesuè L, Castellino P, Cioffi M, et al. Effects of dietary protein restriction on albumin and fibrinogen synthesis in macroalbuminuric type 2 diabetic patients. *Diabetologia.* 2008 Jan;51(1):21–8.

90. Teplan V, Schück O, Racek J, Mareckova O, Stollova M, Hanzal V, et al. Reduction of plasma asymmetric dimethylarginine in obese patients with chronic kidney disease after three years of a low-protein diet supplemented with keto-amino acids: a randomized controlled trial. *Wien Klin Wochenschr.* 2008 Aug;120(15–16):478–85.

91. Jahn H, Rose F, Schmitt R, Melin G, Schohn D, Comte G, et al. Protein synthesis in skeletal muscle of uremic patients: effect of low-protein diet and supplementation with ketoacids. *Miner Electrolyte Metab.* 1992;18(2–5):222–7.

92. Khan I, Nasiruddin M, Haque S, Khan R. Comparative evaluation of efficacy and safety profile of rhubarb and $_\alpha$-keto analogs of essential amino acids supplementation in patients with diabetic nephropathy. *Saudi J Kidney Dis Transplant.* 2016;27(4):710.

93. Mircescu G, Gârneaţă L, Stancu SH, Căpuşă C. Effects of a Supplemented Hypoproteic Diet in Chronic Kidney Disease. *J Ren Nutr*. 2007 May;17(3):179–88.

94. Hansen HP, Tauber-Lassen E, Jensen BR, Parving H-H. Effect of dietary protein restriction on prognosis in patients with diabetic nephropathy. *Kidney Int*. 2002 Jul;62(1):220–8.

95. Mennini FS, Russo S, Marcellusi A, Quintaliani G, Fouque D. Economic effects of treatment of chronic kidney disease with low-protein diet. *J Ren Nutr*. 2014 Sep;24(5):313–21.

96. Bellizzi V, Chiodini P, Cupisti A, Viola BF, Pezzotta M, De Nicola L, et al. Very low-protein diet plus ketoacids in chronic kidney disease and risk of death during end-stage renal disease: a historical cohort controlled study. *Nephrol Dial Transplant*. 2015 Jan 1;30(1):71–7.

97. Wu C-H, Yang Y-W, Hung S-C, Kuo K-L, Wu K-D, Wu V-C, et al. Ketoanalogues supplementation decreases dialysis and mortality risk in patients with anemic advanced chronic kidney disease. Aguilera AI, editor. *PLoS One*. 2017 May 5;12(5):e0176847.

98. David C, Peride I, Niculae A, Constantin AM, Checherita IA. Very low protein diets supplemented with keto-analogues in ESRD predialysis patients and its effect on vascular stiffness and AVF Maturation. *BMC Nephrol*. 2016 Dec 20;17(1):131.

99. Jiang Z, Tang Y, Yang L, Mi X, Qin W. Effect of restricted protein diet supplemented with keto analogues in end-stage renal disease: a systematic review and meta-analysis. *Int Urol Nephrol*. 2018 Apr 3;50(4):687–94.

100. Lima RCP, Camerino SRAS, França TCL, Rodrigues DSA, Gouveia MGS, Ximenes-da-Silva A, et al. Keto analogues and amino acids supplementation induces a decrease of white blood cell counts and a reduction of muscle damage during intense exercise under thermoneutral conditions. *Food Funct*. 2017;8(4):1519–25.

101. Camerino SRA e S, Lima RCP, França TCL, Herculano E de A, Rodrigues DSA, Gouveia MG de S, et al. Keto analogue and amino acid supplementation and its effects on ammonemia and performance under thermoneutral conditions. *Food Funct*. 2016;7(2):872–80.

102. Liu Y, Spreng T, Lehr M, Yang B, Karau A, Gebhardt H, et al. The supportive effect of supplementation with α-keto acids on physical training in type 2 diabetes mellitus. *Food Funct*. 2015;6(7):2224–30.

103. Prado ES, de Rezende Neto JM, de Almeida RD, Dória de Melo MG, Cameron L-C. Keto analogue and amino acid supplementation affects the ammonaemia response during exercise under ketogenic conditions. *Br J Nutr*. 2011 Jun 16;105(12):1729–33.

104. Liu Y, Lange R, Langanky J, Hamma T, Yang B, Steinacker JM. Improved training tolerance by supplementation with $_a$-Keto acids in untrained young adults: a randomized, double blind, placebo-controlled trial. *J Int Soc Sports Nutr*. 2012;9(1):37.

105. Sapir DG, Owen OE, Pozefsky T, Walser M. Nitrogen Sparing Induced by a Mixture of Essential Amino Acids Given Chiefly as Their Keto-Analogues during Prolonged Starvation in Obese Subjects. *J Clin Invest*. 1974 Oct 1;54(4):974–80.

106. Kopple JD, Levey AS, Greene T, Chumlea WC, Gassman JJ, Hollinger DL, et al. Effect of dietary protein restriction on nutritional status in the Modification of Diet in Renal Disease Study. *Kidney Int.* 1997 Sep;52(3):778–91.

107. Cupisti A, D'Alessandro C, Morelli E, Rizza GM, Galetta F, Franzoni F, et al. Nutritional status and dietary manipulation in predialysis chronic renal failure patients. *J Ren Nutr.* 2004 Jul;14(3):127–33.

108. Walser M, Hill S. Can renal replacement be deferred by a supplemented very low protein diet? *J Am Soc Nephrol.* 1999 Jan;10(1):110–6.

109. Teplan V, Schück O, Horácková M, Skibová J, Holecek M. Effect of a keto acid-amino acid supplement on the metabolism and renal elimination of branched-chain amino acids in patients with chronic renal insufficiency on a low protein diet. *Wien Klin Wochenschr.* 2000 Oct 27;112(20):876–81.

110. Bulla M, Bremer HJ, Ronda-Vildozola R, Roth B. The effect of oral essential amino acids and their ketoanalogues on children receiving regular haemodialysis. *Int J Pediatr Nephrol.* 7(2):73–80.

111. Kasiske BL, Lakatua JD, Ma JZ, Louis TA. A meta-analysis of the effects of dietary protein restriction on the rate of decline in renal function. *Am J Kidney Dis.* 1998 Jun;31(6):954–61.

112. Levey AS, Greene T, Sarnak MJ, Wang X, Beck GJ, Kusek JW, et al. Effect of dietary protein restriction on the progression of kidney disease: long-term follow-up of the Modification of Diet in Renal Disease (MDRD) Study. *Am J Kidney Dis.* 2006 Dec;48(6):879–88.

113. Malvy D, Maingourd C, Pengloan J, Bagros P, Nivet H. Effects of severe protein restriction with ketoanalogues in advanced renal failure. *J Am Coll Nutr.* 1999 Oct;18(5):481–6.

CHAPTER 32

Exercise and Kidney Disease

This will be the one of the shortest chapters. We all know exercise is good for us. This has been proven for many decades.

My question is: Does exercise slow the progression of kidney disease in any special way, or are the benefits of exercise the same for us as for everyone else?

The answer was easier than I thought:

A Comparison of Aerobic Exercise and Resistance Training in Patients Abstract[1]

The morbidity and mortality associated with chronic kidney disease (CKD) are primarily caused by atherosclerosis and cardiovascular disease, which may be caused in part by inflammation and oxidative stress. Aerobic exercise and resistance training have been proposed as measures to combat obesity, inflammation, endothelial dysfunction, oxidative stress, insulin resistance, and progression of CKD. In non-CKD patients, aerobic exercise reduces inflammation, increases insulin sensitivity, decreases microalbuminuria, facilitates weight loss, decreases leptins, and protects against oxidative injury. In nondialysis CKD, aerobic exercise decreases microalbuminuria, protects from oxidative stress, and may increase the glomerular filtration rate (GFR). Aerobic exercise in hemodialysis patients has been reported to enhance insulin sensitivity, improve lipid profile, increase hemoglobin, increase strength, decrease blood pressure, and improve quality of life. Resistance training, in the general population, decreases C-reactive protein, increases insulin sensitivity, decreases body fat content, increases insulin-like growth factor-1 (IGF-1), and decreases microalbuminuria. In the non-dialysis CKD population, resistance training has been reported to reduce inflammation, increase serum albumin, maintain body weight, increase muscle strength, increase IGF-1, and increase GFR. Resistance training in hemodialysis increases muscle strength, increases physical functionality, and improves IGF-1 status. Combined aerobic exercise and resistance training during dialysis improves muscle strength, work output, cardiac fitness, and possibly dialysis adequacy. There is a need for more investigation on the role of exercise in CKD. If the benefits of aerobic exercise and strength training in non- CKD populations can be shown to apply to CKD patients as well, renal rehabilitation will begin to play an important role in the approach to the treatment, prevention, and slowed progression of CKD.

This summary is pretty long, so let me summarize here.

Benefits of Aerobic Exercise:

Healthy population	Non-dialysis CKD	Dialysis patients
Reduces inflammation	Decreases microalbuminuria	Improves lipid profile
Increases insulin sensitivity	Protects against oxidative stress	Increases hemoglobin
Decreases microalbuminuria	May increase GFR	Lowers blood pressure
Promotes weight loss		Increases insulin sensitivity
Decreases leptins		Increases quality of life
Protects against oxidative stress		

Benefits of Resistance Training:

Healthy	Non-dialysis CKD	Dialysis CKD
Decreases C-reactive protein	Reduces inflammation	Increases IGF 1
Improves insulin sensitivity	Increases serum albumin	Increases muscle strength
Reduces body fat	Reduces body weight	Increases physical functioning
Increases insulin growth factor (IGF 1)	Increases muscle strength	
Reduces microalbuminuria	Increases IGF 1	Increases GFR

Note: Did you see that increased GFR was listed for both aerobic and resistance training for non-dialysis CKD patients? Increased serum albumin and reduced microalbumin are also benefits, along with reduced inflammation, and the list goes on.

I don't think any other treatment can post these kinds of combined benefits. In addition, we are the highest risk group ever studied for heart disease. There is little doubt that we need physical exercise at least as much as the healthy population, but in reality, we need more exercise or more consistent exercise—to combat heart disease and get the other benefits for our kidneys.

Before I run off to compete in the next ironman competition, I heard from a very qualified person that exercise is bad for your kidneys. Let's address this right now. There was a hint of truth to this, but it is still bad advice. When you break down muscle tissue, your body has to clear the waste products. Heavy workouts may cause your creatinine clearance numbers to rise until your body is better conditioned. This is a warning to us to go easy when starting out with any physical fitness program and get a doctor's approval before starting any physical activity. You have a good excuse not to push too hard when starting out.

Rhabdomyolysis is what they were warning me about. Rhabdomyolysis occurs when muscle is broken down on a large scale. Crush injuries are a common cause, but it can occur if you work out too hard and are dehydrated. Myoglobin (a protein) is released and can damage the kidneys. This condition is pretty rare, with 26,000 cases in the U.S. each year. The reason for my warning is with reduced kidney function, and a very minor case of Rhabdomyolysis might become serious for us. Again, go easy starting out.

A good rule of thumb is you should never be so sore or so tired that you can't do the same workout tomorrow without a struggle. Slow and steady wins the race for us.

Slow and steady is good for us because many of us feel exhausted and tired before we even start exercising. We will have to build up slowly and safely.

The following study is about swimming, but the real message is about regular exercise over a long period.

| Study 32.1 | Regular Aquatic Exercise for Chronic Kidney Disease Patients: a 10-year Follow-up Study.[2] |

Pechter Ü1, Raag M, Ots-Rosenberg M.

Author information

ABSTRACT:

Chronic kidney disease (CKD) patients not yet in dialysis can benefit from increased physical activity; however, the safety and outcomes of aquatic exercise have not been investigated in observational studies. The aim of this study was to analyze association of 10 years of regularly performed aquatic exercise with the study endpoint—that is, all-cause death or start of dialysis. Consecutive CKD patients were included in the study in January 2002. The exercise group (n=7) exercised regularly under the supervision of a physiotherapist for 10 years; the control group (n=9), matched in terms of age and clinical parameters, remained sedentary. Low-intensity aerobic aquatic exercise was performed regularly twice a week; 32 weeks or more of exercise therapy sessions were conducted annually. None of the members of the aquatic exercise group reached dialysis or died in 10 years. In the sedentary control group, 55% reached the study endpoint renal replacement therapy (n=2) or all-cause death (n=3). Occurrence of the study endpoint, compared using the exact multinomial test with unconditional margins, was statistically significantly different (P-value: 0.037) between the study groups. Regular supervised aquatic exercisearrested CKDprogression. There was a statistically significant difference between the sedentary group and the exercise group in reaching renal replacement therapy or all-cause death in a follow-up time of 10 years.

The message here is that regular exercise over a long time wins the race. There were no deaths in the group that worked out regularly. This is pretty big news for us. I just started swimming this week. It's a convincing study, what more can I say.

Let's look at one more large study before ending this chapter. This study is a composite of 45 studies.

Study 32.2	Exercise Training for Adults with Chronic Kidney Disease.[3]

Heiwe S, Jacobson SH.

MAIN RESULTS:

Forty-five studies, randomizing 1,863 participants were included in this review. Thirty-two studies presented data that could be meta-analyzed. Types of exercise training included cardiovascular training, mixed cardiovascular and resistance training, resistance-only training and yoga. Some studies used supervised exercise interventions and others used unsupervised interventions. Exercise intensity was classed as "high" or "low," duration of individual exercise sessions ranged from 20 minutes/session to 110 minutes/session and study duration was from two to

18 months. Seventeen percent of studies were classed as having an overall low risk of bias, 33% as moderate, and 49% as having a high risk of bias. The results shows that regular exercise significantly improved: 1) physical fitness (aerobic capacity, 24 studies, 847 participants: SMD -0.56, 95% CI -0.70 to -0.42; walking capacity, 7 studies, 191 participants: SMD -0.36, 95% CI -0.65 to -0.06); 2) cardiovascular dimensions (resting diastolic blood pressure, 11 studies, 419 participants: MD 2.32 mm Hg, 95% CI 0.59 to 4.05; resting systolic blood pressure, 9 studies, 347 participants: MD 6.08 mm Hg, 95% CI 2.15 to 10.12; heart rate, 11 studies, 229 participants: MD 6 bpm, 95% CI 10 to 2); 3) some nutritional parameters (albumin, 3 studies, 111 participants: MD -2.28 g/L, 95% CI -4.25 to -0.32; prealbumin, 3 studies, 111 participants: MD - 44.02 mg/L, 95% CI -71.52 to -16.53; energy intake, 4 studies, 97 participants: SMD -0.47, 95% CI -0.88 to -0.05); and 4) health-related quality of life. Results also showed how exercise should be designed in order to optimise the effect. Other outcomes had insufficient evidence.

AUTHORS' CONCLUSIONS:

There is evidence for significant beneficial effects of regular exercise on physical fitness, walking capacity, cardiovascular dimensions (e.g. blood pressure and heart rate), health-related quality of life and some nutritional parameters in adults with CKD. Other outcomes had insufficient evidence due to the lack of data from RCTs. The design of the exercise intervention causes difference in effect size and should be considered when prescribing exercise with the aim of affecting a certain outcome. Future RCTs should focus more on the effects of resistance training interventions or mixed cardiovascular and resistance training, as these exercise types have not been studied as much as cardiovascular exercise.

Note: Lower blood pressure and increased physical fitness are expected. Increased albumin or prealbumin is not. There is something else going on here. The most likely explanation is that reduced inflammation and oxidative stress allowed albumin to rise. Remember, albumin is a strong mortality indicator, so anything we can do to increase our albumin is a win.

Okay, I am not going bore you with dozens of studies, as the benefits of exercise are well-known.

However, I do want to say a few things before moving on to the next chapter. Keep these in mind when you start or continue your exercise program.

Regular exercise may be one of the most effective forms of therapy for kidney patients over the long term (years).

The combined effects:

> Lower blood pressure

> Better weight control

> Reduced inflammation

> Increased albumin

> Increased insulin sensitivity

> Reduced oxidative stress

> Increased growth factor (IGF 1)

This combination of factors may result in:

> Slower progression of your disease

> Increased GFR

> Increased quality of life

> Fewer injuries as we age

> A better survival rate if we have surgery or a serious illness

> Lower rates or reduced heart disease factors

Exercise is not a silver bullet or miracle cure, but regular exercise over many years will add up to slower disease progression in many cases. Small benefits over many years end up making a big difference later.

1. Get a doctor's approval before you begin any exercise program. High rates of heart disease make this mandatory. Again, do not start a workout program without your doctor's approval. Some of us are very sick, so go easy, but do something to get moving.

2. Your creatinine clearance numbers will rise if you are breaking down muscle tissue. This will happen when you start exercising after being sedentary or are lifting heavy weights. Your kidneys have to clear the waste products, so your creatinine clearance blood test may look worse for a while. Once your body gets used to the workouts, your numbers will get back to the previous range or very close.

3. With #1, #2, or #3 in mind, go easy when starting out and increase slowly. There is no finish line for breaking a certain time or lifting a certain amount of weight. Your kidneys don't care. Slow and steady progress over 10 years or more is the way to win this race. A good rule of thumb is you should always be able to work out tomorrow without being sore or too tired. If not, you are working too hard.

   Anything is better than being sedentary. If you can walk for only five minutes, then walk for five minutes every day for a month. The next month, go for 10 minutes, and so on. I know we can feel tired and pretty crappy with this disease, but soldier on in small increments and you will be rewarded later; I promise. Do whatever you can to start moving every day.

4. I could find no conclusive data that any one type of workout is better than another. Do whatever you love to do. Play tennis, swim, bike, walk, run, hike, go to exercise classes, go to zumba, jazzercise, dance, yoga, ski, surf, and so on. There is no magic workout, despite what you may see on TV or read on the net. If we want to look younger and feel better, we have to pay for it, 40 to 60 minutes a day. That's the magic. Whatever you like is fine—just get your butt moving five or six days a week for life.

   The only clear message is that you should do both aerobic and resistance training.

5. Track what you are doing. The old saying, "You can't manage what you can't measure" is true. I prefer a heart monitor that automatically records everything. I like to be brain dead when working out and don't want to bother with writing anything down or trying to keep track in my head. Heart rate monitors can be purchased pretty cheaply these days, and you can always check Craigslist or Ebay as well. It is easy to track the amount of calories burned this way. This helps with your diet management as well. You will know how many extra calories to eat to offset your calories burned working out. Fitness watches are more expensive, but if they help you, go for it. Keep increasing month over month in small amounts. Keep track well enough to know whether you are increasing your exercise each month. Going to the gym without a plan equaled goofing off for me.

Part of your treatment plan will be exercising five to six days a week. Again, no ironman competitions or marathons. Start slow and steady with the guidance and oversight of your doctor.

For our purposes, we are going to define a minimum workout as 35 minutes, plus a warm up. No need to go past an hour. It takes about 30 minutes of aerobic exercise to start getting the benefits, but that does not include warm up times. For us, 35 minutes of actual exercise is the minimum goal to start with. Most of us can walk for 35 minutes or more. If you can't, your goal is to work up to 35 minutes of the easiest exercise you can do. Many malls are open early in the morning, and you will find other walkers. It's warm in the winter, cool in the summer, and there's a nice flat surface with no hills if you are just starting out.

In summary, regular exercise over long periods of time may be one of the most effective treatments for kidney disease, and it's good for our hearts and minds too. You will feel better, live longer, look better naked, and make your friends green with jealousy by looking so good. Not to mention giving kidney disease the finger. All you have to do is get moving regularly and make it a habit five or six days a week.

References

1. Moinuddin I, Leehey DJ. A comparison of aerobic exercise and resistance training in patients with and without chronic kidney disease. *Advances in Chronic Kidney Disease.* 2008;15(1):83-96.

2. Pechter Ü, Raag M, Ots-Rosenberg M. Regular aquatic exercise for chronic kidney disease patients: a 10-year follow-up study. *International Journal of Rehabilitation Research.* 2014;37(3):251-255.

3. Heiwe S, Jacobson SH. Exercise training for adults with chronic kidney disease. *Cochrane Database* Syst Rev. 2011;10(10).

CHAPTER 33

Reducing the Cascade Effect of Comorbid Conditions (C³)

This is a short chapter, as we have talked comorbid conditions for hundreds of pages. However, a short chapter does not mean it's not important.

If you get only two things from this book, and nothing else, it should be:

1. Reducing the number of comorbid conditions will extend your life and the quality of it.

2. Reducing the number of comorbid conditions is the best way to slow your disease and go for remission.

By focusing on reducing comorbid conditions, we get concrete steps to work on and our progress can be measured, managed, and evaluated effectively. Setting a goal of getting better won't work. You will have a hard time quantifying "getting better" and won't know what to do first.

This means not living with or being okay with blood tests outside the normal range. The reason this is so important is that every blood test or condition outside the normal range triggers a cascade of other conditions that will speed the progression of our disease. The idea that "Being a little high or low" on a test is okay, should be put to rest. It's not okay if you want to live a long and productive life. It's black and white backed up by dozens, maybe hundreds of studies.

C³

I had my share of doctors tell me it's okay that this or that test is outside the normal range. It's to be expected as a kidney patient. This is complete and utter bullshit! The reason why I think this is incredibly bad advice is something I call C³ for shorthand, "Cascading Comorbid Conditions" aka C³ or the exponential effect of comorbid conditions. The idea of C³ the was basis for my own path towards remission.

In my eyes, C³ is what really kills us. The reason is a single comorbid condition contributes to or causes other comorbid conditions. For each comorbid condition you have, you are contributing to other comorbid conditions as well. As these conditions pile on, you will get sicker and sicker.

The reverse is also true. As you cure conditions, other conditions will get better as well. You will be curing more conditions than you know each time you cure one condition.

Let's use sodium as an example:

High Sodium outside the normal range contributes to or causes:

> High blood pressure
>
> Inflammation
>
> Edema or swelling
>
> And other issues we don't test for

Sodium is just one test on paper, but in reality we have put our foot on the gas for many conditions that speed the progression of our disease.

Next, the first effect of high blood pressure leads to:

> Faster decline and damage to our kidneys
>
> Increased risk of heart attack and stroke
>
> Increased risk of diabetes
>
> And other issues we don't test for

Next, inflammation increases the risk and speed of just about everything. One health condition leads to other health conditions. It's a rule that seemingly can never be broken. Everything is connected and kidney disease is systemic.

Now, let's do the opposite:

Sodium in the normal range leads to:

> Reduced blood pressure which slows the progression of kidney disease
>
> Reduced risk of heart attack and stroke
>
> Lower inflammation
>
> Reduced or eliminated edema
>
> And other issues we don't test for

Now blood pressure, inflammation, and edema all become easier to manage as they should be less severe or maybe eliminated in some cases. The decline in kidney function will slow and heart disease should slow by some amount as well.

This is a very basic list, but the message is clear. One health condition affects many other health conditions. One comorbid condition or health condition has a cascading effect on our health. One condition feeds or fuels another condition and that condition may feed another condition and so on. The effect of one condition is exponential and far reaching. I used sodium as an example, but the same could be said for any blood or urine test outside the normal range. Take your pick of tests and if you look behind the curtains you will always see getting one condition in the normal range affects many other conditions.

As you "cure," which I define as testing in the normal range or completely eliminating the symptoms of one condition, your health will improve at a rate much higher than expected from just one condition. The concept of C^3 is what allowed me to improve my health.

Curing one condition cures or improves several others. Letting tests be outside the normal range is putting your foot on the gas for existing conditions and begging for new ones to pop up.

Albumin is another good example. Albumin rising from one quarter to the next likely means dozens of other issues are improving as well. Again, these issues are not tested and are unseen, but do have a long-term effect on your health. We have overwhelming proof for this concept.

Not as hard as it looks

I remember at the time I felt overwhelmed by diet and treatment plans, but keep it simple. Here is how I thought about diet and tests outside the normal range.

1. I am eating more than my kidneys or body can process, resulting in tests outside the normal range.

2. I am not eating enough of something, so I am low on this test or measurement.

As you will see in the treatment plan section, making steady and small changes up and down to certain factors in your diet leads to success.

If your blood urea nitrogen (BUN) test is higher than the normal range, you are eating too much dietary protein compared to what your body can process because of kidney disease. Lowering your dietary protein intake and nitrogen load on your kidneys will improve your BUN test results. High BUN levels also have a cascade effect on your health, along with every other condition.

Keep it simple while working on comorbid conditions. Being high or low just means we need to eat more or less of something—that's it. Curing these conditions gives us a path and blueprint to slowing or stopping our disease and a way to measure the progress of our treatment plan. The idea that we should be "okay" with tests outside the normal range flies in the face of all available research. Yet, this is still the approach used today, especially for early-stage patients.

The United States is a third world country when it comes to kidney disease outcomes. While there are several reasons for this, a primary reason is lack of early treatments to stop or slow the progression of our disease. Imagine a cancer patient being told, "We can't help you until you are terminal," or a heart disease patient being told to wait until they have a heart attack, and then come back for treatment. The idea that kidney patients can't do anything in the early stages of the disease is dead wrong.

Study after study shows that the number of comorbid conditions is a strong predictor of mortality rates. It makes sense. The more conditions you have, the sicker you are. The more conditions you have today, the more likely you will develop more comorbid conditions until you get to a point you can't recover.

Study 33.1 — Multiple chronic conditions and life expectancy: a life table analysis

RESULTS:

<u>Life expectancy decreases with each additional chronic condition.</u> A 67-year-old individual with no chronic conditions will live, on average, 22.6 additional years. A 67-year-old individual with five chronic conditions and ≥10 chronic conditions will live 7.7 fewer years and 17.6 fewer years, respectively. <u>The average marginal decline in life expectancy is 1.8 years with each additional chronic condition-ranging from 0.4 fewer years with the first condition to 2.6 fewer years with the sixth condition.</u> These results are consistent by sex and race. We observe differences in life expectancy by selected conditions at 67, but these differences diminish with age and increasing numbers of comorbid conditions.

> Let's assume I have 10 comorbid conditions (which I did). Using this study, my lifespan will be anywhere from 18 to 26 years shorter than someone with no comorbid conditions. My expected lifespan would be cut short by 20 to 30 years.

Study 33.2 — Association of Cardiometabolic Multimorbidity With Mortality

CONCLUSION:

<u>Mortality associated with a history of diabetes, stroke or MI was similar for each condition.</u> <u>Because any combination of these conditions was associated with multiplicative mortality risk, life expectancy was substantially lower in people with multimorbidity.</u>

Study 33.3 — Comorbidity as an independent risk factor in patients with cancer: an eight-year population-based study.

ABSTRACT:

This study determined the prevalence of medical conditions in patients with cancer and their impact on outcome. We evaluated a cohort of 37,411 patients diagnosed with cancer between 2000 and 2008 in Taiwan, collecting the cancer diagnosis and chronic disease diagnoses. The severity of the comorbid condition was correlated with the cancer diagnosis and outcome. Overall, 71.9% of the study population had one or more comorbid conditions. <u>Patients with none (n = 10,508), one (n = 8,881), two (n = 6,583), and three or more (n = 11,439) comorbid conditions had mortality rates of 11.49%, 15.99%, 19.61% and 29.39%, respectively. Older patients with comorbid conditions had a significantly higher chance of death. Dementia, heart disease or cerebrovascular diseases were associated with the highest mortality. Cancer patients with comorbid conditions have a significantly higher risk of death. Prevention and better medical management of comorbid conditions is likely to result in improved outcomes for patients with cancer.</u>

To simplify this study, let's list the numbers below:

Number of comorbid conditions	Morality rates
0	11.49%
1	15.99%
2	19.61%
3	29.39%

Notice the jump at three comorbid conditions. This goes hand in hand with other research in this book. Once you get over two comorbid conditions, your odds drop significantly. Most of us can get down to two comorbid conditions if we work hard for a long enough period of time. I will always have protein in my urine, so there is one condition outside the normal range I can't do anything about. My creatinine clearance number fluctuates some with activity and diet. These are two conditions I probably can't cure or change. However, my odds are pretty good with just two conditions.

Now let's look at stage 3 kidney patients.

Study 33.4 **The burden of comorbidity in people with chronic kidney disease stage 3: a cohort study**

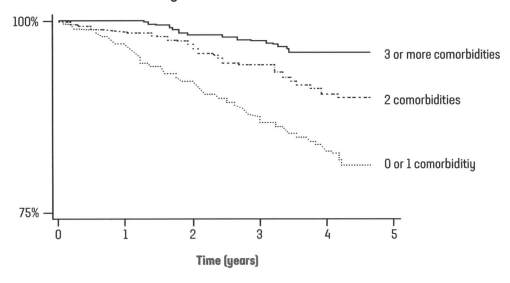

Kaplan Meier plot showing cumulative survival (all-cause mortality) by comorbidity status.

The vertical axis is the percentage of patients of stage three patients who died over a five year period.

The death rate is dramatically higher for patients with three or more comorbid conditions. On this chart lower is better.

DISCUSSION FROM STUDY:

In this cohort study of predominantly older people with <u>mild to moderate CKD we found high levels of comorbidity and polypharmacy and demonstrated that increased comorbidity was associated with reduced survival. While our list of included comorbidities was not exhaustive, our findings demonstrate that, even in a cohort recruited in primary care, CKD rarely occurs in isolation. Virtually all patients were 'multimorbid' according to the usual definition of having two or more chronic morbidities [3]. Our finding that only 4 % of people with CKD stage 3 had no comorbidity is striking and clinically important.</u>

Note: Read that again, only 4% of people with stage 3 kidney disease had no comorbid conditions. Polypharmacy means the use of multiple drugs.

This is why curing comorbid conditions is so worthwhile. As you cure comorbid conditions, you are making life easier on your kidneys and reducing your risk of death. The cascade effect of curing comorbid conditions ended with my disease going into remission. I will never know exactly what combination of factors led to remission. I do know that if I did not cure as many comorbid conditions as possible, I would have never gone into remission. I started improving only as I started wrestling each condition into the normal range. I don't see how remission is possible with four, five, or more comorbid conditions. The reason for this is the cascading effect of any comorbid condition.

This is also the reason low-protein diets have a bad reputation. Using my case as an example, if I treated only protein issues like Blood Urea Nitrogen (BUN), creatinine, and phosphorus, I was treating three of ten conditions. On paper I would still have seven comorbid conditions, which cause a cascade of other health conditions. I would always be struggling in this scenario.

I needed to get the number of conditions down from ten to two in order to really change my future prognosis, and so do you. That is my message to you. Get down to two comorbid conditions if you can.

Treatment Plan and Diet

How does this work for the treatment plan in this book? Let me show you what is treated and how easy it is to knock out a few comorbid conditions.

Comorbid Condition	Treatment
Uremia	Low-protein diet, low-nitrogen protein foods, plant-based diet
Acidosis	Low-protein diet, low-nitrogen protein foods, plant-based diet
Low serum albumin	Low-protein diet, low-nitrogen protein foods, plant-based diet
Inflammation	Low-protein diet, low-nitrogen protein foods, plant-based diet
Proteinuria	Low-protein diet, low-nitrogen protein foods, plant-based diet

Comorbid Condition	Treatment
Sodium	Low-salt diet
Phosphorus	Low-phosphorus diet, use phosphorus binders
Potassium	Low-potassium diet, use potassium binders
Oxidative stress	High-antioxidant diet
Weight	Lose or gain weight
Hypercalcemia	Lower calcium intake
Hypermagnesemia	Lower magnesium intake
Blood pressure	Low-salt diet, exercise, ACE inhibitors
Advanced glycation end products	Low-AGE diet, increase antioxidant and polyphenol intake
Hyperlipidemia	Lower saturated fat and cholesterol intake, exercise, drugs
Depression/anxiety	Medication, therapy
Edema	Low-salt diet, raising albumin and diuretics
Grip strength	Low-protein diet, low-nitrogen protein foods, plant-based diet, exercise

This not a complete list, but as you can see you can measure and manage almost all of the drivers of disease progression.

Ninety percent of the drivers of our disease can be wrestled into the normal range with some effort. Now, we add conditions that decrease the speed of kidney disease progression.

Factors that slow kidney and heart disease progression

Magnesium	Get in the high end of the normal range
Reduce workload on remaining kidney function	Low-protein diet, low-nitrogen protein food
Exercise	Get off your bum and get moving
Reducing comorbid conditions	Diet, drugs, exercise, therapy, etc.
calcium	Reduce or eliminate supplemental calcium

The formula for curing comorbid conditions looks something like this:

low-protein diet +

low-nitrogen protein food +

plant-based diet +

exercise +

drugs +

therapy, medication for anxiety/depression +

routine blood and urine tests to constantly adjust diet and dosage with your doctor's advice = greatly reduced mortality rates, kidneys lasting longer, and a higher quality of life.

Almost all drivers of kidney disease progression can be dealt with in some way, but the cornerstone is a low-protein diet, combined with a low-nitrogen protein food, combined with a plant-based diet. This treats the most symptoms. If we don't treat the main symptoms, then we will never get to two or fewer comorbid conditions. This is why we have to start with a low-protein, low-nitrogen, plant-based diet.

Just "managing" sodium, potassium, and phosphorus won't get you very far if you have other comorbid conditions. You can see why: you are likely leaving too many conditions unchecked to slow the progression of your disease. Research tells us curing three out of ten conditions may not help us much in terms of mortality rates and likely disease progression.

This is yet another reason I am against managing conditions. Numbers outside the normal range still have a cascading effect on other parts of our bodies. It's still the road to hell, just a little bit slower.

Another reason I am such a believer in curing comorbid conditions that drive the progression of our disease is we get a roadmap that didn't exist before. Instead of focusing on hypothetical situations, we focus on concrete items that can be verified with a blood or urine test and our doctor's evaluations.

We don't have to guess if something is working or not. We know without a shadow of a doubt, using blood and urine tests as our guide.

Never forget, we have an incurable disease, but we can dramatically affect the speed of progression by taking out health conditions one at a time. Imagine going from ten conditions to just two. You might be able to slow your disease progression to almost zero. This is a lifesaver for patients who are older and can make their kidneys last an extra 10 years.

Eighteen Months Has Given Me Eleven Years

Curing comorbid conditions, not managing symptoms from the day of diagnosis, should be standard practice. I hope this book will change that fact. Changing your diet and lifestyle, and keeping track of things like diet and exercise takes some effort, but you may be paid back seven to one.

My eighteen months of finally doing everything right paid off in remission, maybe for life, or it could come back at any time. Eighteen months has given me, as of today, eleven years of good health and a high quality of life. Twelve months of this diet and treatment plan could give you ten or more years of high-quality life compared to the alternative of ten years of downward progression. This means for every month I stuck to the plan, I got seven months of good health so far. Seven to one is a pretty good payoff in my opinion.

I beg you to try the upcoming treatment and diet plan in this book for ninety days and see what happens. It may be life-changing for you.

Please remember this: Every time you move a condition into the normal range, your odds get better. Never forget this and make this the basis of your treatment plan.

References

1. Nugent RA, Fathima SF, Feigl AB, Chyung D. The burden of chronic kidney disease on developing nations: a 21st century challenge in global health. *Nephron Clinical Practice.* 2011;118(3):c269-c277.

2. DuGoff EH, Canudas-Romo V, Buttorff C, Leff B, Anderson GF. Multiple chronic conditions and life expectancy: a life table analysis. *Medical care.* 2014;52(8):688-694.

3. Di Angelantonio E, Kaptoge S, Wormser D, et al. Association of cardiometabolic multimorbidity with mortality. *Jama.* 2015;314(1):52-60.

4. Chen C-I, Kuan C-F, Miser J, et al. Comorbidity as an independent risk factor in patients with cancer: an 8-year population-based study. *Asia Pacific Journal of Public Health.* 2015;27(2):NP590-NP599.

5. Fraser SD, Roderick PJ, May CR, et al. The burden of comorbidity in people with chronic kidney disease stage 3: a cohort study. *BMC nephrology.* 2015;16(1):193.

Intro to the Treatment Plan Section

The next section contains the blueprint/ plan I used to get into remission.

We first covered all of the factors that increase the speed of kidney disease progression and factors that slow the progression of kidney disease.

Next is a plan for putting all of these factors together in a way that is measurable and repeatable.

CHAPTER 34

Introduction to the Treatment Plan

A treatment plan for incurable kidney disease is optimistic and ambitious at the same time. It's optimistic because we are trying to do something that is supposed to be impossible. An incurable disease is incurable, after all. The plan is also ambitious because I will be asking for feedback and volunteers to help refine the treatment plan and improve it each year.

Imagine if we had data from thousands of people from all over the world in the upcoming years. We could greatly improve the treatment plan. I hope you will consider helping with this project. We can do great things as a group. I continue to believe that patients helping patients will yield the fastest results for us.

I believe it is very important to understand why you are doing things and what your expectations should be. Understanding and education are power in your hands.

It's all you

First, you will be writing your own treatment plan with your doctor's help and approval. In most cases, your doctor will have already recommended the standard treatments. Many of you will have tried different drugs, or drugs may not be an option for you. You are not trying to replace your doctor's advice, but trying to find a new way to slow or stop your disease. This is going to take some experimenting on your part. This is why you will be writing your own experimental treatment plan.

You will also be asking for help with something that is new to the U.S. and many other countries. Your plan needs to be well-thought-out and well-researched.

You are going to write your plan and get your doctor's blessing and support to follow it. No one else is going to do this for you. It's all on you, and me, and every other patient to do this if we really want to get help. No one is coming to our rescue; we have to rescue ourselves.

You need to think of this as your own personal clinical trial. If you don't stick to your plan, then the results are worthless. The phrase "garbage in, garbage out" (GIGO) comes to mind. If you put bad data in, then you get bad data out. Clinical trials are full of rules so the data extracted from the trial is reliable. Your version is no different.

You will need to follow your plan in order to get reliable data that you can use to make good decisions. Compliance is the holy grail of these treatment plans. Assume you stay on the diet for one week, but tomorrow you pass out in a roadside barbecue joint and wake up covered in barbecue sauce with your pants unbuttoned. (I had this dream once when trying to give up meat.) The data you get back from your blood tests will be unreliable. Yes, none of us are perfect and some failures are expected, but the more you stray from the plan, the less reliable your blood and urine tests will be for future decision-making. This is a big deal! In order to make good decisions, you need good data.

If you are eating a random diet, your results will be random and unreliable indicators for treatment decisions.

What does writing a treatment plan mean?

It means a lot.

While I worked on my own plan, I had to confront a few things. First, what does "experimental" mean in terms of my health and treatment options? What is fair game? What is off limits? What makes sense and what doesn't? What is dangerous and what is safe? What is a wild goose chase and what is sane?

When we are in the fight, we are not the most objective people. Many of us are doing our best to get by, considering our current situation. You need a good plan to guide you and keep you on the straight and narrow path. One of your doctor's jobs is to be the objective one.

I had to come up with a few rules to live by. When the whole world is a treatment option, things get out of control pretty quickly. I needed a few rules to ground me and guide me. I had to stay on the path and stay focused on the most important factors driving my disease and long-term health.

These rules helped guide all of my decisions. If you ever wonder what you should be doing, refer back to these rules.

#1: Aggressively Treat Kidney Disease from Day One and Never Stop Trying to Stop or Slow the Progression of your Disease

Why is this rule number one? Because you never get back lost kidney function. Starting your treatment plan with a GFR of 60 is much easier than starting with a GFR of 20, and your expected outcome will be better. You have more time to try different treatment options, your diet will not be as restricted, your current health is better, and so on.

It is sheer madness not to start, and keep trying, to slow and stop the progression of your disease from the day of diagnosis. Monitoring progression is not a treatment. Monitoring progression is the road to dialysis. Don't ever fall for the idea that monitoring your decline is a form of treatment. The gamble here is whether your kidneys will hold out long enough. Long enough for what? Dying young, dialysis, transplant? What are we supposed to wait on? Don't take this gamble; it's just too risky.

You should always be going for remission. Why, you ask? Because the process of going for remission will yield the most benefits, even if you don't actually go into remission. How are we going to try for remission? By removing every driver of kidney disease progression and adding everything that slows disease progression. We are going to systematically stop, cure, or manage every single driver of progression we can find. In addition to stopping every driver of progression, we are going to add as many factors that slow disease progression as possible.

I gave up on remission, but still tried to stop every driver of my disease. This process ended with my disease in remission. I followed a system to slow my disease for over a year before I went into remission. The systematic process of stopping every driver of kidney disease progression may result in stopping the progression of your disease.

Think about it like a scoreboard. You are the home team and your disease is the bitter rival team you always hated.

Assume you currently have ten drivers of kidney disease (like I did) and you are not doing anything to slow your disease.

Right now, the scoreboard reads 0 to 10, and you are going to lose the battle if nothing changes. Odds are your disease is going to keep progressing at 100 mph if nothing changes.

Now, let's assume you lower the drivers of kidney disease progression to two comorbid conditions, and now you have added two conditions that slow disease progression. The scoreboard is now 2 to 2. Now it is all but guaranteed that your disease progression will slow.

Now, assume the score is 3 to 1, and you are doing everything you can to slow the disease. You have wrestled every driver of kidney disease into submission, except for one you can't seem to cure. Do you think your outcome will be better? Damn right it will be better! Your mortality odds will drop dramatically. In 99% of patients, disease progression will slow dramatically.

Remember, the time between diagnosis and stage 5 is years, if not decades. How you manage your disease this decade will likely determine your odds of survival in the next decade. If you want to be doing well in your 70s, then do well in your 60s first. Slowing your disease this decade equals better health and a better quality of life the next decade. Going for remission by systematically taking out the drivers of the disease gives you the best odds for the upcoming years. Remission is not possible for many people with chronic kidney disease, but going for remission will still yield the best results.

Mortality rates drop dramatically when you have only one or two comorbid conditions. You can live longer with a high quality of life, even if you can't cure every condition.

Years of doing nothing to slow your disease will yield nothing and may well rob you of years of life. It's a hard truth, but it is the truth.

#2: Everything Is on the Table, From a Treatment Perspective, If Your Doctor Feels It Is Worth the Risks

You have an incurable disease. This means you have a right to try all forms of treatment as early as possible (in my opinion). Treatments like drugs, diet, exercise, and any other therapies are going to be part of the plan, but you have to know the limits. You need a strategy to work through all of your viable options.

By viable options, I mean treatment plans and strategies if your doctor feels the possible benefit is worth any risks. Remission may not be possible, but it is possible to wrestle every condition that contributes to disease progression into the normal range. A combination of diet, exercise, supplements, and drugs is very effective at controlling blood pressure, cholesterol, etc. Getting into the normal range on every blood test is one of our goals. Combine all kinds of treatments if needed.

Trying everything does not mean flying to a third world country for some expensive, completely unproven treatment or using a homeopath who is treating you with arsenic (this is a true story). I mean evidence-based medicine, treatment plans your real medical doctor approves, and ways to measure the effectiveness of the treatment plan.

This next story is true and, sadly, happened to a couple I know. On vacation, both became very ill. After coming home, they were both diagnosed with kidney disease. After a traditional MD told them nothing could be done, they understandably sought out alternative treatments. A homeopathic doctor tested their hair and found arsenic. This made sense, as both became ill at the same time. They must have been exposed to something on vacation. He treated the couple with low doses of arsenic. They felt the homeopathic doctor had more answers than the MD. Needless to say, the outcome was not good. The wife died the next year and the husband is still struggling with his disease. I am not saying the treatment killed her. My point is that they did not seek a real medical doctor and did not have regular blood tests while going through this treatment.

They were taken in by the idea that someone could help them, and they ignored all of the available evidence. We are suckers when we are sick and it seems that no one can help us. I know firsthand how easy it can be to be taken in. Be careful and always be under the care of a professional medical doctor. If everything evidence-based has failed and the outlook is still bad, you can ask your doctor about treatments that alternative medicine may be promoting. However, even if you pursue alternative medicine, you should always be under a medical doctor's care.

When you see phrases like these, be careful:

> Ancient healing or ancient treatments
>
> The healing power of the body and mind
>
> Secrets of some past person, tribe, or event
>
> And other similar concepts.

Don't send me hate emails about alternative medicine. I do believe in a few ancient things like meditation, but we have a life-threatening illness. We can't be screwing around with celebrity or hipster trends while we are driving 100 mph toward kidney failure.

I completely understand the idea that traditional medicine may not know everything and we should be open-minded. To be honest, I am sympathetic to this concept and in some ways I agree. However, the idea that ancient medicine knows something that we don't know today can be put to the test using life expectancy.

Year	Average life expectancy
0-1900's	30 -40 *
1950s	48
1970s	67
1990s	71
2018	80ish

*Human life expectancy stayed the same for about 2,000 years until the widespread use of antibiotics in the 1940s. Clearly, the idea that tried and tested ancient medicine is superior to modern medicine doesn't pass the smell test; in fact, it stinks. Give me modern cutting-edge medicine, 24/7, 365 days a year.

I say this because I looked into alternative medicine to try to cure my disease as well. What I found was upsetting. The placebo effect is very real. Much of the supplement and alternative medicine business is based on getting us to believe something is working for you, whether it's working or not. It's true that if we believe something will help us, it just might. However, sometimes we want to believe something will help us, so we overlook all available evidence to the contrary. It's hard to face the fact that we are out of options. I hear you. I have been there too.

This includes well-meaning advice from family and friends. The crazy advice I have gotten over the years is, well, just that—crazy.

Let me say this another way:

> **Writing a treatment plan and trying every available option is not a license to do crazy shit!**

It's the opposite of this. The key is using well-thought-out treatments with ways to measure effectiveness that your real medical doctor feels are worth any risks. You have a duty to yourself and your loved ones to start with low risk treatments and then work down the list towards higher-risk treatments.

Any good treatment plan has three basic components:

1. Includes your medical doctor and regular blood and urine tests

2. Has an accurate way to measure dosage and evaluate results over a set period of time

3. Risks are understood

You may receive pushback from doctors saying things like, *"Let's just monitor this for now and see what happens"* or *"You're early stage 3—no need to try all kinds of treatments."* This is standard medical practice and does not make your doctor a bad person. However, this is just plain bad advice. Everything should be on the table from day one. Even if your GFR is 70-plus, you should consider all of your options and not relent. Keep this in the front of your mind: You don't get back lost kidney function, so don't wait on treatments just because you feel okay today.

Don't forget kidneys with GFR around 60 start having real problems handling protein and things go downhill from there.

You should work through all of your options with your doctor. This can be frustrating, but good communication on your part is key. Always think about being a strong, but patient and persistent advocate for yourself when working with your doctor or any medical staff. Good communication is essential, and in this scenario, good communication is your responsibility, not your caregiver's.

You should start with the most proven and lowest-risk treatments first and then work your way down the list until the risks are not worth the possible benefits. Some treatments may be low-risk, but unproven. Others may be high-risk, but more proven. You and your doctor need to work through your options.

You may be able to combine therapies for a better outcome. Combinations that have not been tried before are fair game. However, they need to be based on good science and the potential risks need to be understood.

Here is an example of combining therapies that I feel could be very valuable:

> A small fire is easier to put out than a big fire, a small infection is easier to treat than a large one, and so on. I tried drugs when my disease was at its worst. Everything was bad and getting worse, despite drug therapy. Using the fire example, I had a fire that was out of control before I started drug therapy. On a scale of 1 to 10, 10 being worst, my disease was 10.

What if I had tried the diet and treatment plan here first? What if my disease severity had dropped from 10 to 5? What if I had been able to remove most of the drivers of my disease? My inflammation had dropped and my overall numbers were much better, but still no remission. Drug therapy could be used to push me over the remission finish line. These drugs should be more effective if inflammation is lower. These drugs may also be safer to use if we are in better health.

Diet is about as low-risk as you can get, especially compared to drugs. Based on everything I know, this should be a viable treatment plan for the right people. Use the diet and treatment plan in this book to get as close to remission as possible. Then bring out the big guns to push you over the line. In theory, this should work for some people with autoimmune-related kidney disease. If you try it, please let me know about your personal plan so we can build a database of these treatments to share with others.

We don't know if this one-two punch would increase the rate of remission or not. Hypothetically, the remission rate could be worse. We just don't know for now. However, combining therapies may be better than one therapy alone. For example, the combination of a low-salt diet, exercise, and blood pressure meds is very, very effective at lowering blood pressure.

My point here is to think outside the box if needed. You and your doctor may find something better than the rest of us have thought of. The treatment plan in this book is a combination of the latest research, combining therapies, and innovative thinking.

Don't Automatically Say No to Anything

Many patients will want to take drugs and not go on a special diet. This is understandable and a decision each patient has to make with his/her doctor's advice and guidance. Compliance with taking a pill is much higher than dietary compliance. However, we may be missing out on a valuable treatment opportunity. We should never rule out anything. Sure, try the easiest treatment first, but don't shut the door on anything. It's perfectly viable to try strong drugs first, then if those fail, try to change your diet and lifestyle.

In your treatment plan, you may be asking to do things that are new to your doctor or counter-intuitive. Magnesium is a good example. Large single doses of magnesium are bad for late-stage kidney patients. However, magnesium also improves our survival advantage, reduces inflammation, and reduces vascular calcification. You should have an open conversation about these issues. Be prepared to educate your caregivers as needed and back up any requests with research.

You should be prepared to listen to any concerns they have as well. Their concerns are valid in almost every case. Again, it's up to you to be a good communicator and advocate for yourself.

Experimental drug or dietary trials should also be on the table if everything else fails.

The benefits of trying several treatments are unknown, but likely beneficial. The more treatments you try, the better your odds of something good happening. I will use my case as an example. After drugs failed, I searched for clinical trials and found Dr. Walser at Johns Hopkins. While I wasn't cured in the trial, I was exposed to new ideas and treatment plans I had never heard of or considered. I had to find the trials on my own, just like you will.

If you don't like your MD or find that he/she is resistant to trying different options, then find another MD and get a second opinion, but do not start messing around with alternative forms of medicine that may not be founded on evidence-based science. It's not a risk worth taking. Well-thought-out treatment plans supervised by a real doctor are the only way to go.

In many areas, nephrologists are in short supply and it takes several months to get an appointment. Your family or primary care doctor works just fine, but nephrologists are ideal. I used my regular doctor for ongoing testing and evaluation because it took months to see my nephrologist. The key here is that you should always be in the care of a qualified physician.

#3: You Need a Repeatable and Measurable Treatment Plan with Feedback Built In

Random, scattershot, and short-term treatments will yield random results, and you won't be able to trust your blood and urine tests. I wasted years jumping from one treatment to another because I had no help and didn't know what I was doing. Looking back, I see that I never had a great plan or one that was well-researched. I wasted years and tens of thousands of dollars. Please learn from my mistakes.

The key here is to follow a structured plan so you know if it's working or not. I will use pills as an example.

Instructions:

1. Take one pill daily.

2. Get blood test after x days to see if pill is working as predicted.

3. Use test results to determine if pill is working and if dosage should be changed.

4. Repeat until the correct dosage is found or try a new medication and repeat the same process.

Pretty simple and common sense, right? This is fine for high blood pressure or cholesterol meds, but we are starting from scratch when no standard treatment plan exists. We need a plan that greatly increases our odds and prognosis. Pills are not an option for us, so we have to be a little more creative.

#4: Kaizen for Kidneys

I don't remember where I first heard the term kaizen. Maybe it was in Japan in 1989 or 1990. For some reason, when I thought about how I was going to deal with writing an experimental treatment plan for myself that I could manage and measure, kaizen came to mind.

Kaizen is Japanese for "good change" or "change for the better." The roots of kaizen came into the American consciousness after World War II. Dr. William Deming was working to help improve Japanese manufacturing processes.

The Deming Improvement Cycle acronym, PDCA, stands for Plan, Do, Check, and Act. It's been proven for over 70 years. The name may change, but the basic principles do not.

The basic Deming improvement cycle is as follows:

1. **Plan:** Gather information and ideas on something you would like to improve.

2. **Do:** Implement the change you researched in Step 1.

3. **Check:** Did the changes implemented in Step 2 bring the expected improvements?

4. **Act:** Lock in the change you were able to prove by checking the results against past data or a baseline number. If the change did not work, then start the process over again with a new plan.

Deming's genius is standard practice today, but it gives a proven structure for our treatment plan and incremental improvement.

I will add one more step to Deming's list for those of us trying to cure an incurable disease.

Simple

Simple means keeping things easy for yourself. There is no award for the most complicated plan or strategy. The more complicated your plan, the less likely you are to follow it. Your test results may be confusing. You won't know what part of the complicated plan worked and what part was a waste of time. Simple, clear, and measurable plans and treatment goals are part of an effective treatment plan.

Make it easy on yourself whenever you can. I came to hate mixing powders three times a day. I used the blender to mix the powders with juice or water. It ended up taking fifteen minutes to measure the powder, mix, and then clean the blender. Last, I would have to check to see how much of the measured dose was stuck to the side of blender or my glass after drinking. This is one of the reasons Albutrix is in a pill form, to make dietary compliance easier, faster, and more exact. When you have the opportunity to make things easy and simple, do so.

#5: Treat Heart Disease as Aggressively as Kidney Disease from Day of Diagnosis

After you are diagnosed with kidney disease, you become a member of a group nobody wants to be in, the highest risk group ever studied for heart disease. You and I very likely already have heart disease to some extent by the time we are diagnosed. Yes, it's a depressing thought, but information is power. Now we can do something about it.

Accelerated heart disease brought on by kidney disease is what most kidney patients actually die from. Kidney disease is a perfect storm for heart disease. Vascular calcification may be the exact factor that causes deaths from heart disease, but anything we can do to improve heart health has got to be part of the plan.

I was eating very bad foods, from a nutritional point of view, in the name of low protein. I felt bad, I was not exercising, and so on. If any treatment, drug, diet, or therapy adds to your risk of heart disease, then you have to question it.

Think About It

Accelerating or increasing heart disease risk in the name of kidney disease treatment is a very questionable practice. You and your doctor should think long and hard about any treatment that may increase heart disease risks.

The opposite is also true. Accelerating kidney disease progression in the name of heart disease treatment needs to be questioned as well.

For example, you could eat a very low-protein diet using fake foods made of oils and starches. Cornstarch and palm oil are low-protein sources of calories, but these foods are questionable from a heart health point of view. Yes, you would treat uremia, but at the expense of everything else. Increasing oxidative stress by lowering your intake of antioxidants, increasing your saturated fat intake, and maintaining poor nutrition from low-protein foods may be counterproductive. You may lower symptoms of uremia only to worsen other symptoms or conditions.

Reducing heart disease risk and vascular calcification has to be part of any well-thought-out treatment plan.

#6: Have a Meaningful and Emotional Goal

Let me say this upfront. "Half ass motivation, leads to half ass results," you need gut-wrenching emotional goals to stay the course. Ok, back to goals.

I floundered around for years jumping from one idea to the next. Changing your goals constantly just leads to more chaos. When we are trying to slow or stop an incurable disease, goals are harder because there are so many unknowns.

I set a goal of remission, but how to get to remission was unknown and still is. We can't set a goal of stopping or slowing our disease unless we know how to do it.

The second part is it's hard for all of us to change. A emotional goal is needed to help with change. You are going to need **sufficient motivation** to make these changes and stick to your plan.

If you don't have a goal set or to strive for, your next year or two will be harder than it has to be. Having a concrete goal allows you to refocus when doubt sets in or something doesn't go as expected. Goals allows you to measure your progress so you can feel good about what you are doing or know you should be trying something different.

Goals can be anything from avoiding dialysis, or moving from dialysis three times a week to once a week. It maybe going for remission or slowing the progression to a rate that's so slow you can't even measure it.

Some of these goals have problem though, they are hard to measure. How are you going to avoid dialysis or how are you going to slow the progression of your disease?

A goal of slowing disease progression is a great goal, but how do you measure when there is no test for remission? Who defines what is slow, medium, or fast in terms of progression? You know the saying, "You can't manage what you can't measure." These goals have one problem: They are difficult to measure or the measurements are debatable.

To avoid this, I recommend that you create simple, measurable, and verifiable small goals that lead to you a big emotional goal. Going this route really improved my mindset and allowed me to have a better focus.

My two cents is your goals should be as follows:

1. Eliminate all comorbid conditions that contribute to kidney and heart disease progression.

2. Add all conditions that slow the speed of kidney and heart disease progression.

3. Once this has been taken as far as you can go, reevaluate your options.

These are trackable and objective in most cases. They are meaningful because every time you eliminate a condition, your odds get better. The odds of your disease slowing get better and your health gets better.

Keep score like you are the home team and kidney disease is the hated rival you are dying to beat. I mentioned this before, and you will be hearing about this again.

After you have eliminated all comorbid conditions and added conditions that slow kidney disease, then optimize your numbers.

This process resulted in my best gains and ended with remission. Even if you don't go into remission, you will have concrete goals to work with that your doctor can evaluate with you.

If you want to avoid dialysis, this is the best way, in my opinion. It is also the best way to go for remission.

Think about it this way, if every ninety-day or quarterly cycle you eliminate one health condition and add one that slows your disease or increases your quality of life, after a year or two, your life is going to be pretty great and your disease is going to slow or maybe even stop.

How should we keep score?

It doesn't matter how you keep score, what matters is you keep some kind of score to track your progress. If you blood or urine test is outside the normal range, it's a point for kidney disease. If you have a visible symptom like edema, it's a point for kidney disease.

Every time you wrestle a condition into the normal range or a condition disappears, you get a point. Every time you knock out a condition, your odds get better.

Don't count current conditions that are already in the normal range.

For most of us, the score will be something like 0 to 10 when we start. That's okay as we are all starting from behind. We are going to be the comeback kings and queens.

At the end of a year, your score will likely go from 2 to 4 or maybe even better. Add another few cycles and many of you may have a scores of 4 to 2.

This is a simple system that keeps you focused. Every time you eliminate or wrestle a condition into the normal range, your odds just got better. Rember the concept of C^3. Tying eliminating conditions to your emotional goal is key.

You can use anything to get into the normal range. Drugs, diet, therapy, and exercise can all be used together to get into the normal range. This speeds your progress and likely improves your outcomes faster.

The second part of this is knowing that this goal is worth the effort. Again, my guess is no therapist or psychologist would advise this, but remember "moderation kills." This is also true for your motivation. Go for gut-wrenching or deliriously happy goals to stay motivated. Weak emotions get weak results.

You need to connect to something that motivates you to work hard and change. For me, it was the angst and shock of burying a younger sister and watching the horrible pain my parents never really recovered from. I vowed they would not let them bury me. No way was I going to put them through that again. I was sure it would kill them. To this day, I have never told my wife, twin sister, or my family about this goal. I have kept it to myself until know. I don't know why, but I have never felt comfortable sharing this before. If they don't read this page, they will still never know.

If I picture the pain of my parents burying me, tears still well up in my eyes instantly. My message to you is to choose a motivation that will bring you to tears, knock you to your knees, or take your breath away. That's when you know you are getting close to a meaningful goal that will work.

It may be staying in good enough health to be a grandparent, or taking care of a loved one like a parent or special needs child. It could also be fear of dying, fear of dialysis, fear of dying waiting on a transplant.

If unicorns and butterflies do it for you, great. Use it. If picturing your kids crying and throwing dirt on your grave does it, use it. If picturing yourself old, frail, and sickly does it, use it. Don't judge what works for you; you don't have to share it with anyone unless you want to. Like I said, I never shared what worked for me until writing this page. Do whatever it takes to find a crippling emotion and use it to your advantage.

If you don't tap into this kind of emotional hardcore motivation, you are unlikely to change or stay with the program. From the bottom of my heart, I hope you don't need a death in your family to get you on board and moving in the right direction.

For me, this book, Albutrix, and clinical trials have always been about family. More time with family, less pain in our lives, more happiness is what we all want and it's what your loved ones want as well. My kids will certainly bury me someday, but I had better be at least a hundred years old. They will say things like " He was too stubborn to die" or "He never gave up." They won't say "He didn't try" or "He is gone too soon."

Find emotions that make you scream for joy or scream in pain, but find a primal emotion and tap into it. It may not fun, but it is extremely effective. You will need daily emotional reminders to stay on track.

Dietary compliance is only about 10% to 15%, which is depressing as hell from my point of view. The real reason is motivation in survival situations, people will eat or drink just about anything to live. We have hardcore motivation of dying in a few days if we don't find a way to eat and drink. While we are not stranded on a desert island, we are in a survival situation in many ways. Find that motivation that moves you and think of it daily to stay on track. They say kidney disease is the "silent killer," as it is painless.

I have lost too many people I loved due lack of early intervention or putting their head in the sand. You are going to deal with your disease or your disease is going to deal with you.

I watched an uncle I dearly loved succumb to cancer. To say he was good to me is an understatement. Near the end he told me "I killed myself by being an idiot. I knew something was wrong years ago, but I was afraid to go the doctor." He had symptoms for years, but ignored them. By the time the symptoms could not be ignored, it was too late. The cancer had already spread. His grandchildren will never know one of the greatest guys in the world.

Don't wait until it's too late just because you don't feel bad today. Don't ignore your diagnosis and the facts surrounding this disease. I promise that no matter how cranky and cantankerous you can be sometimes, there are a lot of people whose lives will be poorer if you are not around.

A Quick Summary of this Chapter

1. You are going to have to write your own treatment plan because a standard treatment plan does not exist for your incurable kidney disease. I have been your guinea pig, but you are still going to have to write and customize a plan for your current situation.

2. Aggressively treat your disease immediately after diagnosis. You don't get kidney function back once it's lost. Do not settle for managing symptoms or monitoring your decline. Focus on curing or stopping every driver of kidney disease you can.

3. Everything should be on the table, from a treatment point of view. This doesn't mean you will try everything on your list, but you need to make educated choices. Leave no stone unturned, including new therapies and experimental drug or diet trials.

4. Follow a system so you can trust the result and understand exactly what is working or not working. Garbage in, garbage out.

5. Keep it as simple and easy as possible.

6. Don't forget about the impact of any treatment plan on your heart. Accelerating heart disease and/or vascular calcification may not be worth the risks.

7. Use measurable goals and emotional motivation to keep going for the first ninety days.

Never forget that you should always be under the care of a licensed physician. Your doctor is the most important part of your treatment plan in many ways.

The first step in PDCA is planning. This is the hardest part, but the right plan yields the most benefits. Planning will take some prep work and time, but I promise it is worth it. Bad plans just lead to wasted time and money, and blood test results you can't trust. I lost a decade, learn by my mistakes.

We will tackle planning next.

CHAPTER 35

Planning Your Treatment

The first step of PDCA is plan. Planning well sets you up for success and good decision making. I did the research in this book over the first 20-plus chapters trying to figure out what issues were making my disease unstoppable.

I had to find out every possible contributing factor or cause and address each one if I wanted to take a real shot at a cure, remission, or slowing my disease to a snail's pace. We are going to take out every factor we can that contributes to disease progression.

Based on the 20-plus factors that can contribute to kidney disease progression, we need to plan for the following:

1.   A low-protein diet with the lowest nitrogen protein source I could find.

2.   A diet high in antioxidants, fiber, nitrates, and overall nutrition.

3.   Diet should be net alkaline (low acid or negative PRAL) each day, or at least neutral from an acid point of view.

4.   Diet should also be low in cholesterol and saturated fats.

5.   Get enough calories to maintain my weight.

6.   Reduce (or maybe increase) intake of sodium, potassium, phosphorus, calcium, and/or food that might contribute to any of the conditions on the list depending on blood test results.

7.   It was clear that I had to exercise regularly.

8.   I would have to make my own food/recipes in order to control these factors. Packaged foods are typically high in salt and may have added phosphorus.

9.   Take any and all prescribed medications that help with the above conditions.

10. Don't take any over-the-counter supplements, high-dose vitamins, herbs, or other unregulated supplements unless my doctor prescribes them and are tested regularly for effectiveness and toxicity.

11. Stay on the plan well enough and long enough to get real, measurable results that I can use for the next step, which is to actually do or execute the plan. This leads to quarterly or 90-day cycles.

12. Treat for depression and anxiety as needed.

13. Track and measure my progress.

This is the basic plan. It sounds complicated, but it's really not. Now, let's go over the first checklist you need to start with.

The Planning Checklist

A great book titled "The Checklist Manifesto" by Atul Gawande provides evidence of thousands of lives being saved by checklists in hospitals. So, a checklist it is.

Some of the items in this checklist may seem obvious, but based on hundreds, no, thousands of emails over the past year, you need to follow the checklist just to be sure. We are all starting from different stages and types of diseases. A checklist allows us to standardize the first step in planning.

Everyone should start with this checklist. This is our first stop before starting your treatment plan.

Step 1 Checklist

1. Make an appointment with your doctor and get updated blood and urine tests.

    A few things: Get your blood and urine taken a week or so before your doctor's appointment. You want to have results in your hands during your doctor's appointment, not a week or two later.

    Ask for the following blood and urine tests and any other tests your doctor wants.

    Blood Urea Nitrogen (BUN)

    GFR or eGFR

    Creatinine Clearance

    Serum Albumin

    Magnesium

    Calcium

    Phosphorus

    Potassium

    Cholesterol

    Complete blood panel (CBC)

    C-reactive protein

    Vitamin D

Parathyroid hormone or PTH

Urine protein

Get your bloodwork done before your doctor visit. Always do this.

These are standard blood tests, but you will have to ask for some, like magnesium.

Go to our site, **www.stoppingkidneydisease.com**, to get a printout.

2. Once you have test results and meet with your doctor, ask your doctor about the most proven treatments for your type of kidney disease.

    Find out if you are a candidate for any therapies to treat your disease that you may not be aware of or have not tried.

    If you have treatment options, then make a list from the lowest-risk therapies to the highest risk. You can also make a list of the most proven to the least proven or experimental.

    I didn't have this at the time, but here is what my list would have looked like after the first meeting with my doctor.

    Drug options:

    Cyclosporine or similar immune-suppressing drug

    Prednisone or similar steroid

    Experimental trials:

    Experimental drug or diet trials

    You can add:

    Kidney Factors diet, a low-protein kidney- and heart-healthy diet, and working on curing comorbid conditions.

This gave me four options in this example.

Next, ask your doctor to help you rank your options in terms of risk, from the lowest-risk to the highest-risk.

Different doctors may rank treatments differently.

Ranked low-risk to high-risk:

1. Diet and exercise-based plans

2. Prednisone

3. Cyclosporine

4. Experimental drug trial risk may not be fully known and/or you could be in the placebo group (if they have one).

You always want to the try the lowest-risk therapies first if you are willing to do them. It doesn't matter if it is a drug, diet, or medical procedure. If the first one fails, move on to the second one, and so on. After proven drugs, you can ask about experimental treatments or drugs or newer therapies.

Another aspect to treatments is time frame. How long will it take to judge effectiveness?

You could add time frame to help guide your decisions:

1. Diet and exercise-based plan   90 days

2. Prednisone   4 to 6 months

3. Cyclosporine   4 to 6 months

4. Experimental drugs   unknown

You could also add cost, insurance coverage, and so on to build your list.

Feel free to ask about newer or different therapies, like incremental dialysis, depending on your disease stage.

While diet will almost always be the lowest-risk and fastest, some patients will not want to change their diet/lifestyle and will opt for drugs first. There's nothing wrong with this; you are being honest with yourself. If you can't or won't stick to a change in lifestyle and diet, it's not a potential cure for you. You can always come back to diet if higher-risk treatments fail.

The key here is you know all of your options and you work through these options systematically with your doctor from low-risk to high-risk. This is the sane and rational way for you to think about your options. Don't say "no" to any option; keep it on your list and come back to it later if you need to. Always keep your options open.

3. If you want to pursue the diet and treatment plan in this book, ask for your doctor's support with the following:

    You want to pursue a heart- and kidney-healthy low-protein diet to reduce the load on your remaining kidney function and also try to cure or manage any conditions that contribute to kidney disease progression.

    The treatment plan will consist of:

    Blood/urine tests and doctor visits to evaluate results every 90 or so days

    A low-protein diet to reduce the workload on your remaining kidney function

    Diet is heart-healthy and high in fiber, antioxidants, and nutrition

    Regular exercise

    Over time you are going to try to manage all of your health conditions into the normal range through diet, supplements, exercise, and drugs.

Of course, you will continue to take all prescribed medications or other prescribed therapies during this time.

Tell your doctor you would like to try this for a minimum of 90 days and then come back in to see how you have improved. After the first 90-day period, you would like his/her help evaluating the effectiveness of the diet and treatment plan. This is key; you are asking for an objective opinion, which is an important part of any treatment plan. You want to make good, fact-based decisions with your doctor's help.

If after 90 days, you and your doctor don't see any improvement, then you can move on to trying a different treatment.

After explaining, ask your doctor: Will you support me on this treatment plan to see how much I can improve? If you have a paper version of this book, take it with you.

This is important because your doctor is your biggest ally in this fight.

In 99% of cases, you will get an enthusiastic "yes." Your doctor really wants to help you. For the other 1%, don't be afraid to ask "Why?" For me, I had no other viable options, so my doctor felt it was fine to pursue diet-based strategies as long as I had regular blood tests.

Get your doctor's approval and support

4. Before you leave the doctor's office, list your comorbid conditions, diet restrictions, and supplements that are needed to cure, manage, or treat your disease with your doctor.

You need a list of the following:

1. Any blood or urine tests that are outside the normal ranges.

2. List other health conditions like high blood pressure, diabetes, acidosis, and so on.

3. Ask if you need to be on a restricted diet for any issues. Potassium is an example.

If so, what is the recommended restriction?

My list looked like this:

Cholesterol

Serum albumin

Potassium

Creatinine clearance

Blood urea nitrogen

C-reactive protein

High blood pressure

Edema

Red blood cell count	
Muscle cramps at night	
Diet restrictions	
Potassium	4,000 mg a day

If you are not treating these conditions, ask your doctor:

"Can any drugs help me get these numbers into the normal range, or do I need to adjust the dosage of current drugs to lower my risk?"

If your blood pressure, or cholesterol, or whatever, is too high or too low and drugs will help you get in the normal range and the risks are worth the expected benefit, then ask your doctor to prescribe the medication or change the prescription as needed. We want to start knocking out comorbid conditions right now. Don't wait. You want to start getting better today, not next week.

The list of numbers outside the normal range is part of what's driving your disease progression. We will evaluate this list every 90 days to judge the efficacy of your treatment plan.

The result you want is a list of everything you need to address on one simple page. Put the list on your fridge or someplace you will see it every day. It may look a little depressing, but don't worry; it's going to get better.

Make a list with your doctor of all of your health conditions you need to cure, treat, or manage, and any recommended dietary restrictions/recommendations. Get any prescription needed to treat conditions.

5. Get your body mass index (BMI) from from your doctor.

Your doctor/nurse will normally calculate this at your appointment. If not, you can find BMI calculators on the internet. Your BMI is a measurement of your body fat adjusted by your gender and height.

BMI is for tracking our progress at this point. Don't worry about the number yet. (Yes, I understand BMI is not perfect, but it works well enough and is easy to get.)

6. Get your doctor's approval for exercise.

You want to know what level of exercise is safe for you. Some doctors will recommend an electrocardiogram, EKG, or maybe a heart stress test before you start exercising. Remember, heart disease is the number one killer of kidney patients. You can't be too careful here. Get your doctor's approval before beginning any exercise program. Get any needed tests to clear you for exercise, and when you start exercising (if you are not already), start slowly.

This is a good time to ask for a coronary artery scan if you have a family history of heart disease. This scan tells you how much calcium has built up in your arteries and is a good indication of heart disease risk. If you can get one, do it. Finding out your risk ahead of time is a million times better than finding out during or after a heart attack.

7. Make your next appointment before you leave the doctor's office, no less than 90 days out and no more than 120 days.

Summary of first steps:

1. Make an appointment to see your doctor and get your blood and urine tests done ahead of the appointment.

2. Ask your doctor if any drug therapies exist that may cure or slow the progression of your disease. Do you have any options you are not aware of?

3. Get your doctor to buy into your new treatment plan if drugs are not an option.

4. Make a list of all of your blood/urine tests that are outside the normal ranges, and another of other health or comorbid conditions and diet restrictions. Get prescriptions as needed.

5. Get your BMI from your doctor or calculate it online.

6. Get your doctor's approval/recommendation for exercise.

7. Go ahead and make your next appointment for 90 to 120 days out.

After leaving your doctor's office, you should have the above steps completed. You will have gotten your current results or baseline data, explored your options, gotten your doctor's blessing to try the diet and hopefully his/her approval for exercise.

You will feel better after completing these steps because you are taking control of your future and making the choice to fight.

We have a little more planning to do in the next chapter, but this checklist is a good start.

CHAPTER 36

Planning the Details

We need to finish our planning stage with a few more details. We need to know what to eat, how much to eat, and so on. We have to plan this in advance so we know what are doing and can shop appropriately.

Remember, we are going to keep things as simple as possible the first cycle.

The treatment plan is based on ninety-day or quarterly checkups and adjustments, I refer to it as cycles. A cycle is ninety days on the treatment plan ending with an evaluation using blood/urine tests and your doctor to judge results. It takes this long for change to occur that we can count on. We are not going to attempt too much change during the first ninety-day cycle.

The big picture treatment plan is pretty simple and is based on the following:

1. Every ninety-day/quarterly evaluations and corrections

2. Eliminating comorbid conditions

3. Adding conditions that slow your disease

4. Use every tool in the toolbox (diet, drugs, therapy, medical foods, supplements, exercise, etc.)

5. Go from baseline to baseline (Goldilocks) to get the best results.

These are pretty self explanatory except for number five, so let me explain.

Hindsight is 20/20 and looking back, let me give you one version of kidney hell. I changed plans, diets, drugs, and supplements every 30 days and was ending up in a kidney disease hell. What I didn't know at the time was thirty days was too short to get any real changes. I chased ghosts many times these improvements did not stick or gains stopped. These changes were short-term and easily lost.

The hell I refer to is getting test results the opposite of what I thought should happen after changing everything around based on the last test results. It's chaos and an emotional roller coaster that none of us need. We are just spinning our wheels and wasting time.

Going from baseline to baseline is the way to go and the road to kidney disease ass kicking. Remember, we are trying to slow an incurable disease, wins are hard won and don't always come easily, and any win is a victory and likely improves your odds.

Going from baseline to baseline means staying with the same diet until your gains stop coming. Any gain is a big deal so why would you change a diet and treatment plan that is working? You shouldn't. If something is working that's amazing considering the cirucmstances. Don't mess it up by trying to change a bunch of things after you have a few wins. It's a miracle anything is working for an incurable disease, don't mess it up or second guess. PDCA says we have to "lock" in any improvements. PDCA saved me from kidney disease hell by giving me a system to lock in changes that allowed me to improve.

The second reason is you don't know how far these changes can take you. For some, just staying on the diet and treatment plan will lead to remission or a dramatic slowing of disease progression and a solid increase in GFR. You may not have to do anything else, but you won't know this if you keep changing or jumping around from one thing to another. Staying on course allows you to find out how far you can go with the diet and treatment plan. It may take you all the way or maybe not, but the only way to know is to stay on the same diet and treatment plan without any major changes. You will never know what is possible if you keep changing everything or go off and on the diet and treatment plan.

A new baseline will be established when you have two ninety day cycles in a row with no meaningful change. This took me five cycles. Cycles six and seven were almost identical, but cycle seven ended with my doctor announcing remission. You know you have taken the basic plan as far as you can go if you have two cycles in a row with no improvement. Two cycles in a row with no change equals a new baseline.

We are using facts to make decisions, not guesses.

After two cycles in a row with no improvement, it's time to make a few changes to keep the gains coming. We have the new results from two cycles in row as a new baseline. The stubborn issues that still won't change will be the focus of the next cycle. However, any changes before two cycles with no gains should be avoided in almost all cases. You want to reach the "Goldilocks zone" we will talk about later.

Keep this in mind: any gain on an incurable disease is amazing, awesome, incredible, unbelievable, fantastic, mind-blowing, and life affirming. Don't screw it up by making a bunch of changes. Ride the diet and treatment plan into the dirt before making any changes.

It took years if not decades of something to bring on your disease, you are not going to solve it in a week and modern science hasn't solved it yet either. Changes take time and in our case these changes likely take more time as our bodies are compromised already. It likely took fifteen+ years of abusing my body for it to rebel. If it takes a year to make up for fifteen years, that's a pretty good trade.

Back to Planning

For the first 90 days, we are not going to worry about anything but three things:

1. Staying on the diet.

2. Exercising 5 days a week.

3. Taking any and all prescription drugs and keeping all doctor's appointments.

Before you ask, yes, there are more things we could be doing, but we want to focus on the high impact items first. We want to master the highest impact items first, then we will add or tweak issues down the road. So for the first 90 days, Nothing else in your life matters except these three things. The first two are the only ones that require any work, planning, or time.

For the first ninety days, we need to establish the workout habit and learn how to eat so we can do as much work for our kidneys as possible. That's plenty for the first ninety-day cycle.

Calculating Your Nutritional and Protein Needs

I hope one thing has been made clear in this book: nutrition matters. Proper nutrition is critical to everyone's health.

One more time so we are clear: you cannot be on a low protein (LPD) or very low protein diet (VLPD) without supplementing protein to ensure adequate nutrition. If you are eating less than .8 grams per kg of body weight you have to supplement protien in some way.

Let's go over the basic rules of the diet plan:

1. No calorie restrictions, eat as much as you want given the restrictions for the first ninety days.

2. .4 grams of dietary protein per day per kg of bodyweight limit for the first ninety-day cycle

3. Use a low nitrogen protein food to supplement protein designed for your stage of kidney disease to reduce nitrogen load to the lowest possible amount.

4. Follow any restrictions you may have, like potassium, which are individual to each patient.

5. Focus on eating whole plant-based foods prepared at home. No meat or dairy or grains unless they have a negative potential renal acid load (PRAL) and are low-protein.

6. If you are underweight, ensure you get enough calories each day to start gaining weight. If you are overweight, don't worry about counting calories. Just make sure you count the restricted items like protein and potassium, and don't go over.

Let's go over the reasons for these rules.

1. No calorie restrictions is one of the keys to making this transition. I was much more successful with this approach. I didn't feel deprived or starved. One hint is eat at regular times and eat before you are hungry. Potassium, protein, or other dietary restrictions are strict enough to ensure we don't get too many calories each day. In addition, fruits and veggies are naturally low calorie. Eat as much as you want of healthy foods given your restrictions. We will deal with weight later unless you are underweight. You can't eat too many healthy foods.

2. The .4 gram restriction is higher than traditional .3 gram per kg associated with very low-protein diets (VLPD) for a reason. The reason is I found it very hard to eat healthy with a .3 gram restriction. To get adequate calories, you have to supplement with foods that are not healthy and or increase fat and sugar calories (which have no protein) to a questionable amount.

For example, one cup of broccoli has 4 grams of protein but only 45 calories. 4 grams is almost 20% of the daily protein restriction using the .3 gram(VLPD) model. Yet, it has only 2.2% of the needed calories (assuming 2,000 calories per day).

Going with .4 grams to start allows us to eat a wider variety of foods and consume more calories than the .3 grams. We are getting half of our protein nutrition from food and the other half from a product like Albutrix. The chance for malnutrition also decreases compared to a .3 restriction. The type of protein matters, so by going all plant-based we get a little more room to increase protein as well. Plant based protein is easier on our kidneys and we don't absorb plant based phosphorus as much as phosphorus in meat or inorganic phosphorus. Plant based allows us to increase our protein just a little to .4 per kg.

.4 grams per kg will be our baseline for now.

3. Each patient's dietary restrictions will be different. For example, one patient with a GFR of nine had no potassium restriction, but another with a GFR of 50 did have a potassium restriction. You and your doctor will have to address these issues. Know and calculate any daily restriction that applies to you.

    An example, your potassium restriction maybe almost zero, allowing for 4,700 mg a day or the normal recommended amount. Other patients may be down to 2,000 to 3,500 mg a day.

    Know or use you current blood work to estimate personal restrictions before starting the diet.

5. Plant based diets are proven to slow, stop, or reverse heart disease, type 2 diabetes and even prostate cancer. We are going down the proven route with some changes to take the workload off of our kidneys. Whole foods means unprocessed. Eating a raw apple is better than applesauce. Processing rarely if ever adds good calories to food: the exception might be fortified foods, which is another debate. Stick to simple foods as close to the natural form as possible.

6. Calculate your minimum daily calories needed to maintain a healthy body weight. For our purposes, we are going to use a target BMI of 25. You will have to play with the inputs to arrive at a BMI of 25. It's simple if you are over 25, keep reducing your weight until you hit a BMI of 25. If you are underweight, work on increasing your weight until you hit a BMI of 25.

You want to estimate your calories for your target weight, not your current weight. If you are 300 lbs and have a BMI of 35, then you need to calculate your calories based on a BMI of 25, not 35.

If you are underweight with a BMI of 15, then you need to calculate your calories based on a BMI of 25, not 15.

Link to free BMI calculator on the National Institute of Health website:
https://www.nhlbi.nih.gov/health/educational/lose_wt/BMI/bmicalc.htm

Or you can do it by hand.

BMI Formula

1.   Divide your weight in kilograms (kg) by your height in metres (m).

2.   Then divide the answer by your height again to get your BMI.

Example: 75 kg male / 1.82 meters= 41.20, next divide 41.20 by 1.82 again which equals 22.63

Either way is fine, but you want a hard number of calories per day.

Next take your body weight and calculate the amount of calories per day to maintain your ideal body weight for a BMI of 25.

Calorie Intake Formulas

12 calories per lb is a ballpark number. If your weight at a BMI of 25 is 170 lbs, then 170 x 12 equals 2,040 calories per day.

In KG, 26.4 x your BMI in KG will yield the same number. 77 x 26.4= 2032 calories

In this example, I want to ensure I am getting a minimum of 2,040 calories per day to maintain my weight. If you get 2,100 or 2,200 calories or even 2,500 calories that's fine for now for the first ninety days. You may need more calories to feel satiated the first ninety days, just don't break any dietary restrictions for protein or others.

2,000 calories a day is easy to get in a normal american diet. Most meals at restaurants are between 700 and 1300 calories for one meal.

However, in our case healthy foods tend to be lower calorie, so we have to be smart about our food choices to get 2,000 healthy calories or as close to healthy as we can get with the limitations.

Next calculate your protein needs per day

.8 grams per kg or .36 per pound of body weight will tell us the minimum amount of protein we need per day.

In kg, using the same 77 kg example, 77 x.8 = 61.6 grams of protein per day

In lbs, .36 x 170 lbs = 61.2

In this example, we need to get 61 grams a day or protein. Use your current weight if you are overweight and use your ideal weight at a BMI of 25 if you are underweight to calculate protein.

Now calculate your daily protein limit from dietary sources. At .4 kg per kg, your dietary protein limit will be half your normal protein needs, 30.5 to 31 grams per day from your diet.

Now we know a few things:

1.   Our target weight based on BMI of 25.

2.   Estimated daily calories needed to maintain a BMI of 25.

3.   Daily dietary protein limit based on .4 grams per kg of body weight or 30 grams per day.

Now, we need to solve for the remaining protein from our supplement, drug, or medical food.

Low Nitrogen Protein Foods

Now, that you know how much protein you need, you need to find the best protein supplement. You will need to order whatever you decide to use before starting the diet.

What is available to each patient will depend on what country they currently live in. One of the reasons we are shipping Albutrix free to almost anywhere in the world is the fact that I was not able to access life saving or life extending treatment that was available in other countries. No one should be in that position. As I said before, everything is on the table, so the next step is finding out what is available in your country, insurance coverage, cost, and issues like nitrogen and calcium content.

Remember, one of the main reasons we are using a protein food or supplement to address issues like uremia and lowering our blood urea nitrogen (BUN) and creatinine levels. The lowest nitrogen sources will reduce the workload on your kidneys the most.

A simple checklist will help you decide. You want to choose based on the following criteria from most important to least important:

1. What is available in your country locally or what can shipped to your country?

2. Does a special option exist for your specific stage of kidney disease?

3. Lowest nitrogen in milligrams

4. Lowest potential renal acid load (PRAL, negative numbers are better)

5. Lowest calcium in mg

6. Highest magnesium you can tolerate depending on your disease stage/GFR/blood tests

7. Does it lower phosphorus or act as a phosphorus binder?

8. Price

9. Insurance coverage (This is not an option in many countries, but you might as well check). You can use a medical spending account in the U.S. in some cases.

10. Is a prescription required?

Only one option may be available in your country, but it's worth checking to see if you can import as well. Laws differ by country and you will find (like I did) what is a food in one country is a drug in another. Generic amino acids are sold everywhere in the U.S., but are considered drugs in other countries.

For other countries, we are building a list on **www.albutrix.com**. Albutrix may not be available in all countries but other keto/amino acid supplements may be. We are building a list of price and availability by country.

For the U.S., Canada, Australia, U.K., Japan, and most others, Albutrix can be shipped for free worldwide without a prescription.

This chart will help you choose from the options that we are aware of today. We will add to this list in the future. The chart below is based on the recommended daily amount of each. This is the total from the recommended dosage, not from each pill.

	Stage of Kidney disease	Nitrogen load in mg (lower is better	Potential Renal Acid load (PRAL) lower is better	Calcium (lower is better)	Magnesium (higher is better)	Phosphorus binding (yes is better)
Amino acids blends	not stated	1,283	8.8	0	0	no
Calcium based keto/amino acids	GFR below 15	870	-0.83	1,200	0	yes
Albutrix S3 (Stage 3)	Stage 3, GFR greater than 40	223	-8.96	114	399	yes
Albutrix S4 (Stage 4)	Stage 4, GFR 20 to 39	225	-8.67	278	284	yes
Albutrix S5 (Stage 5)	Stage 5, GFR below 20	238	-7.17	729	3.8	yes

See the back of the book for sources.

You can see right away, big differences exist. Nitrogen load in one may be 600% + more than another. The same is true for Calcium, 1,200 mg for another and 114 mg for another. It pays to look at the differences and understand what you are buying and why you are buying it.

Number one tip: You should always be taking the highest magnesium and lowest calcium combination that you can safely tolerate. You want to start slowing or stopping vascular calcification as soon as possible and get the other benefits of magnesium without adding to the amount of supplemental calcium you are taking. If you can tolerate 400 mg vs 300 mg and your magnesium levels are in the normal range, always take the higher dose of magnesium.

This will take a little trial and testing; if you are unsure, start with the product that is below your current kidney function. For example, if your GFR is 42, but you are unsure, then move down to the S4 formula with lower magnesium and check your results after the first ninety-day cycle. You can move up and down as needed. Protein nutrition will be provided both ways, you shouldn't be locked in to any one product. Use the one that works best for you.

Calculating the Amount

Now take the RDA for protein and combine with the diet to see how many pills you need to order or take per day.

Using Albutrix as an example, the dietary protein equivalent is on the box. 1 pill = 4 grams of dietary protein.

This is an estimate for planning purposes as every food has a different amino acid profile. Using the same example, of 61 grams of protein per day and getting 30-31 grams from our diet, we need another 30-31 grams of protein equivalent from our protein food.

30 grams/4 grams per pill = 7.5 pills per day. I recommend rounding up to 8 just to make sure you are getting adequate protein each day. Not to mention, keto acids taste bad; the pills are coated to block the bad taste, but if you break the pills up, you lose the coating.

Some supplements will suggest taking a fixed amount per day regardless of diet and others will suggest a wide range of numbers with no information on how to decide which recommendation to use. You need an exact formula to ensure nutrition with the lowest nitrogen and acid load.

Again, you should always understand what you are doing and why you are doing it. If you are not sure, contact the manufacturer or ask your doctor.

Now, let's list our dietary restrictions

Everyone's restrictions will be little different, but this should be pretty close for most patients. Let's start with the basics you will need to account for every day. You will have to customize this for your current situation. Your potassium restriction or other restrictions will be different.

Here is an example:

Basics:

.4 grams of protein per kg per day, .4 x 75 kg male = 30 gram of dietary protein limit

Remaining 30 grams from low nitrogen protein food

8 low nitrogen protein food pills, take two to three pills with each meal.

3,500 mg potassium restriction (yours will be different, we will use this an example)

2,200 mg sodium limit

1,200 mg plant based phosphorus (we absorb less from plants, so we can have more)

No charred or blackened foods to reduce AGE intake

Dietary nitrate intake greater than 150 mg per day or higher (nitrates from plants, whole foods)

Daily polyphenol intake greater than 1 gram per day (no supplements, whole foods, juices)

Limit saturated fats, healthy fats are fine.

Antioxidant intake per day based on ORAC score greater than 30,000, 30,000+ is even better

Dietary fiber intake per day greater than 30 grams

Negative renal acid load per meal (not per food)

All foods/meal should be heart healthy or at least heart neutral.

Eating as many different foods as possible, a diverse diet is better for you.

No meat, dairy, or soy, but we are going to allow the occasional one egg omelette every once in a while and yes, you can make an omelette using one egg. Make sure you are on the email list and you will get a copy.

In simple terms (for this example):

1. 30 grams of dietary protein or less

2. Low nitrogen protein supplement equal to 30 gram of dietary protein

3. Your personal potassium limit (assume 3,500 mg for this example)

4. 2,200 of sodium limit

5. 1,200 mg plant based phosphorus

6. Limit saturated fats

7. ORAC intake greater than 30,000—higher is better

8. Consume 150 mg of dietary nitrates each day

9. Consume 1 gram of polyphenols each day

10. Fiber intake greater than 30 grams

11. Negative renal acid load

12. Heart healthy

13. Be as diverse as possible given your limitations.

Note: We can't really say anti-inflammatory as no standard has been established for this. In general, food high in fiber and high in antioxidants are considered anti-inflammatory. Same for fruits and veggies. We are also eliminating items that are known to cause inflammation like meat and grain flours.

A Little Extra Motivation Before Going Further

Admittedly, I am willing to say or do just anything to get you to try the first ninety day cycle.

If you won't make some changes in name of stopping your disease, living longer, and feeling better, let's look at some of the other benefits of following this plan:

1. **Increased sex drive**—While this diet is not a vegan/vegetarian diet, it does lean in that direction and research shows that these diets improve sex drive in men by increasing hormones related to sex drive as long as calorie intake is high enough.

2. **Decreased erectile dysfunction**—Diets similar to this diet reduce the odds, frequency and severity of mild erectile dysfunction. If you won't do it for yourself, do it for Willy.

3. **You will be more attractive**—Yes, it's true, studies have linked attractiveness to a diet high in fruit and vegetable consumption. Eating this kind of diet can lead to a skin "glow," as it can change the color of your skin tone. A diet low in salt will also help you get rid of that bloated look and decrease the swelling around your eyes.

4. **You will look younger**—Studies show a diet high in fruits and veggies may slow the appearance of wrinkles and skin aging. I have a twin sister, trust me it's true. (I hope she doesn't read this page.)

5. **You will be more fun to be around**—Feeling and looking better, knocking out a few comorbid conditions will do wonders for your outlook on life. You will be more positive, upbeat, and generally more fun to be around. My wife has mentioned this to me a few hundred times over the years. It's more fun to be having a few wins and trying new things than the alternative. Feel free to be the life of the party instead of sitting around waiting for bad things to happen.

6. **You will feel less emotional stress**—Less stress equals better health. Changing your lifestyle may be a little stressful the first week or two, but after that it's all downhill. Slowing your disease and improving your health will dramatically lower your anxiety and worry. I actually cried a little after my first blood test on this plan and then demanded a second test to make sure the results were real. The emotional release I felt after getting great test results after ten years of failure took me by surprise. You can drop some of the heavy load you have been carrying all of these years. Trust me, dropping that load and knowing you are getting better is just about the best feeling in the world. The reason it feels so good is it's not random. You know exactly what you are doing. What you are doing is kicking kidney disease's ass and that always feels good.

If having more sex, stronger erections, looking younger, having more fun, feeling less stress, and dumping that huge load you have been carrying while stopping or slowing an incurable disease doesn't sell you on trying 90 days on the plan, then nothing will. Ok, maybe stretched a few things here, but you get my point. You will feel and look better ninety days from now. Everything is on the table to get you through the first ninety days. Take a picture before and after so you can see the results.

You can choose to drive 100 mph toward kidney failure and keep your current diet and lifestyle or you can try to stop or slow the disease. It's your choice. Nobody can make this decision for you and nobody can force you to do it either. It's all you and you only.

The attitude that ninety days is nothing is a good one. You should be saying "I could stand on my head for ninety days if I had to" or "boot camp was almost 90 days and that didn't kill me and went by in the blink of an eye" or whatever metaphor makes sense to you. Ninety days is the same as a normal summer and look how those fly by. Ninety days is less than .2% of an average life.

One more word about dietary compliance. Research shows that even eating one bad meal a week can set you back from a kidney perspective. Research also shows that lowering protein intake by a small amount benefits kidney patients. Can you get a benefit from partial diet compliance?

Maybe, but that is the road to hell in my eyes. However, we have to deal with reality. Most, if not all, of us will fail a few times during the ninety days. It's what makes us human.

If you falter during the first 90 days, you can get back on the diet the next meal three or four hours later. Forget about the bad choice and move on to getting back on the diet. Don't beat yourself up, it's a waste of time and energy. The bad meal is already in the past, let it go. Just know, your next round of tests may not be as good as they could be. You will have to take this into account when looking at your results. Get back on the diet the next meal and go forward. None of us are perfect, you are in good company. I have fallen off the dietary wagon hundreds of times, maybe thousands, but starting over a few hours later at the next meal is the solution.

Bottom line: Don't let past habits send you to an early grave. It's crazy when you think about it to choose a food for 5 minutes of fleeting pleasure or a past robotic habit over future years with your family and loved ones. Think about this when you are going through the drive-through at a fast food restaurant and that bacon cheeseburger is calling your name. Think about your kids throwing dirt on your casket or meeting your first grandchild for the first time while you are waiting in a fast food line. You will change your order if you have harnessed the right motivation. If you don't change your order, you know didn't pick a strong enough emotion for motivation.

You only need 90 days to know if it's working or not!

What I came to love about this plan is the idea of measurable results that mattered. I felt like I finally had some control over my future. Gone were the days of random results that didn't make sense. Results I could control, change, and adjust by following a repeatable plan. If I followed the plan, I could trust the results and make the next decision with confidence.

If at the end of the ninety days, your blood and urine tests have not improved (and you didn't cheat), then you will have solid information that the diet and treatment plan may not work for you. You can move on to the next treatment option.

If you did improve by any measure you owe me, everyone that loves you, and yourself another 90 day cycle. This is why planning "The Doing" stage or execution part of your treatment plan is so important, you want results you can believe in and trust. Remember, GIGO.

Now, that we have plan, let's talk about the "Do."

CHAPTER 37

The "Doing"

The "Do" part of PDCA is now the easy part, at least from a writing point of view. A better word may be execution. We just have to execute or "do" the plan we put together in the planning phase. Planning allowed us to put together a measurable plan and start down the road of kicking kidney disease's ass.

Let's say it again. You are going to focus on only three things for the first ninety days:

1. Staying on the diet.

2. Exercising five days a week.

3. Taking all prescription meds and keeping all doctor's appointments.

The hard work of planning is done, but now the hard work of change in lifestyle and diet is the issue we have to deal with daily.

So let's think about a few things as we think about the "do." Good execution of your plan will help give you good data for your next appointment and will be the best way to judge the effectiveness of the plan. Always remember: GIGO, GIGO, GIGO.

Before we go into the diet, let's talk one more time about dietary compliance.

It is hard to stay on a new diet and change your lifestyle. As a species, we suck at dieting or keeping to special diets.

A few hints about the "do" part of the plan:

1. Take it one meal at a time. Don't worry about tomorrow, next month, or even the next meal.

   I would say things to myself like, "Okay, just this meal I am going to stay on plan. I am not going to worry about lunch right now." Take it one meal at time. You eat an elephant one bite at time. The execution of the diet is no different. Diets are made and broken on 1,000 tiny decisions, not one big one.

   I took a rock climbing class many years ago. The instructor pointed out that the only thing that mattered was a small circle around you. The area you could reach with your arms and legs. The rest of the mountain was completely meaningless. You couldn't do anything about what was ten feet or a hundred feet away. The secret was focusing on what you could reach right now with your hands and feet.

The same principle applies for long distance swimming; focus on getting to the next buoy, don't worry about the entire race. Breaking the plan into tiny goals and tiny victories is easier than thinking about the whole ninety days.

One more analogy from the shooting world: Lanny Bassham is a ten-time world champion and a gold and silver medal Olympian in shooting. I am paraphrasing: "If you can shoot a ten once, then you can do it a second time or a thousand times. You already have the skill." For us, all you have to do is put together one good meal or day on the diet and treatment plan and you know you can do tomorrow, or a thousand more days. You already have the skill.

You can control what you are putting in your mouth this minute—not tomorrow, next week, or an hour from now. Forget about future and past meals. They are completely meaningless. This approach takes a lot of stress and pressure off.

2.   Special diets are made and broken on Sundays and at breakfast.

I was almost always successful when I cooked and did meal prep on Sunday afternoons. I would make most of my meals for the week and put them into containers. My cravings were always overpowered by my laziness. I would always eat whatever was already made rather than cooking something new. I would shop early Sunday when the stores were empty and cook Sunday afternoon. This became a habit; I still do it more than ten years later.

This is also helpful if you are making meals for the family. Your special meal will already be prepared and you can focus on your family.

You should focus on making breakfast a win every morning. If you screw up breakfast, the rest of the day will be hard. Assume a 30 gram dietary protein restriction. Eating 5 or 7 grams for breakfast sets you up for an easy day. Eating 15 grams at breakfast means you have to really plan lunch, dinner, and snacks. There is no law that says you have to evenly space 30 grams into three meals. The same is true for any restriction, whether it's sodium, potassium, or phosphorus. Make it work for you, but if you knock it out of the park at breakfast, your dietary day is all downhill from there. You will be coasting the rest of the day. However, if you bomb at breakfast, your day will likely get more complicated.

Be flexible about your dietary limits and make them work for you.

Set up whatever system works for you, but breakfast should always be a win, and you should always make and plan your meals on one day a week. Two to four hours of meal prep makes the week easier.

On the website, we have had hundreds of questions on meal prep and maybe thousands on meal plans. A new book will be out in early 2019 with meal plans and recipes. It's too much to put in this book.

3. Keep a record of your daily intake and your goals.

You have to keep track of protein, calories, potassium, and so on. You need to write it down so you have a record to evaluate. It is also helpful to write your emotional motivating goal at the top of the page.

I would write "My parents are not going to bury me today" on the top line of the legal pad when I was preparing breakfast and taking notes on my intake. You can do it on a legal pad, notebook, smartphone, or laptop; just make sure you calculate your intake every day. This will be very valuable information ninety days from now.

I swear this works. Reminding yourself why you are doing this as you start the day works. This makes breakfast an easy win and the rest of the day is easy. Keep track on paper, phone, computer, or whatever; just keep track of your daily dietary stats. It takes five minutes a day once you get the hang of it.

To beat this disease, you are building a system you can trust. If you go off the plan for a meal or a day—okay it happens—write it down and keep track of it. I would feel such horrible guilt writing that I gave into a steak burrito at Chipotle. Listing the protein, sodium, and everything else helped me resist the urge in the future.

The reason you need to keep track is that when you evaluate your results, you need to know how many times you fell off the wagon and how many times you missed your goals for the day. These will have a big impact on your test results. Small changes can make big differences. Be honest about it so your test results can be honestly evaluated.

In just a week or two, as you remember the stats of your favorite meals, it will get pretty easy. The truth is most of us eat the same foods over and over again. We don't eat hundreds of different foods. After the first two weeks, it will be easy to keep track of everything. Getting the habit is the hard part.

"Do" Your Exercise

Exercise takes a little time, so planning has to be done, especially if you work and have a family. You may have to be a little creative. My wife tracks her steps every day. She walks during lunch at work when the weather is decent and finishes any remaining steps in the neighborhood.

I gave myself the goal of passing the military physical fitness test. It was meaningful to me to be in similar shape as when I was in the military. Your fitness goal should be pretty easy for the first ninety days. There is no award for being sore and tired every day.

A few guidelines to help you plan and do your exercise:

1. Make your first ninety-day goal very easy. Walking for 35 to 45 minutes a day is a good start. You can walk inside or outside; you don't need any special equipment or gym memberships.

2. Take a class or classes. Gyms, the YMCA, community colleges, and so on have exercise classes. These keep you on a schedule and some research indicates working out with a group is better in terms of social support. There's dancing, Zumba, jazzercise, water aerobics,

Crossfit, yoga, and the list goes on and on. Be creative. You can walk on your off days from your exercise class.

3. Don't kill yourself. You should always be able to do the same workout tomorrow. This means you should not work out so hard that you can't do the same workout tomorrow with ease. If you are too sore or tired to do the same workout the next day, back off and go easier.

4. The "doing" is more important than what you do. No miracle exercise exists, just moving and lifting a few things on a regular basis works better than some exercise fad. Do what you love and/or do what's easy. Again, there is no award for the hardest or most complicated plan.

5. Exercising at the same time every day makes it easier to start building a habit.

6. No excuses. I used every excuse in the world not to work out, but they were all lies I was telling myself. You can find 35 to 45 minutes a day to get moving. You are a liar if you say you can't. This is a priority for you. You have time to watch TV or do other things, so put a treadmill or bike in front of the TV and pedal away.

7. Measure the amount of exercise you do every day. It can be calories burned, distance walked, or the number of steps, laps, or pushups. Over time, we want to increase our ability to exercise. If we don't have an accurate way to measure, it will be hard to know if we are really improving. Pedometers, heart rate monitors, smart watches, and so on are getting lower and lower in price. You can find relatively affordable ways to monitor your exercise on Amazon, eBay, or Craigslist.

I always feel and sleep better after exercising, but I will admit that setting the habit has been hard for me. It's good for my heart, kidneys, and mind. Working out also allows me to try to keep up with my kids.

So "doing" is about taking it one meal or workout at a time. The hard work was planning; now you just have to execute or "do" your plan.

In the next chapter, we get to the really fun and rewarding part: checking your progress after ninety days. I dreaded my blood and urine tests in the past, but now they are the best part. Trust me, good things are about to happen on your first evaluation.

CHAPTER 38

The Ninety-Day Progress "Check"

Somewhere between ninety and one-hundred-twenty days from your first appointment, you'll go back to your doctor for a check to see how you are progressing and if the diet and treatment plan is working for you.

The "C" in PDCA is "check." We are now to going to check to see if your diet and treatment plan is working.

Start with the same drill as before:

1. Get your blood and urine tests done a week or two before your appointment so you have them in hand when you see your doctor. (These are the same blood and urine tests as the last time.)

2. Have your original list of issues that were outside the normal range on your first appointment and your current BMI.

The most common question is "How do we interpret the results?" It might not be what you think.

The temptation is to start troubleshooting each test outside the normal range, expecting everything to be cured or to go more extreme on the diet. This is a mistake if it's your first evaluation. In a world where millions of people could have any of hundreds of different forms of kidney disease, it's impossible to say what numbers will improve first. We are all unique and will respond a little differently. If you focus on increasing a certain number or blood test, you might start chasing ghosts and erase some or all of your gains. By chasing ghosts, I mean trying to impact a certain blood test or condition only to have it cured later by just sticking to the diet and treatment plan. The other way to chase ghosts is to try to improve one test at the expense of another one. Again, this leads to chaos and uncertainty we don't need.

What we are looking for is a trend in the right direction. Are a few things getting better? Hopefully nothing is getting worse. Remember, kidney disease is systemic and affects many body functions. We need to treat the whole person, not just one symptom or blood test. You will get knocked off track if you obsess about one test or another. The first ninety-day evaluation is a big picture evaluation.

It took six months for my inflammation markers to start falling, and when that happened everything started improving. Avoid the temptation for sudden or extreme changes, and give it time. At nine months, everything was starting to improve for me across the board.

You have to give your body time to start fixing itself and adjusting to the new plan on a level. That's where real change comes from. Some things have to be in the normal range long enough for your body to respond. Getting one test into the normal range this cycle will make it easier to get another one into the normal range the next cycle. One thing this book has shown over and over again is that everything in kidney disease is related.

What to Say and What to Ask on Your First "check"

We want to ask the doctor a series of simple questions that give us black-and-white facts to act on. Before your doctor evaluates your results, you need to announce the following:

"I was x% compliant with the diet."

This is very important to think about before evaluating results. If you were 100% compliant, you'll evaluate your results a little differently than if you were 50% compliant. Be honest. I always exaggerated my compliance at first, until I realized the only person I was screwing was myself. I also found that 99.9% of doctors expect 0% dietary compliance. (If you don't believe me, ask your doctor.) So even if your compliance was 10%, your doctor will be very happy. He or she will be thrilled with any improvement. If you are not honest, you are hurting only yourself. Many of us struggle with a new diet and lifestyle, so don't sweat it. I asked Dr. Walser if he had tried the diet he recommended. He said, "Yes, I lasted eight days." Don't freak out, get upset, or feel guilty if your compliance was less than you wanted. We will deal with this later, and it's hard, so don't feel bad. Being honest allows you and your doctor to accurately evaluate your results, and you need to make fact-based decisions.

Now, ask your doctor the following:

1. Considering all of my results, have I improved since my last visit?   Yes/No/Maybe

2. Has anything gotten worse since my last visit? Yes/No/Maybe

Answers and Actions

For #1

If the answer is a resounding "yes," great job on your part. Think about what just happened. Your incurable disease just got better! This is a f--king miracle and shouldn't be possible, but it is and you are starting to kick kidney disease's ass. It's okay to scream for joy or kiss your normally reserved doctor on the lips. Your odds are going to get better every ninety days. You have also answered the question of whether the diet and treatment plan will work for you. You have a black-and-white answer, no guessing needed. You know that if you stay on this diet, you have a good chance of improving your health and slowing your disease progression.

If your compliance was low and you still improved by some amount, that's an even better indicator that the diet and treatment plan will work for you. If you improved and were 50% compliant, then you know for sure the diet and treatment plan will work for you.

Now that the big picture items are out of the way, you need to ask two more questions:

1. What is my BMI? Am I gaining or losing weight?

2. Is it safe for me to increase my exercise intensity or duration by 10% or 20%?

Let's go over the possible scenarios and what to do next.

We want to make as few changes as possible going forward. As they say, "Don't look a gift horse in the mouth." Be grateful, don't question it, don't try any dramatic changes and, by all means, send me an email at **l.hull@kidneyhood.org** and share the news with me. But, for God's sake, don't change anything except for the items on this list:

1. Update any prescription meds at this time. Increase or decrease the doses as needed to get any issues into the normal range, or to stay in the normal range.

2. If your albumin is low, increase your dosage of keto or amino acids. Do not increase your dietary protein intake. See **www.albutrix.com** for the exact formula.

3. Check your magnesium and calcium levels, and adjust your keto or amino acid supplements as needed. You may need a higher or lower dose of magnesium. If you are in the normal range, you can increase magnesium or move to a different product. For example, you might go from Albutrix S4 to S3. Ask your doctor for their advice, but you always want to take the highest magnesium dosage you can safely tolerate and the lowest amount of supplemental calcium.

4. Update your diet if you are outside the normal range on things like potassium, phosphorus, sodium, and so on. Make small changes, not big ones. If your potassium is still too high, reduce your intake, and so on. Make small changes 100 or 200 mg at a time. You can also increase your intake if you are below the normal range. This happened to me with sodium. After a year, I had to increase my sodium intake to get into the normal range.

5. You may want to decrease your protein intake very slightly if your creatinine and blood urea nitrogen (BUN) numbers have not improved improved at all. If they have improved by a measurable, but small amount don't change anything yet. Your number may improve as inflammation or other conditions are cured or reduced. If you do make a change, make it small, a small change is all that is needed. I would keep changes to 10% or less. If you are not getting results, you can move to 27 instead of 30 grams of dietary protein a day, but don't forget to increase your protein supplement to compensate.

Again, let me know about your success at **l.hull@kidneyhood.org**. Just remember it's the first quarter and we haven't won the game yet.

Troubeshooting

If the answer to question #1 was "maybe" and you got mixed results, ask yourself and your doctor a few questions:

1. Did you really stick to the diet? It's time to be honest. If you didn't really stay on the diet, welcome to the club. If you got mixed results and were less than 80% compliant, then your job now is to go another ninety-day cycle on the plan and *really* do it this time. Everyone is different and some need to ease into change. I think the "moderation kills" approach is best, but we are all different. The first ninety days is gone, so forget about it and focus on getting it right the next ninety days. You get a mulligan or a do-over.

    This will be a very common outcome for patients whose diet varied during the ninety-day cycle. It's okay, just get going on doing better the next ninety days. You have an indication it will work for you now.

2. If you stuck to the diet and treatment plan, ask what got worse and what got better. If the things that got worse are diet-related like phosphorus, you can decrease your phosphorus limit by a small amount to deal with these kinds of issues. If things like inflammation, aka C-reactive protein, or GFR/eGFR got worse and you stayed on the diet, you should do one of two things. 1) If you don't have any other treatment options, try another ninety-day cycle with very good compliance. 2) If you have other treatment options, you and your doctor may want to pursue them.

If the answer is "things got worse" and you stayed on the diet:

1. Stop the treatment and diet plan immediately and pursue other treatment options.

Hopefully, this won't happen to anyone, but if you are not getting better, then you need to pursue other treatment options. You can cross this treatment off your list.

I want to make a point here about treatment plans. Any recommended treatment plan that is open-ended and doesn't have a way to gauge effectiveness should be strongly questioned and evaluated before use. My suggestion is to look elsewhere if this is the case.

BMI Answers

If you are underweight, then you need to be gaining weight. If you lost weight or stayed the same and you are underweight, increase your daily calories by 10%.

If you are overweight, then you need to be losing weight. If you did not lose weight during the first ninety days, reduce your daily calorie intake by 10%.

If you are close to a BMI of 25, then keep everything the same.

You want to start moving towards your target BMI of 25 after the first ninety-day cycle.

Exercise Answers

Ideally, we want to be increasing our capacity to exercise. The ability to increase our exercise duration or intensity is a sign our bodies are working correctly and likely we are getting healthier.

Increasing your exercise intensity or duration every ninety days is a very slow way to increase your exercise capacity, but it's enough for us to get a benefit. Remember, slow and steady is going to win this race. No need for marathons or crazy workouts, just small increases every cycle.

Increase your exercise amount or intensity by at least 10% or 20% if you can. If you were taking 8,000 steps a day, increase it to 9,600 steps a day, or at least 8,800 steps a day. I can't advise on each issue, but you get the point. If you were walking at 3 mph for 45 minutes, increase your speed to 3.5 mph for 45 minutes, and so on. Swim 10% more laps, polka 10% longer, and so on.

Increasing our exercise capacity helps us fight heart and kidney disease, but it also helps us keep up with our kids, grandkids, spouses, and life in general.

If you weren't lifting some kind of weight before, now is the time to start lifting weights once a week. I don't mean lifting weights like a bodybuilder.

Don't worry about a certain fitness routine; some cheap dumbbells from Craigslist will do. Push-ups and body weight squats are free. The key here is to stop the loss of any muscle and maybe even grow your muscles by a small amount. You want to lift weights once a week to maintain your muscle mass and strength. Once a week will do it and, again, go slowly and easily when you start.

We have a few reasons to wait until the second cycle to start lifting weights. First, the workout habit is hard; walking or some other easy exercise makes it easier to get in the habit, and keeps it simple when we are starting out. The second reason is we need to check albumin levels and adjust if we are too low. We need to ensure we are getting adequate protein nutrition before we work on building muscle. Third, we want to make sure we are getting adequate calories before adding more exercise. After the first check, you will adjust your protein supplement and calories as needed.

Time to keep score and update the scoreboard.

1. Did any condition move into the normal range? If so, update the scoreboard.

2. Make sure to count the things you are doing to slow the disease as well.

Keeping score allows you to track your progress and it feels good. Don't expect miracles at every evaluation, especially your first one. If you move one test into the normal range each visit, it's a huge win for someone with an incurable disease. You are beating the odds, one ninety-day cycle at a time. If you can move one test into the normal range every ninety day cycle, you are dramatically changing your future odds. Here is what happened to me.

Serum Albumin	no change, increased intake of low nitrogen protein food
Cholesterol	Normal range with increased dose of statins, diet, and exercise
Potassium	Improved slightly
Sodium	Moved into normal range
Creatinine Clearance	No real change
Blood Urea Nitrogen	Improved slightly
C-reactive Protein	Very little change
High Blood Pressure	Normal range with increased dose of blood pressure meds, diet, and exercise
Edema	Better, but still pretty bad
Red Blood Cell Count	Same as before
Muscle Cramps at Night	Better, but still not gone

Let's check my score. Before, the score was 0–10 for me. After the first ninety days, I moved three drivers of kidney disease progression into the normal range: blood pressure, sodium, and cholesterol.

The combination of increased dosage of statins and blood pressure meds with diet and exercise easily moved these into the normal range. Now, the score is 0 to 7 but I also get to count what I am doing as well.

Now the score has changed to 2–8, in my case. This is a pretty big deal in terms of slowing your disease. Remember, any gain is a big deal for you. Going from 0-10 to 2-8 in score is pretty great and the next ninety-day cycle the score will get better. You already know the diet and treatment plan is working for you.

A question here has been "Why don't you count things that improved or got better?" Because they still contribute to disease progression, just at a slower rate. Improving symptoms is nice, but still a B.S. goal in terms of our health and outcome. We want to cure conditions; that's how we are going to get better. Driving to hell at 70 mph vs 100 mph stills ends up in the same place. We always want to be curing conditions, and by cure, I mean get into the normal range or 100% elimination of a condition like edema. A symptom must be cured in order to count it. By the way, your doctor is the one who gets to say if a condition has been cured or not—not you. It's too easy to delude ourselves and tell ourselves what we want to hear.

You can keep score any way you like, but don't you dare count anything that is not cured or in the normal range. Symptom reductions are nice, but worthless in my eyes if you want to really slow your disease.

Ok, so your appointment is done, Let's go over a few scenarios for you and your doctor to consider:

1. If your compliance was 80% or less, I would focus on getting close to 100% on the next cycle and not worry about everything else for now. You are likely going to get a bigger benefit by nailing the diet and exercise habit than doing other things. Just repeat the first cycle with better compliance. Don't add anything, as you haven't mastered the basics yet. This is also true for exercise. Master the basics of diet and regular exercise before adding items to your treatment plan.

2. If your compliance was over 80% and you improved, then go for at least 90% compliance (or whatever is higher than your current compliance) next cycle. Start working on getting to your target weight by increasing or decreasing calories and start lifting some kind of weight once a week, if you are not already.

Remember, Deming's genius was constant improvement—not settling if things could be improved. We have to master the basics and focus on the high-impact items first before we start adding things.

Changes to make after your first successful cycle:

1. Update prescription meds dosage

2. Update low-nitrogen protein supplement dosage

3. Update supplemental magnesium and calcium dosages

4. Make tweaks to your diet in small increments

5. Get approval from your doctor to increase exercise intensity or duration (10% increase is enough)

6. Add some kind of weight lifting to your exercise routine at least once a week.

7. Increase or decrease calories to work towards a BMI of 25. No more unlimited calories unless you are underweight.

What to Do On Your Next Ninety-Day Checks

The assumption by the second "check" is you have mastered the basics or at least getting pretty close with diet and exercise compliance. You are in the groove and doing well.

If you are still struggling with compliance, then go back to the first cycle goals of a low-protein diet and regular exercise. Many of us will struggle for a few quarters. I know I did. Keep at it and change will come. Keep repeating the first cycle over and over until you get to 80%+ compliance with the diet and treatment plan. This will give you the biggest benefit.

Second, Third, Fourth, Fifth, Sixth, or Seventh Ninety-Day "Checks"

It's exactly the same as the first cycle in terms of blood and urine tests. Ask the same questions, check your BMI, update prescriptions, and so on.

Check your score and make small adjustments to your diet.

You are going to do everything exactly the same as before as long as things are improving. As long as you are improving, don't make any big changes.

The lesson here is to make small changes as we go so we can trust our results. Wild swings in diet lead to test results you can't trust. Steady diets lead to test results we can use to make good decisions.

Keep making small changes in diet, drugs, and calorie intake each cycle until you move the numbers into the normal range. Slow and steady gives us good data to act on: this is another reason for small and steady changes.

Stress Reduction

Make an effort to reduce stress in your life. We know stress speeds disease progression, so take some time to reduce stress in your life. On one corner, you have things like daily meditation, prayer, time spent in nature, or even some "me" time away from everything. On the other end of the spectrum, you can automate some activities that are a pain in rear. Try automatic bill pay or investing, get some help around the house, or change your work environment.

Stress reduction might also be under the heading of treating anxiety or depression. A book called *10% Happier- How I tamed the voice in my head* by Dan Harris offers a great example. Dan took up meditation and came to the conclusion he was about 10% happier when he meditated. I think Dan's summary of being 10% happier is on the mark. Nothing earth-shaking happened, but his life is generally better. My experience is about the same. Incorporating stress reduction has made it easier for me to stay on my diet and life is generally less stressful.

Keep Repeating

You will keep repeating the cycle of ninety-day checks and constant small improvements. It sounds boring, and it can be, but keep in mind, you are slowing the progression of a disease that is not supposed to be curable or treatable. Any gain is a big win.

Over time, as you bring things into the normal ranges, your body will start working better again. Each part will start working better with the other parts. You won't be back to normal, but much better than before. At some point, you will enter the "Goldilocks" zone. We will talk about this zone after the last step in PDCA.

Now for the next step of PDCA: Act

CHAPTER 39

The A in PDCA

A stands for act, but let me give you another word in instead: "lock." Deming wants us to act and lock in our improvements after we have executed a good plan and checked the results. Locking in improvements is a make-or-break issue for us.

Assume you ran a factory and you developed a technique that increased the life of your product by 10%, and lowered the costs to maintain it. Would you keep this technique, or would you go back to the old way?

What if you were 65-years-old, looking to retire, and one portfolio allowed you to live ten years before going broke while another option allowed you to live twenty-five years before having money problems?

Of course, we choose the better technique and the better portfolio. This is no different than locking in the changes that help our kidneys last longer. We want to get the maximum life out of our already-damaged kidneys. We also want to live the maximum life while fighting and beating this disease.

By locking in the good changes and focusing on getting everything in the normal range, we are dismembering our disease one driver at a time. If we keep taking away conditions that drive the progression of our disease, we will slow it down. This is why we have to lock in changes as we go and find the sweet spot for our own individual situations.

This may seem like common sense, but being the idiot I am, I went back to my old lifestyle after being in remission for about a year. Needless to say, my symptoms started coming back. The first thing I noticed was my feet swelling (edema) so I call the doctor and found out that my GFR had dropped five points.

While my disease is in remission, it could come back tomorrow. I live with that fear every day. There is no guarantee that I will stay in remission.

The reason we fail at locking in positive changes is we are creatures of habit. I guess convenience is part of it as well. Locking in the changes is what is going to save you. This is one of the reasons why we don't want to make any big changes after the first ninety days. We are locking in what is working for us and continuing to refine the program each cycle.

We want to lock in the changes that improve our outcomes. We are locking in these changes until we get to a new baseline so we can see how far we can go. If any one thing helped me, it was the idea of going until I hit a new baseline.

These changes have to become permanent to keep slowing your disease progression. You want to keep locking in postive changes until you hit the "Golidlocks" zone.

CHAPTER 40

A New Baseline, aka Goldilocks Zone

A new baseline occurs when you have two ninety-day cycles with no real improvement. Basically, your blood and urine test does not improve or stay the same for two cycles in a row.

This is uber important, let us count the ways:

1. A new baseline tells us we have taken the current diet and treatment plan as far as it will go.

2. A new baseline allows us to judge how successful the diet and treatment plan has been. We can compare the new baseline to the old one, or first one we started with.

3. A new baseline allows us an end point to the diet and treatment plan to evaluate what we should do next.

4. We have likely established the "Goldilocks zone" for maximizing the life of our kidneys.

Going long enough to hit a new baseline is one of the pillars of this approach. It may be the most important part of the treatment plan. If I didn't take this approach, I am sure I would never have gone into remission. I can't stress the importance of this enough. A new baseline will take five to eight cycles in most cases.

I had never stayed with an approach long enough and in an organized enough manner to get real results before. I have jumped back and forth and all over the place with no results to show. Learn from my mistakes.

What Do you Do When You Hit a New Baseline?

When you hit a new baseline (and you have followed the diet and treatment plan), you and your doctor need to ask several questions to decide what to do next. You have several ninety-day cycles to evaluate at this point.

You and your doctor should think and talk about the following questions:

1. Has my disease progression slowed like we expected?

2. Am I healthier today than when I started?

3. What health conditions do I still have left to treat?

4. Now that that I have likely received at least 90% of the possible benefit for the diet and treatment plan, what do I do next?

Let's talk about basic outcomes.

You should stay on the diet and treatment plan if the following is true:

Your disease progression has slowed and/or you are healthier than before with no other options for treatment.

You should consider doing something different if:

You have treatment options you have not tried, your disease progression has slowed, and you are healthier, but not in remission. At this point, you may want to try other treatments or a combination of treatments to try and get into remission. You may want to try a new or different drug now that you are healthier and your disease is not as bad. Remission is not an option for everyone, but if it is an option for you, go for it.

Here's another option, but only if everything is now in the normal range:

This will be possible only for those who start early in stage 3. You may consider expanding your diet a little to make dietary compliance easier and make your diet more varied. For example, if your limit was 30 grams of dietary protein a day, you may want to try 33 grams a day and see what happens using the same ninety-day cycles. You may also be able to expand your limits of potassium, phosphorus, or sodium. Again, just like before, make small changes and check your progress. You may find now that you are healthier you can expand your diet a little and still keep your numbers in the normal range.

Never, ever go above 0.6 grams of protein per kg per day. We know that above this, kidney disease progression starts again

After a successful ninety-day cycle, you can make another small increase and see what happens. You can always go back to your old diet as needed. Stop if any conditions come back or if your numbers go outside the normal range. Go back to the diet you used when everything was in the normal range.

You now have a system for making these changes. Making small changes and measuring the effects will be a habit by now.

Maximizing the life of your kidneys, the Goldilocks zone (the 100 year old kidney patient)

We all know the story of Goldilocks, who wandered into the bears' house and tried everything. She tried the porridge, chairs, and beds until she found one that was just right. When the economy is perfect, it's a "Goldilocks" economy. Planets in the habitable zone are referred to as "being in the Goldilocks zone." It's not too hot or too cold, so life could exist on these planets.

For us, being in the Goldilocks zone means we have done and are doing everything we can to slow the progression of our disease, and we have found what is possible and what we can maintain. We have taken the diet and treatment plan until we have hit a new baseline, with two cycles in a row of steady results and little to no improvement.

You have optimized your diet, prescription drugs, protein supplements, exercise, etc. in a measured manner to arrive at your current state. You are now in the "Goldilocks" zone where you have improved your health and slowed or maybe even stopped the progression of your disease the maximum amount possible given your disease, current health, and compliance with the treatment plan.

The "Goldilocks" zone is where your disease will progress the slowest and you are the healthiest version of you, given your personal situation. This zone is possible only if you lock in the good changes as you go. Eventually you will find the ideal diet and treatment for you.

You are very likely going to get the maximum life out of your kidneys in this zone.

What Is Ideal

Ideally, everything will be in the normal range and related conditions will be cured, but this is pretty rare.

We know that if we can get the comorbid conditions down to two, we have greatly improved our odds. If your scorecard is something like 4–2, your disease progression is going to be much slower than when you started with a score of 0–10.

I still have protein in my urine and my creatinine clearance is not always where I would like it to be. A portion of my kidneys are fried and not coming back, but everything else is in the normal range. You will likely have one or two conditions that refuse to go away. Once you hit the "Goldilocks" zone after two cycles with no improvements, you can decide if you want to work on the remaining conditions.

You and your doctor need to decide what is next, but do your best to stay in the "zone" where your disease progression is greatly slowed. In this zone, you are extending the life of your kidneys to the maximum amount. This is a permanent change in lifestyle for us. We can't ever go back to our previous life of dietary and lifestyle debauchery.

Now that you are in the "zone," you can take one more step to optimize your blood tests to give yourself the best odds. We have a pretty good blueprint for what it takes to live a long time as a kidney patient; I refer to it as the 100 year old kidney patient.

Here is what we are shooting for in an ideal scenario:

Two or fewer comorbid conditions or tests outside the normal range

A BMI around 25

Blood pressure 120/80 or slightly below

Phosphorus in the lower half of the normal range, below 3.5 mg/dl

Potassium above 4.0 Meq/l but still the normal range

Magnesium in the upper end of the normal range, 2.0 to 2.5 mg/dl

Sodium in the normal range

Total Cholesterol below 150 and HDL greater than LDL

Blood PH normal, no acidosis

Calcium in the normal range and no or minimal supplemental calcium

C-reactive protein or inflammation markers in the normal range

Albumin greater than 4.0 g/dl, higher is better

Blood urea nitrogen in the normal range (This may not be possible, but you need to get it as low as possible)

Creatinine clearance in the normal range (Again, this may not be possible, but you need to get it as low as possible)

No protein or albumin in urine (Again, this is not likely, but is still the goal)

Many issues like renal hypoxia, AGEs, and endotoxemia are not commonly tested, so these are left out from the list. They are still important, but difficult to measure.

Living longer and better

We know that if you can achieve these goals, you are very likely, I mean 99.9% more likely to live longer by slowing the progression of your disease. You will be healthier and happier as well. You may never cure your disease, but you can stop many of the drivers of kidney disease, which helps you slow its progression.

If our goal is to maximize the remaining life of our kidneys or to take the load off the remaining kidney function, we have a pretty good idea of what this looks like:

A plant-based, low-protein diet high in antioxidants and fiber

A diet with a negative potential renal acid load (PRAL)

A low-nitrogen protein food to supplement protein nutrition

Regular exercise

Using drugs, diet, supplements and exercise to bring tests into the normal range

Blood pressure monitoring and treatment

Keeping phosphorus levels under control

Reducing or eliminating supplemental calcium

Magnesium in the upper end of the normal range

Treating for depression or anxiety

Reducing stress

Regular checks and small corrections

Staying on a diet and treatment plan long enough to get results

There is no need to guess about what you should be doing to increase the life of your kidneys. We have good research that gives us a picture of how to slow the progression of our disease. The only catch is we have to do most of it ourselves. No one is going to knock on your door to solve your health problems. You are going to have to do it for yourself.

I really think doing for ourselves is the way we can improve kidney outcomes the fastest.

We don't have to guess at what we should be doing. We know from hundreds of studies what the 100-year old kidney patients looks like and what they should be doing. I will keep saying it, "We don't have to guess." We know what we need to do to live the longest based on hundreds of studies.

It's time for us and our caregivers to stop guessing and start acting to live longer and better lives.

CHAPTER 41

Crowdsourcing 850 Million Kidney Patients for a Better Treatment Plan and Diet

"Patient to Patient" is the philosophy I adopted after working on this project for the past two years. When I started this project, I met with numerous companies, consultants, and doctors thinking I would find a better approach.

It became clear very early that I was on a different page, or maybe a different planet, from this industry. In fact, my goals were so different, we might as well have been speaking a different language. As a patient, father, husband, brother, and son, I had strong feelings about healthcare that were very different from the companies I spoke with.

One CEO said I had a fiduciary duty to the company to charge the highest prices possible. Other suggestions were all at the patients' expense as well. I explained that I was a patient myself and I would be taking the same protien foods, but I don't think I got through to any of these people.

Time was the second issue aside from costs. Time estimates were always in years to get something done, tested, or developed. No one seemed to understand the urgency I felt, despite being very clear on this issue at every meeting.

For this reason, I started Kidneyhood.org. Our goals as people with an incurable disease and the clock ticking are night-and-day different from the goals of big companies or government agencies. We need easy and fast access to foods, drugs, and therapies that could slow our disease, and we need it today. These products also need to be affordable, high-quality, and based on the latest research not the 1970s "current" options.

Kidneyhood.org is a social benefit company, which means profits don't have to come first. We can come first. We still have to make a profit to keep going, but we can be guerilla or lean and mean about it. As someone who worked for Fortune 500 companies, the amount of overhead that is required to keep everything going is tremendous. The pressure to produce profits every quarter is tremendous. A common joke among investment professionals is "You never want to be a client of a publicly traded company." Those new profits come from existing clients in almost all cases.

As a patient, I don't want to pay ten times the cost for something so a CEO can have a second or third home or for outdated and complicated distribution systems. I don't want to pay for layers of overhead and management when I am slowing dying. It still pisses me off to no end that we consider this acceptable. The idea of maximizing profit off of sick people makes my blood boil, but it is the system in which we currently live.

I am not blaming companies or government agencies, they are playing by the current rules and regulations. If the rules were different, the results would be different. However, they are not different and unlikely to change in time to save any of us.

Crowdsourcing For a Better Treatment Plan and Diet

Until a cure is found for dozens of different kinds of kidney disease, all we can do is manage our disease and our kidneys so they last as long as possible. However, if a few of us or hopefully thousands of us pull together, we can find the best possible ways to extend the life of our kidneys.

I am an imperfect man (just ask my wife) and this book is the worst version that will ever be published. I wish this book had better answers and was written better. The next versions will get better and better. The next version will have input from more paitents, doctors, nutritionists, dieticans, etc....

Let me show you what happens when a patient who understands what really happens to us decides to take action.

1. Published the largest and most complete guide to slowing kidney disease progression, available in dozens of countries for less than ten dollars for the ebook.

2. Researched and produced the lowest nitrogen protein supplement for fellow patients.

3. The resulting protein food is 60% cheaper than the average cost of a comparable product. This saves patients $3,000 a year compared to current prices of comparable products.

4. First product to provide nutrition for each stage of kidney disease.

5. First product to focus on raising albumin levels to reduce mortalty rates and improve nutrition.

6. First try to slow the progression of heart and kidney disease at the same time.

7. Two medical trials in are 2019—one animal and one human—to improve treatment plans and our knowledge base.

8. Able to ship the book and supplements worldwide so that anyone in the world can get educated and try to slow the disease, if they choose.

I am just one individual, but can you imagine what would happen if all of us got engaged and became part of the solution? There are 850 million people with kidney disease around the world. That's twenty times more kidney patients than cancer patients. What if we all contributed something tiny to the cause? The results would be unbelievable.

We don't need to be constrained by traditional rules. We can communicate instantly around the world via the internet. We are not bound by boards of directors trying to maximize profits, and we can move much faster than government organizations.

Imagine if we had treatment data on 1,000 patients to improve the treatment plan in this book? What if we updated the book and treatment plan several times a year as we validated better or improved treatment options?

We can do more, faster, better, and cheaper than large corporations or governments, but it only works if everyone will contribute. I am very excited about what we can do. It is time for us to stop waiting and start acting to save our lives.

No one is ever going to care about slowing or stopping kidney disease as much as a patient with the clock ticking.

Stand up and help.

I am going to be asking a lot and I want you to answer.

I am not asking you to protest in the streets. I am not asking for money. I am asking you to participate and act when you get an email from me asking for help. I believe we have more power than any similar group in history. We can conduct our own research programs, and educate doctors, dietitians, and other caregivers on the best ways to help us. We can build the biggest database of possible treatments to slow and stop incurable kidney disease. We can also build the biggest database of healthy, kidney-friendly recipes. The possibilities are endless, but for it to work, you have to give a damn about yourself and your fellow man or woman. I am sorry, but I don't know how else to say it. This book and related projects have taken years of my life and almost all my life savings. Trying to stop my disease also stole a decade of my life. I hit my breaking point after watching someone die doing nothing because that's what their doctor recommended. He never questioned anything or tried to find a better answer. This person passed away never trying to fight because their doctor said nothing could be done. There are tens of thousands (maybe millions) of cases just like this.

Our only choice is to band together and come up with our own research and treatment plans. We don't have decades to wait on traditional medicine.

My First Ask

If you are showing improvement for what is supposed to be an incurable disease, please become an advocate of this diet and treatment plan. Please contact me and make a short video. For me, there is nothing better than hearing about the success of another patient. Many of us suffer in silence and give up once the doctor gives us the speech that there is nothing that can be done for us until dialysis or a transplant.

Be a source of information and inspiration to another patient who may be struggling and not understand they may have another option to slow or stop their disease.

Tell your doctor what you are doing, so he can witness first hand your progress and spread the news to other patients. Same for nutritionists and dieticians.

Word of mouth from fellow patients is a great way to spread the word. You may help someone in a desperate situation add years to their life.

My Second Ask

Help me build a better treatment plan and diet to slow the progression of kidney disease.

Contribute to the base of knowledge by submitting improvements and catching any errors in the treatment plan or diet. I have never claimed to be perfect, but I am determined to build a better treatment plan and diet.

I have set up a series of email addresses to direct the improvments to the right people.

1.   If you find something wrong in the book for any reason or you feel you have better research to support a change, please submit to:

   skdimprove@kidneyhood.org

   Keep in mind, any submission needs to be supported by at least three research studies or clinical trials. Please also understand, we are a low budget operation, we don't have a large staff. Please only submit only real-life ideas that are backed by science.

   If you are a licensed physican, please use this email address:

   drimprove@kidneyhood.org

2.   Submit recipes or improvements to recipes

   Again, please submit only new recipes or major revisions to existing ones. A good rule of thumb would be if you would serve it to your family or make it for a first date. If not, maybe you shouldn't send it in.

   Recipes should include nutritional information. Recipes are sent to real kidney patients who are acting as test cooks. If they give it a thumbs up, we will add it to the recipe list, give you credit for it, and send it out to thousands of patients for free.

   Please use **dietimprove@kidneyhood.org** for submissions.

   Do not submit more than two recipes per month; we don't have the staff to evaluate hundreds of recipe submissions.

   Recipes should conform to the basic rules of the diet and protein restrictions.

3.   Be part of submitting your data for a clinical trial

We need to better validate this approach. I am only one person, so my experience or the hundreds of studies in this book are not enough to validate this approach yet. We need data from other paitents so the data can be analyzed by an objective third party.

Please email: **ctrials@kidneyhood.org** for more information.

My goal is to add at least 100 patient histories and results each year to the database. Please sign up if you are willing to help improve and validate a better treatment plan for all of us.

Crowdsourcing a Cure is Ambitious, but Worth It

The idea that thousands or even millions of patients can work together to slow or stop the progression of a deadly disease is an experiment. I don't know if it's going to work or not. I believe that most people will help given a chance.

I am betting that we as a group can move faster, cheaper, and more effectively because no one cares more than us. We are going to start small and slow , but hopefully build steam over the upcoming years.

We can document the best treatment plan and the best diet to share with patients around the world.

The only reason this won't work is if we don't care about our own future and about the future of our fellow man/woman.

In summary, we are 850 million strong worldwide and no one is going to care more than us. We can move faster, cheaper, and improve our lives and the lives of thousands of other patients if will all contribute something to the cause.

Please be a part of improving the lives of fellow patients and building a better treatment and diet plan for all of us.

CHAPTER 42

Conclusion

I will keep this brief, as you have already suffered through my writing for hundreds of pages.

In 2019, we have a good blueprint and plan for slowing or maybe stopping the progression of incurable kidney diseases. This blueprint is based on up-to-date research and common sense. The research here contradicts current treatment in many ways, but many current treatment philosophies are still based on research that is fifty years old. The plan here is not perfect or without flaws, but it is the best available today and will get better each year with your help.

I am maybe one of the few people in the world to take a protein supplement of some kind and be on dozens of different diets for a little over ten years. Let my "lost" ten years add ten or more years of life to your kidneys. The plan in this book worked when everything else failed and it worked after almost fifteen years of disease symptoms started. It's never too late to start trying to slow your disease.

We are going to dismember our disease by taking out the drivers of our disease one by one and adding factors that slow our disease. One ninety-day cycle at a time, we are going to cure conditions and wrestle as many tests as possible into the normal range using everything in our arsenal. Nothing should be off limits when you have an incurable disease. Just remember, you can't go crazy or take questionable supplements with things with questionable ingredients. Less is more when it comes to impaired kidneys.

Your doctor is your ally in the fight and whatever is suggested in the book, you and your doctor have to make all of the final decisions.

Our goal is remission, partial remission, or getting and staying in the "Goldilocks" zone to maximize the life of our kidneys and likely our lives as well.

Please get on the list at **www.stoppingkidneydisease.com**, and stay up to date and informed on new data.

Look for the recipe and meal planning guide with recipes. It was too much to put in this book. If you are on the list at **www.stoppingkidneydisease.com**, you will get free recipes.

I hope this book helps you improve your health dramatically, and give you many more decades of quality life with your family and loved ones.

Do one last selfish thing for me

Send me a picture of yourself holding your improved blood and urine tests. Even better, send me a pic of before and after showing your improvments. I want to wall paper my office with pictures of people beating the odds and kicking kidney disease's ass. If you read this far, you already know I'm a little warped. You can send it to **l.hull@kidneyhood.org**.

In conclusion

Go give it hell and never give up on yourself and treating your disease. You have a good blueprint in the book to start slowing and possibly stopping your disease.

One things you may not know, there are tens of thousands of us rooting for you and we will all be thrilled and inspired by your success. Our email list has grown from zero to a little over 20,000 patients in one year. We can't cheer or be inspired by you unless you let us know how you are doing. We are waiting to hear about your success.

Lee

P.S. Don't forget about the selfie with your results, send it to l.hull@kidneyhood.org.

INDEX

D

L

M

N

22971127R00299

Made in the USA
San Bernardino, CA
18 January 2019